Study Guide to accompany Linton & Maebius

Introduction to Medical-Surgical Nursing

Third Edition

Nancy K. Maebius, PhD, RN
Instructor
The Health Institute of San Antonio
San Antonio, Texas

SAUNDERS
An Imprint of Elsevier Science
Philadelphia London New York St. Louis Sydney Toronto

W.B. SAUNDERS COMPANY
An Imprint of Elsevier Science (USA)
The Curtis Center
Independence Square West
Philadelphia, Pennsylvania 19106-3399

 ISBN 0-7216-9530-2

Vice President, Publishing Director: Sally Schrefer
Senior Editor: Terri Wood
Associate Developmental Editor: Teena Ferroni, Sophia Gray
Developmental Editor: Catherine Ott
Project Manager: Gayle Morris

Printed in the United States of America.

Last digit is the print number: 9 8 7 6 5 4 3 2 1

Contents

To the Student

This study guide was created to assist you in achieving the objectives of each chapter in *Introduction to Medical-Surgical Nursing*, Third Edition, and establishing a solid base of knowledge in medical-surgical nursing. Completing the exercises in each chapter in this guide will help to reinforce the material studied in the textbook and learned in class. Such reinforcement also helps students to be successful on the NCLEX-PN.

Study Hints for All Students

Ask Questions!

There are no stupid questions. If you do not know something or are not sure, you need to find out. Other people may be wondering the same thing but may be too shy to ask. The answer could mean life or death to your patient. That is certainly more important than feeling embarrassed about asking a question.

Chapter Objectives

At the beginning of each chapter in the textbook are objectives that you should have mastered when you finish studying that chapter. Write these objectives in your notebook, leaving a blank space after each. Fill in the answers as you find them while reading the chapter. Review to make sure your answers are correct and complete. Use these answers when you study for tests. This should also be done for separate course objectives that your instructor has listed in your class syllabus.

Key Terms

At the beginning of each chapter in the textbook are key terms that you will encounter as you read the chapter. Text page number references are provided for easy reference and review, and the key terms are in color the first time they appear in the chapter.

Phonetic pronunciations are provided for terms that students might find difficult to pronounce. The terms that were assigned simple phonetic pronunciations were selected because they are either (1) difficult medical, nursing, or scientific terms or (2) other words that may be difficult for students to pronounce. The goal is to help the student reader with limited proficiency in English to develop a greater command of the pronunciation of scientific and nonscientific English terminology. It is hoped that a more general competency in the understanding and use of medical and scientific language may result.

Key Points

Use the Key Points at the end of each chapter in the textbook to help with review for exams.

Reading Hints

When reading each chapter in the textbook, look at the subject headings to learn what each section is about. Read first for the general meaning. Then reread parts you did not understand. It may help to read those parts aloud. Carefully read the information given in each table and study each figure and its caption.

Concepts

While studying, put difficult concepts into your own words to see if you understand them. Check this understanding with another student or the instructor. Write these in your notebook.

Class Notes

When taking lecture notes in class, leave a large margin on the left side of each notebook page and write only on right-hand pages, leaving all left-hand pages blank. Look over your lecture notes soon after each class, while your memory is fresh. Fill in missing words, complete sentences and ideas, and underline key phrases, definitions, and concepts. At the top of each page, write the topic of that page. In the left margin, write the key word for that part of your notes. On the opposite left-hand page, write a summary or outline that combines material from both the textbook and the lecture. These can be your study notes for review.

Study Groups

Form a study group with other students so you can help one another. Practice speaking and reading aloud. Ask questions about material you are not sure about. Work together to find answers.

References for Improving Study Skills

Good study skills are essential for achieving your goals in nursing. Time management, efficient use of study time, and a consistent approach to studying are all beneficial. There are various study methods for reading a textbook and for taking class notes. Some methods that have proven helpful can be found in *Saunders Student Nurse Planner: A Guide to Success in Nursing School.* This book contains helpful information on test-taking and preparing for clinical experiences. It includes an example of a "time map" for planning study time and a blank form that the student can use to formulate a personal time map.

Additional Study Hints for English as a Second Language (ESL) Students

Vocabulary

If you find a nontechnical word you do not know (e.g., *drowsy*), try to guess its meaning from the sentence (e.g., *With electrolyte imbalance, the patient may feel fatigued and drowsy*). If you are not sure of the meaning, or if it seems particularly important, look it up in the dictionary.

Vocabulary Notebook

Keep a small alphabetized notebook or address book in your pocket or purse. Write down new nontechnical words you read or hear along with their meanings and pronunciations. Write each word under its initial letter so you can find it easily, as in a dictionary. For words you do not know or for words that have a different meaning in nursing, write down how they are used and sound. Look up their meanings in a dictionary or ask your instructor or first-language buddy. Then write the different meanings or usages that you have found in your book, including the nursing meaning. Continue to add new words as you discover them. For example:

primary
- of most importance; main: *the primary problem or disease*
- the first one; elementary: *primary school*

secondary
- of less importance; resulting from another problem or disease: a secondary symptom
- the second one: *secondary school (in the United States, high school)*

First Language Buddy

ESL students should find a first-language buddy—another student who is a native speaker of English and who is willing to answer questions about word meanings, pronunciations, and culture. Maybe your buddy would like to learn about your language and culture as well. This could help in his or her nursing experience as well.

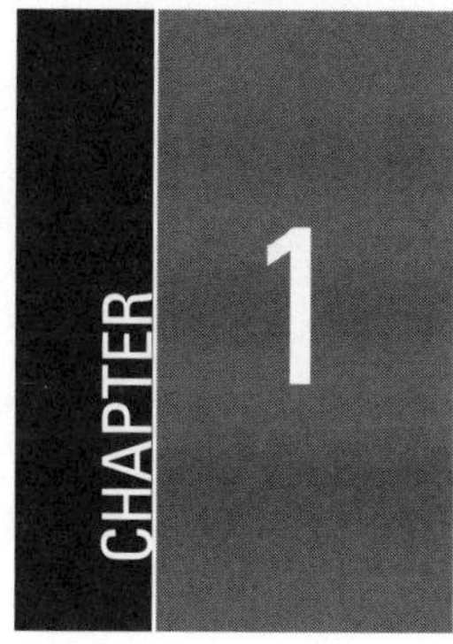

Student Name ____________________

The Health Care System

Answer Key: Textbook page references are provided as a guide for answering these questions. A complete answer key was provided for your instructor.

OBJECTIVES

1. Describe the organization of the health care system in the United States.
2. Describe the focus of public health services.
3. Define the three levels of prevention.
4. Discuss financing of health care in the United States, including Medicare and Medicaid programs.
5. Describe the components of the health care system that provide both outpatient and inpatient care and the types of service each provides.
6. Describe the impact of cost-containment measures on the delivery of care.

LEARNING ACTIVITIES

A. Match the example in the numbered column with the most appropriate term in the lettered column. Answers may be used more than once.

(2)	**1.**	________	Providing Pap smears at reduced cost	A. Primary
(2)	**2.**	________	Efforts to educate people to wear seat belts	B. Secondary
(2)	**3.**	________	Teaching a diabetic proper diet and foot care	C. Tertiary
(2)	**4.**	________	Reduced-cost mammograms	

Continued next page

(2) **5.** ________ Use of physical therapy to prevent contractures in a stroke patient

(2) **6.** ________ Campaigns in schools to prevent children from smoking

(2) **7.** ________ Exercise programs to increase strength and cardiovascular fitness

B. Match the definition in the numbered column with the most appropriate term in the lettered column.

(1, 2) **1.** ________ Branch of the Department of Health and Human Services (DHHS) of the U.S. government whose chief purpose is to provide better health services for the American people

(1) **2.** ________ Provision of comprehensive health care at a reasonable cost through enrollment in an HMO, PPO, or similar plan, with incentives to save costs

A. Public Health Service
B. Diagnosis-related group (DRG)
C. Managed health care
D. Older Americans Act
E. Skilled nursing facility
F. Long-term care facility
G. Primary prevention
H. Secondary prevention
I. Tertiary prevention

Continued next page

Student Name____

(8) **3.** __________ Law passed in 1965 to ensure that elderly persons have an adequate income and suitable housing, physical and mental health services, community services, and the opportunity to pursue meaningful activities

(3) **4.** __________ System of reimbursement standards for hospitals for care based on a fixed fee for a diagnostic category, regardless of cost

(9, 10) **5.** __________ A level of residential care that includes medical, nursing, social, and rehabilitative services to individuals who cannot manage independently

(9) **6.** __________ Nursing home that provides care for people who are unable to care for themselves because of chronic illnesses and physical impairments

(2) **7.** __________ Steps taken to prevent disease recurrence or complications of diagnosed disease or injury

(2) **8.** __________ Steps taken to improve health and prevent disease and injury

(2) **9.** __________ Steps taken to detect disease early and begin treatment as soon as possible

Continued next page

C. Match the definition in the numbered column with the most appropriate term in the lettered column.

A. Medicare
B. Medicaid
C. Health maintenance organization (HMO)
D. Preferred provider organization (PPO)
E. Fee-for-service
F. Capitation
G. Point of service (POS)

(2) **1.** ________ Accepting a fixed amount of money to pay for health care services to all health care plan members with no additional billing

(2) **2.** ________ An established fee set by physicians or health care providers for services or procedures actually provided

(1, 2) **3.** ________ System that uses a network of independent physicians, hospitals, and other providers who provide services to a pool of patients for a discounted fee

(3) **4.** ________ Program that provides health care services for needy, low-income, and disabled individuals with funds distributed at the state level

(3) **5.** ________ Health insurance program administered by the federal government that is funded by Social Security payments

(2) **6.** ________ Coverage that blends multiple options and enrollees select which option they want to use

(4, 5) **7.** ________ Health care organization that provides health care and services through group practice for a membership fee

Student Name____

D. Match the description in the numbered column with the most appropriate term in the lettered column. Answers may be used more than once.

(9)	**1.**	__________	Provide skilled care from a licensed nursing staff, including rehabilitative care
(9, 10)	**2.**	__________	Nursing homes, skilled nursing facilities, and extended-care facilities
(9)	**3.**	__________	Provide specialized services for people unable to care for themselves
(10)	**4.**	__________	Provide care for those who need observations during acute or unstable phase of illness
(9)	**5.**	__________	Permit a high degree of independence with limited access to nursing care
(9)	**6.**	__________	Residents' units have kitchens, but group meals are typically provided
(7)	**7.**	__________	Purpose is to care for and provide palliative care to dying persons
(9)	**8.**	__________	Extended care for people who have the potential to regain function

A. Long-term care facilities
B. Intermediate care facilities (extended care facilities)
C. Skilled nursing facilities
D. Assisted living centers
E. Hospices

E. Match the description in the numbered column with the most appropriate term in the lettered column. Answers may be used more than once.

A. Medicare
B. Medicaid

Funding

(3) **1.** ________ Monthly premium from paycheck; funds matched by federal government

(3) **2.** ________ Federal, state, and local taxes

Eligibility

(3) **3.** ________ Needy, low-income, and disabled persons and their dependent children younger than 65 years

(3) **4.** ________ All persons older than 65 years plus disabled persons younger than 65 who qualify for Social Security benefits

How Administered

(3) **5.** ________ Federal government

(3) **6.** ________ Both federal and state governments

Student Name ____________________

MULTIPLE-CHOICE QUESTIONS

F. Choose the most appropriate answer.

(4) **1.** Which is an example of outpatient care?

1. hospital operating room
2. acute care hospital
3. physician's office
4. long-term care facility

(4) **2.** HMOs provide health care and services:

1. through group practice.
2. through solo practice.
3. to all older Americans.
4. to all physically and mentally challenged (disabled) persons.

(3) **3.** Which system groups patients according to the medical diagnosis so that hospitals receive a fixed payment based on the patient's diagnosis?

1. HMOs
2. DRGs
3. PPOs
4. CQIs

(8) **4.** Physicians are now discharging patients as early as possible to:

1. improve care, because the focus is on primary prevention.
2. improve care, because hospice can take care of patients needing extended nursing services.
3. reduce costs, because hospitals only receive a fixed amount of money as a results of DRGs.
4. reduce costs, because hospitals can refer patients to home health and long term care facilities.

(8) **5.** Which of the following conditions is one of the five most frequent reasons for hospitalization?

1. surgery for fractures
2. congestive heart failure
3. trauma from accidents
4. osteoporosis

(2) **6.** Which term describes the collection by physicians of a fixed amount of money each month for each member enrolled in the plan?

1. HMOs
2. capitation
3. PPOs
4. fee-for-service

(5) **7.** The demand for professional home health care services continues to increase for all age categories because:

1. ambulatory surgery center services are decreasing.
2. health care costs are decreasing.
3. managed health care is focused on acute care.
4. hospitals are reducing the length of hospital stays.

(1) **8.** What concerns do health insurance companies, HMOs, and PPOs have in common?

1. health care service delivery for low-income persons
2. delivery of health care services at a reasonable cost
3. establishment of ambulatory care centers
4. diagnosis-related groups (DRGs)

(2) **9.** Which is an agency that carries out the activities of the Public Health Service?

1. Social Security Administration
2. Centers for Medicare and Medicaid Services
3. Food and Drug Administration
4. Office of Human Development

(8) **10.** In which setting is the number of patients decreasing?

1. ambulatory care
2. home health
3. clinics
4. hospitals

(7) **11.** A stroke patient who is aphasic will need the services of a(n):

1. occupational therapist.
2. physical therapist.
3. speech therapist.
4. social worker.

(7) **12.** Patients and their families needing assistance to manage chronic illness in the home will need the services of a(n):

1. speech therapist.
2. social worker.
3. occupational therapist.
4. physical therapist.

(1) **13.** The effects of managed care include:

1. increase in fee-for-service.
2. decrease in home health care.
3. decreased focus on wellness.
4. increased focus on prevention.

(2) **14.** In public health, the focus of attention is on:

1. emphasizing patients' rights.
2. improving health of aggregates.
3. increasing cost sharing.
4. decreasing home health care.

(2) **15.** One aim of primary prevention is to:

1. promote health.
2. detect disease early.
3. treat disease to improve patient outcomes.
4. prevent complications of disease.

(2) **16.** *Cost containment* refers to:

1. reducing costs.
2. increasing fee-for-service plans.
3. decreasing third-party reimbursements.
4. controlling rates of increasing costs.

(2) **17.** A strategy designed to control costs is:

1. capitation.
2. fee-for-service.
3. retrospective payment.
4. voluntary enrollment.

(8) **18.** The "revolving door syndrome" occurs when patients return to the hospital for care because:

1. hospice services were not available at home.
2. high-technology services were needed.
3. the emphasis was on preventive health care at home.
4. they did not fully recover at home.

(3) **19.** Which statement is true regarding the way DRGs have affected hospital finances? If the patient:

1. gets better faster, the hospital loses money.
2. gets better faster, the hospital makes money.
3. requires a longer stay, the hospital makes money.
4. requires a shorter stay, the hospital loses money.

Student Name ____________________

(5) **20.** Cost-effective health care methods began with DRGs. What method of health care delivery today is aimed at cost-effective health care delivery?

1. primary prevention
2. long-term care
3. managed health care
4. extended care

(8) **21.** The focus of hospice care is to:

1. extend life of the terminally ill.
2. provide a better quality of life for dying persons and their families.
3. provide assistance to families trying to manage chronic illness in the home.
4. provide emergency care to dying patients at home.

(7) **22.** Assessment and intervention used by hospice nurses are centered around:

1. palliative care.
2. treatment of disease.
3. preservation of life.
4. infection control.

CHAPTER 2

Student Name ______________________________

Patient Care Settings

Answer Key: Textbook page references are provided as a guide for answering these questions. A complete answer key was provided for your instructor.

OBJECTIVES

1. Describe the role of the nurse in community and home health, rehabilitation, and long-term care settings.
2. Differentiate community health and community based nursing.
3. Describe the types of specialty care that nurses may provide in home health care.
4. Describe the principles of rehabilitation.
5. List the four levels of disability.
6. Discuss legislation passed to protect the rights of the disabled.
7. Identify the goals of rehabilitation.
8. Name the members of the rehabilitation team.
9. List the types of extended care facilities.
10. Discuss the effects of institutionalization on the elderly person.
11. Describe the principles of nursing home care.

LEARNING ACTIVITIES

A. Match the definition in the numbered column with the most appropriate term in the lettered column.

(16) **1.** __________ Measurable loss of function, usually delineated to indicate a diminished capacity for work

(14) **2.** __________ Certain nursing procedures, such as dressing changes, Foley catheter insertions, and venipuncture

A. Impairment
B. Skilled observation and assessment
C. Rehabilitation
D. Handicap
E. Skilled procedures
F. Disability

Continued next page

(16) **3.** ________ Physical or psychological disturbance in functioning

(16) **4.** ________ Inability to perform one or more normal daily activities because of mental or physical disability

(14) **5.** ________ Used to determine adequacy of home environment, knowledge level of the patient and family regarding care procedures and side effects of treatment, and family's level of comfort in performing specific procedures

(16) **6.** ________ Process of restoring individuals to best possible health and functioning following physical or mental impairment

B. Match the description of disability in the numbered column with the level of disability in the lettered column.

(16) **1.** ________ Severe limitations in one or more ADL; unable to work

(16) **2.** ________ Slight limitation in one or more ADL; usually able to work

(16) **3.** ________ Total disability characterized by near complete dependence on others for assistance with ADLs; unable to work

(16) **4.** ________ Moderate limitation in one or more ADL; able to work but workplace may need modifications

A. Level I
B. Level II
C. Level III
D. Level IV

Student Name____

C. Match the definition in the numbered column with the most appropriate term in the lettered column.

(18) **1.** __________ Person who assists the patient in regaining swallowing or speaking functions

(18) **2.** __________ Person who assists patient with regaining fine motor skills necessary for dressing, eating, and grooming

(18) **3.** __________ Person who assists with coordinating resources for placement in the home or convalescent facility after discharge

(18) **4.** __________ Person who assists patient in all aspects of mobility

A. Physical therapist
B. Occupational therapist
C. Speech therapist
D. Social worker

D. List two goals of rehabilitation.

(16) **1.** ____

(16) **2.** ____

E. What are five basic criteria for home health care that must be met to receive Medicare reimbursement?

(13) **1.** ____

(13) **2.** ____

(13) **3.** ____

(13) **4.** ____

(13) **5.** ____

F. List five of the most common intravenous therapies that can be given at home.

(15) **1.** ______________________________

(15) **2.** ______________________________

(15) **3.** ______________________________

(15) **4.** ______________________________

(15) **5.** ______________________________

G. Match the descriptions in the numbered column with the five common effects of institutionalization in the lettered column.

(20) **1.** __________ Patients are treated in light of their diagnosis or dysfunctional behavior patterns.

(20) **2.** __________ Behaviors considered normal at home are labeled abnormal or are unacceptable in the institution.

(20) **3.** __________ Family visits are few and include little discussion of the outside world.

(20) **4.** __________ A patient's physical, mental, and social abilities are lost because of disuse.

(20) **5.** __________ Residents of long-term care facilities are exposed unnecessarily when caregivers enter rooms without knocking.

A. Depersonalization
B. Indignity
C. Redefinition of "normal"
D. Regression
E. Social withdrawal

Student Name____

H. Match the nursing interventions in the numbered column with the appropriate principle of long-term residential care in the lettered column.

(21) **1.** __________ Place a urinal near to the bed, for immobile patients with incontinence.

(21) **2.** __________ Allow nursing home residents to assist in establishing care goals.

(21) **3.** __________ Give long-term care residents choices in activities.

(21) **4.** __________ Explore factors that may be responsible for the patient's incontinence.

(21) **5.** __________ Set specific goals for each resident that encourage independent functioning.

A. Maintenance of function
B. Promotion of independence
C. Maintenance of autonomy

MULTIPLE-CHOICE QUESTIONS

I. Choose the most appropriate answer.

(16) **1.** The process of restoring an individual to the best possible health and functioning following a physical or mental impairment is called:

1. independent function.
2. home health care.
3. rehabilitation.
4. autonomy.

(16) **2.** A disturbance in functioning that may be either physical or psychological is called:

1. rehabilitation.
2. impairment.
3. restoration.
4. independence.

(16) **3.** People born without arms can perform ADLs by using their feet and assistive devices. These people are said to have a:

1. disability.
2. handicap.
3. paralysis.
4. return of function.

(16) **4.** A measurable loss of function, usually indicating diminished capacity for work, is called:

1. impairment.
2. alteration to integrity.
3. compensation.
4. disability.

(16) **5.** An inability to perform daily activities is called:

1. impairment.
2. disability.
3. handicap.
4. paralysis.

(18) **6.** The ultimate goal of rehabilitation is to live with:

1. assistance.
2. modification.
3. independence.
4. adaptation.

(20) **7.** Which effect of institutionalization is diminished by not knocking before entering the room and not draping patients during care activities?

1. redefinition of "normal"
2. social withdrawal
3. indignity
4. regression

(17) **8.** The first comprehensive approach to problems experienced by people with disabilities was the:

1. Vocational Rehabilitation Act of 1920.
2. Social Security Act of 1935.
3. Medicare Act of 1965.
4. Rehabilitation Act of 1973.

(17) **9.** Which act began affirmative action programs to assist in the employment of disabled people and prohibited discrimination against them in programs receiving federal funds?

1. Vocational Rehabilitation Act of 1920
2. Social Security Act of 1935
3. Medicare Act of 1965
4. Rehabilitation Act of 1973

(16) **10.** The focus in rehabilitation is to:

1. promote self-esteem.
2. assist with activities of daily living.
3. restore maximal possible function.
4. eliminate impairment.

(16) **11.** An example of mental impairment is:

1. loss of memory.
2. paralysis of an arm.
3. brain hemorrhage.
4. fractured neck.

(16) **12.** Moderate limitation in one or more ADLs resulting in a person's being able to go to work, but requiring modifications in the workplace, is classified as:

1. Level I disability.
2. Level II disability.
3. Level III disability.
4. Level IV disability.

Student Name ______________________________

(14) **13.** Which of the following is an example of a skilled procedure?

1. Foley catheter insertion
2. enema administration
3. mouth care
4. ear drop administration

(16) **14.** An individual with an injured back who has a diminished capacity for work is classified as:

1. handicapped.
2. impaired.
3. disabled.
4. dependent.

(16) **15.** Return of function and prevention of further disability are goals of:

1. community-based nursing.
2. public health nursing.
3. rehabilitation.
4. long-term care.

(19) **16.** Nursing homes and skilled nursing facilities are types of:

1. domiciliary care facilities.
2. outpatient facilities.
3. long-term facilities.
4. health maintenance organizations.

(14) **17.** By providing clear documentation of functional losses and goals for care, the nurse is meeting the Medicare criterion of:

1. skilled care.
2. reasonable and necessary care.
3. homebound patient care.
4. intermittent care.

(18) **18.** What percentage of elderly persons live in institutions?

1. 5%
2. 10%
3. 15%
4. 20%

(19) **19.** What percentage of persons 85 and over reside in nursing homes?

1. 1%
2. 6%
3. 10%
4. 20%

(19) **20.** The best indicator of who will need nursing home placement is:

1. age.
2. ADL dependency.
3. presence of handicaps.
4. severity of infectious disease process.

(19) **21.** Which type of facility provides basic room, board, and supervision, where residents come and go as they please?

1. domiciliary care facilities
2. sheltered housing
3. intermediate care
4. skilled care

(19) **22.** Facilities that contain modifications to provide care for the frail elderly and usually provide community dining are called:

1. domiciliary care facilities.
2. sheltered housing.
3. intermediate care.
4. skilled care.

(20) **23.** Treating patients primarily in light of their diagnoses or dysfunctional behavior patterns is an example of:

1. indignity.
2. regression.
3. social withdrawal.
4. depersonalization.

(24) **24.** Being left in bed a great part of the day, finding it difficult to walk, and losing skills of conversation are examples of:

1. social withdrawal.
2. indignity.
3. regression.
4. depersonalization.

CHAPTER 3

Student Name ____________________

The Leadership Role of the Licensed Practical Nurse

Answer Key: Textbook page references are provided as a guide for answering these questions. A complete answer key was provided for your instructor.

OBJECTIVES

1. Differentiate leadership from management.
2. Describe leadership styles.
3. Discuss management theories.
4. List tips for effective management.
5. Describe the role of the licensed vocational nurse as a team leader.

LEARNING ACTIVITIES

A. Match the definition in the numbered column with the most appropriate term in the lettered column.

(25) **1.** __________ Authoritarian, directive, or bureaucratic types of leadership

(25) **2.** __________ Mixture of autocratic and democratic leadership; feedback from group members is used by the leader to make a final decision

(25) **3.** __________ Achievement of goals through participation by all group members

A. Autocratic leadership
B. Theory X
C. Laissez-faire leadership
D. Democratic leadership
E. Participative leadership
F. Theory Y
G. Theory Z

Continued next page

(25) **4.** ________ Nondirective type of leadership

(26) **5.** ________ Management by autocratic rule with little participation in decision making by workers

(26) **6.** ________ Democratic style of management with some participation in decision making by workers

(26) **7.** ________ Management with full participation in decision making by workers

B. Match the definition in the numbered column with the most appropriate term in the lettered column.

(30) **1.** ________ Turning over part of one person's responsibility to another person with that person's consent

(30) **2.** ________ Identification and delegation of specific tasks to a specific person who is hired and paid to perform these tasks

(24) **3.** ________ Guidance, or showing the way to others

(24) **4.** ________ Effective use of selected methods to achieve desired outcomes

A. Leadership
B. Management
C. Assignment
D. Delegation

Student Name____

C. Following are characteristics of people in their work environment. Mark an "X" before the characteristic if it refers to the theory X classical management theory, a "Y" if it refers to the theory Y classical management theory, and a "Z" if it refers to the Z classical management theory.

(26) **1.** __________ Work together for the good of the company

(26) **2.** __________ Care about what they are doing

(26) **3.** __________ Find no pleasure in work

(26) **4.** __________ Constantly striving to grow

(26) **5.** __________ Naturally lazy and prefer to do nothing

(26) **6.** __________ Work mainly for the money

(26) **7.** __________ Do not want to think for themselves

(26) **8.** __________ Mature and responsible

(26) **9.** __________ Self-directed

(26) **10.** __________ Work only because they fear being fired

(26) **11.** __________ Childlike and like being told what to do

(26) **12.** __________ Work for rewards other than money

(26) **13.** __________ Active and enjoy setting their own goals

(26) **14.** __________ Not capable of making decisions for themselves

(26) **15.** __________ Based on mutual trust and loyalty

(26) **16.** __________ Dislike responsibility

(26) **17.** __________ Accept responsibility

(26) **18.** __________ Dynamic, flexible, and adaptive

D. Match the description of conflict in the numbered column with the related stages of conflict in the lettered column.

(28) **1.** ________ The conflict leads to various behaviors that may or may not resolve the conflict

(28) **2.** ________ Reformulation of goals that is acceptable to all parties

(28) **3.** ________ People believe their goals are being blocked

(28) **4.** ________ Each party formulates a view of the basis of conflict

A. Frustration
B. Conceptualization
C. Action
D. Outcomes

E. Match the characteristic of leadership style in the numbered column with the leadership style in the lettered column. The answers may be used more than once.

(25) **1.** ________ Leader provides little or no directive leadership

(25) **2.** ________ Leader turns problems over to the group to manage

(25) **3.** ________ Leader leads by suggestion rather than domination

(25) **4.** ________ Opposite of autocratic

(25) **5.** ________ Cross between autocratic and democratic leaders

(25) **6.** ________ Authoritarian, directive, or bureaucratic

(25) **7.** ________ Leader analyzes feedback from the group and then makes decisions

A. Autocratic
B. Democratic
C. Laissez-faire
D. Participative

Student Name____

F. Match the outcomes and uses of conflict resolution modes in the numbered column with the related mode of conflict in the lettered column.

(28, 29)	**1.**	__________	Generates commitment to work together	A.	Accommodation
				B.	Collaboration
				C.	Compromise
				D.	Avoidance
(28, 29)	**2.**	__________	Produces mutually acceptable solutions	E.	Competition
(28, 29)	**3.**	__________	Agreement is reached		
(28, 29)	**4.**	__________	Reflects strong stance to defend principles		
(29)	**5.**	__________	Temporarily defuses highly charged emotional disagreement		

G. List four essential elements of effective delegation.

(30) **1.** ____

(30) **2.** ____

(30) **3.** ____

(30) **4.** ____

H. List six tips for effective management.

(29) **1.** ____

(29) **2.** ____

(29) **3.** ____

(29) **4.** ____

(29) **5.** ____

(29) **6.** ____

MULTIPLE-CHOICE QUESTIONS

I. Choose the most appropriate answer.

(25) **1.** Which of the following methods does the democratic leader use to make decisions?

1. Participation of all group members and group consensus
2. Nondirective style, letting group members decide
3. Makes decisions independently from group
4. Presents personal views to group members for comments before making final decision

(25) **2.** Four basic types of leadership are autocratic, participative, democratic, and:

1. authoritarian.
2. bureaucratic.
3. directive.
4. laissez-faire.

(25) **3.** Individuals who achieve their goals by setting objectives and having them carried out without input or suggestions from others display what style of leadership?

1. democratic
2. autocratic
3. laissez-faire
4. cooperative

(25) **4.** Individuals who encourage people to provide input into problem-solving and come up with group consensus display what style of leadership?

1. democratic
2. autocratic
3. laissez-faire
4. authoritarian

(25) **5.** Individuals who lead by suggestion rather than by domination exhibit what style of leadership?

1. autocratic
2. laissez-faire
3. authoritarian
4. democratic

(25) **6.** A leadership style where individuals are allowed to do whatever they want is:

1. democratic.
2. autocratic.
3. authoritarian.
4. laissez-faire.

(26) **7.** Which style do leaders who use the Y theory of management usually have?

1. autocratic
2. democratic
3. bureaucratic
4. laissez-faire

(27) **8.** Which management step includes making assignments and explaining what needs to be done?

1. coordinating
2. directing
3. planning
4. controlling

(27) **9.** The process of selecting one course of action from alternatives is:

1. coordinating.
2. decision making.
3. directing.
4. evaluating.

Student Name ____________________

(27) **10.** Once the problem is identified, the next step in decision making involves:

1. choosing the most desirable solution.
2. evaluating the best response.
3. coordinating the representative ideas.
4. exploring all possible solutions.

(28) **11.** The management step that helps overlap, duplication, and omissions is:

1. organizing.
2. directing.
3. coordinating.
4. controlling.

(29) **12.** The benefit of taking an active approach to planning is that the nurse is likely to:

1. emphasize the importance of documentation.
2. avoid conflict before it occurs.
3. make employees accountable for their actions.
4. treat other employees with respect.

(25) **13.** Which leadership style provides the quickest response?

1. laissez-faire
2. democratic
3. participative
4. autocratic

(25) **14.** Which leader is described as multicratic or situational?

1. laissez-faire
2. democratic
3. participative
4. autocratic

(27) **15.** In making assignments, an attempt should be made to match the skills of the assigned personnel with:

1. patient personalities.
2. nursing needs.
3. patient needs.
4. institutional needs.

(28) **16.** When making assignments for patient care, which approach encourages cooperation and tends to get more work done?

1. direct ordering that a task be done
2. requesting that a task be done
3. delegating tasks to more than one person
4. asking to see the staffing plan

(27) **17.** Which step of the management process involves developing objectives, policies, and procedures?

1. directing
2. planning
3. organizing
4. coordinating

(28) **18.** Controlling is basically a form of:

1. evaluation.
2. assessment.
3. planning.
4. implementation.

(30) **19.** Which should *not* be delegated to unlicensed personnel?

1. making a bed
2. weighing a patient
3. writing a nursing care plan
4. feeding a patient

(28) **20.** *Continuous quality improvement* (CQI) is a term frequently used in relation to:

1. organization.
2. direction.
3. coordination.
4. control.

(25) **21.** Which of the following is likely to occur when an autocratic leader hires an autocratic manager?

1. group concerns
2. problem solving
3. power struggle
4. confusion

(25) **22.** Which type of leadership style requires a highly motivated, focused group to work well?

1. democratic
2. laissez-faire
3. autocratic
4. participative

(25) **23.** Group members assist the participative leader with setting goals, achieving for themselves a sense of:

1. empowerment.
2. structure.
3. domination.
4. creativity.

(31) **24.** Characteristics of an effective team include:

1. continuous quality improvement (CQI).
2. established standards.
3. clear goals.
4. active listening.

(29) **25.** When the other person really does have a better idea than you, an effective mode of conflict resolution is:

1. accommodation.
2. collaboration.
3. compromise.
4. competition.

(29) **26.** A mode of conflict resolution that wastes time if used for resolution of trivial issues is:

1. accommodation.
2. collaboration.
3. compromise.
4. competition.

CHAPTER 4

Student Name ______________________________

The Nurse-Patient Relationship

Answer Key: Textbook page references are provided as a guide for answering these questions. A complete answer key was provided for your instructor.

OBJECTIVES

1. Define holistic view of nursing.
2. Define the concept of *self.*
3. Discuss the use of self in the practice of nursing.
4. Compare the meaning of the terms *patient* and *client.*
5. List commonly held expectations of patients and families.
6. Describe the meaning of the Patient's Bill of Rights.
7. Describe guidelines for nurse–patient relationships.
8. Describe basic components of communication.
9. Describe four basic principles of ethics.

LEARNING ACTIVITIES

A. Match the definition in the numbered column with the most appropriate term in the lettered column.

(34) **1.** __________ Principles or standards shared by members of a society that determine what is desirable or worthwhile

(39) **2.** __________ Ethical habits of a person

(34) **3.** __________ Convictions or opinions

(34) **4.** __________ Feelings toward persons or things

A. Attitudes
B. Values
C. Beliefs
D. Morals

B. List six characteristics the nurse must have to assume the helper role.

(36) **1.** ______________________________

(36) **2.** ______________________________

(36) **3.** ______________________________

(36) **4.** ______________________________

(36) **5.** ______________________________

(36) **6.** ______________________________

C. List seven examples of nonverbal communication.

(36) **1.** ______________________________

(36) **2.** ______________________________

(36) **3.** ______________________________

(36) **4.** ______________________________

(36) **5.** ______________________________

(36) **6.** ______________________________

(36) **7.** ______________________________

D. Fill in the blank.

(37) Observation is to nonverbal language as listening is to ______________________________.

E. List four tips for effective listening.

(37) **1.** ______________________________

(37) **2.** ______________________________

(37) **3.** ______________________________

(37) **4.** ______________________________

Student Name____

F. Indicate by an X in the appropriate column whether the description refers to a helping person or a friend.

		Helping Person	Friend	
(36)	**1.**	__________	__________	Shares personal information
(37)	**2.**	__________	__________	Responsible to client
(37)	**3.**	__________	__________	Sexual overtones or a sexual relationship may develop
(37)	**4.**	__________	__________	Both individuals express feelings, attitudes, and opinions
(37)	**5.**	__________	__________	Attitude is nonjudgmental
(37)	**6.**	__________	__________	Relationship is goal-directed
(37)	**7.**	__________	__________	Individuals meet each other's needs
(37)	**8.**	__________	__________	Relationship is time-limited
(37)	**9.**	__________	__________	Objective of relationship is to meet client's needs
(37)	**10.**	__________	__________	Relationship may continue
(37)	**11.**	__________	__________	No plan involved
(37)	**12.**	__________	__________	Discourages any sexual overtones in relationship
(37)	**13.**	__________	__________	Try to influence each other in discussing issues
(37)	**14.**	__________	__________	Does not keep secrets
(37)	**15.**	__________	__________	Attempts to influence patient to his or her way of thinking

G. Match the example of communication technique in the numbered column with the proper label in the lettered column.

(38) **1.** ________ Fight urge to fill quiet periods with conversation.

(38) **2.** ________ "Tell me your reactions to your new treatment."

(38) **3.** ________ "You say you're feeling better since your brother has returned?"

(38) **4.** ________ "So, you have decided to have surgery, but delay it until after Christmas."

(38) **5.** ________ "I hear you say you're concerned about your son."

(38) **6.** ________ "Do you mean 'sad' when you say 'upset'?"

A. Reflecting
B. Clarifying
C. Silence
D. Restating
E. Summarizing
F. Open-ended statement

H. Match the example of nontherapeutic communication technique in the numbered column with the proper label in the lettered column.

(39) **1.** ________ "You shouldn't worry about the new treatment."

(39) **2.** ________ "Try to think positively."

(39) **3.** ________ "If I were you, I would take your sleeping pill now."

(39) **4.** ________ "You must quit smoking immediately."

(39) **5.** ________ "It's surprising that your doctor did not tell you when you could get out of bed."

A. False reassurance
B. Premature advice
C. Commanding
D. Communication cut-off
E. Assuming truth of statements rather than checking them out

Student Name____

I. Match the basic concept of ethics on the left with the proper label in the lettered column.

(39) **1.** __________ Do no harm

(39) **2.** __________ Obligation to do good

(39) **3.** __________ Obligation to be fair to everyone

(39) **4.** __________ Right to make one's own decisions

(39) **5.** __________ Obligation to be faithful to agreements

(39) **6.** __________ Telling the truth

A. Veracity
B. Beneficence
C. Justice
D. Nonmaleficence
E. Fidelity
F. Autonomy

MULTIPLE-CHOICE QUESTIONS

J. Choose the most appropriate answer.

(36) **1.** The ability to be open and honest about one's feelings is characteristic of:

1. self-image.
2. self-esteem.
3. self-disclosure.
4. self-trust.

(36) **2.** Exchanging ideas, beliefs, thoughts, and feelings between two or more people is:

1. empathy.
2. caring.
3. self-disclosure.
4. communication.

(37) **3.** An active process that involves trying to understand what is being said is:

1. listening.
2. talking.
3. explaining.
4. self-awareness.

(38) **4.** Understanding another's feelings and becoming immersed in the situation is:

1. empathy. 2. helping.
3. sympathy. 4. apathy.

(37) **5.** The main difference between a therapeutic relationship and a social relationship is that the therapeutic helping person:

1. has a spontaneous approach.
2. discusses own beliefs.
3. shares feelings and opinions.
4. is responsible to the client.

(39) **6.** The obligation to be fair to everyone is an ethical concept called:

1. fidelity.
2. veracity.
3. justice.
4. beneficence.

(39) **7.** What is the meaning of the ethical concept of autonomy?

1. obligation to be fair
2. the right to make one's own decisions
3. obligation to be faithful to agreements
4. telling the truth

(39) **8.** The professional duty to help others is an example of:

1. veracity.
2. beneficence.
3. fidelity.
4. autonomy.

(39) **9.** A system or code of behavior related to what is right is known as:

1. ethics.
2. empathy.
3. caring.
4. empowerment.

(39) **10.** Which ethical concept is applied when the nurse provides quality care to patients, regardless of their socioeconomic status?

1. justice 2. veracity
3. autonomy 4. fidelity

(39) **11.** What is the ethical concept applied when the nurse reports substandard nursing practice?

1. beneficence
2. veracity
3. fidelity
4. nonmaleficence

(35) **12.** Encouraging patients to be active participants in their own care is called:

1. empowerment.
2. veracity.
3. fidelity.
4. empathy.

(35) **13.** According to the Patient's Bill of Rights, a basic right of patients is the right to:

1. complete medical care regardless of the ability to pay.
2. choose the best method of health care delivery.
3. considerate and respectful care from all health care providers.
4. determine treatment for medical care.

(35) **14.** Protection of the patient's confidentiality is stated in the:

1. Joint Commission of Accreditation Act.
2. Social Security Act.
3. Patient's Bill of Rights.
4. Right to Privacy Act.

(39) **15.** Which ethical concept refers to the patient's right to make his or her own decisions regarding treatment?

1. beneficence
2. autonomy
3. fidelity
4. veracity

CHAPTER 5

Student Name ______________________________

Cultural Aspects of Nursing Care

Answer Key: Textbook page references are provided as a guide for answering these questions. A complete answer key was provided for your instructor.

OBJECTIVES

1. Describe cultural concepts related to nursing and health care.
2. Identify traditional health habits and beliefs of major ethnic groups in the United States.
3. Explain cultural influences on the interactions of patients and families with the health care system.
4. Discuss cultural considerations in providing culturally sensitive nursing care.
5. Discuss ways in which planning and implementation of nursing interventions can be adapted to a patient's ethnicity.

LEARNING ACTIVITIES

A. Match the definition in the numbered column with the most appropriate term in the lettered column.

(41) **1.** __________ A group of individuals within a culture whose members share different beliefs, values, and attitudes from those of the dominant culture

(41, 50) **2.** __________ Replacing values and beliefs with those of another culture

(41) **3.** __________ The existence of many cultures in a society

A. Cultural diversity
B. Enculturation
C. Subculture
D. Culture
E. Assimilation
F. Ethnic group

Continued next page

(41) **4.** ________ Learned values, beliefs, and practices that are characteristic of a society and that guide individual behavior

(41) **5.** ________ Integration of cultural considerations into all aspects of nursing care

(42) **6.** ________ Group of individuals with a unique identity based on shared traditions and customs

(41) **7.** ________ The process of learning to be part of a culture

B. List the three basic characteristics of all cultures.

(41) **1.** ____________________

(41) **2.** ____________________

(41) **3.** ____________________

C. Match the healers in the numbered column with the ethnic group that may be likely to use them in the lettered column. Answers may be used more than once.

(51) **1.** ________ Spiritualists

(51) **2.** ________ Curanderos

(51) **3.** ________ Root doctors

(51) **4.** ________ Medicine men

(51) **5.** ________ Herbalists

(51) **6.** ________ Acupuncturists

A. Asian
B. Native American
C. Latino
D. African-American

D. List the three phases of culture shock associated with hospitalization.

(51, 52) **1.** ____________________

(51, 52) **2.** ____________________

(51, 52) **3.** ____________________

Student Name____

MULTIPLE-CHOICE QUESTIONS

E. Choose the most appropriate answer.

(41) **1.** The ideas, beliefs, values, and attitudes that a group of people possess represent:

1. race. 2. religion.
3. ethnicity. 4. culture.

(41) **2.** The effort of many immigrants to assimilate into society is known as:

1. salad bowl.
2. melting pot.
3. cultural diversity.
4. true ethnicity.

(41) **3.** The way in which new arrivals seek to maintain individual differences while acclimating to new surroundings is termed:

1. melting pot.
2. salad bowl.
3. cultural diversity.
4. true ethnicity.

(41) **4.** The Latinos are examples of a:

1. salad bowl. 2. melting pot.
3. subculture. 4. democracy.

(42) **5.** What percentage of households in the United States are single-parent families?

1. less than 1%
2. 10%
3. 20%
4. 50%

(50) **6.** People who claim that illness is a result of punishment for a sin that an individual has committed believe in:

1. divine punishment.
2. corporal punishment.
3. legal punishment.
4. ethnic punishment.

(50) **7.** People who believe that health and illness are influenced by four humors that regulate body function believe in:

1. divine punishment theory.
2. cultural diversity theory.
3. salad bowl theory.
4. hot-and-cold theory.

(52) **8.** Culture shock associated with hospitalization occurs in three stages. They include asking questions, being disenchanted, and:

1. generalization.
2. denial.
3. adaptation.
4. bargaining.

(41) **9.** The integration of cultural considerations into all aspects of nursing care is called:

1. cultural diversity.
2. transcultural nursing.
3. enculturation.
4. subcultural nursing.

(43) **10.** Kosher dietary laws which state that there is no mixing of milk and meat at a meal is a belief of which religious group?

1. Seventh-Day Adventist
2. Eastern Orthodox
3. Judaism
4. Protestant

(51) **11.** Which ethnic group values self-respect, respect for elders, and pride?

1. whites
2. african-americans
3. latinos
4. asians

(43) **12.** Which religious group believes that the body should not be left alone until buried?

1. Judaism
2. Protestant
3. Eastern Orthodox
4. Mormon

(49) **13.** Which religious group believes in reincarnation and calls in a priest at the time of death, who ties a thread around the neck of the dead person as a blessing?

1. Mormon
2. Hinduism
3. Eastern Orthodox
4. Judaism

(48) **14.** Which religious group believes that the body should be washed, prepared, and placed in a position facing Mecca following death?

1. Judaism
2. Eastern Orthodox
3. Catholic
4. Muslim

(53) **15.** Which ethnic group responds better to diuretics for hypertension?

1. african-americans
2. latinos
3. native americans
4. whites

(53) **16.** A 24-year-old woman has been given an antidepressant for depression. Which ethnic group will respond better to a lower dose of antidepressants?

1. whites
2. african-americans
3. europeans
4. asians

(53) **17.** Why are antihypertensive drugs less effective in Japanese patients?

1. They metabolize the drug more quickly.
2. They eat Kosher foods.
3. Their diet is high in salt.
4. They are at greater risk for drug toxicity.

(51) **18.** Utilizing interpersonal skills to adapt nursing care to the cultural differences of your patients is called:

1. holistic care.
2. complementary care.
3. cultural competence.
4. cultural diversity.

CHAPTER 6

Student Name ______________________

The Nurse and the Family

Answer Key: Textbook page references are provided as a guide for answering these questions. A complete answer key was provided for your instructor.

OBJECTIVES

1. Describe the concept of family and its relationship to society.
2. Compare various family structures or lifestyles that characterize modern American families.
3. Discuss the family from a developmental perspective.
4. Describe roles and communication patterns within families.
5. Describe adaptive and maladaptive mechanisms used by families to cope with various stressors.
6. Describe the role of the nurse in dealing with families experiencing various stresses.
7. Identify community resources that may help to meet the family's needs.

LEARNING ACTIVITIES

A. Match the type of family in the numbered column with the most appropriate term in the lettered column.

(55)	**1.**	__________	Nuclear family	A.	Cohabiting couples
				B.	Blended family
(55)	**2.**	__________	Extended family	C.	Relatives of either spouse who live with the nuclear family
(55)	**3.**	__________	Step-parent	D.	Biologic or adoptive mother and father and their children
(55)	**4.**	__________	Nontraditional		

B. Match the developmental task in the numbered column with the correct stage of the family life cycle in the lettered column.

(56) **1.** ________ Establish mutually satisfying marriage; make decisions about parenthood

(56) **2.** ________ Set up young family as a stable unit; socialize children

(56) **3.** ________ Balance freedom with responsibility for children; communicate openly between parents and children

(56) **4.** ________ Expand family circle to include new family members acquired by marriage; assist aging and ill parents of husband or wife

(56) **5.** ________ Maintain a satisfying living arrangement; adjust to loss of spouse; maintain intergenerational family ties

A. Launching children and moving on
B. Families with adolescents
C. Families with young children
D. Families in later life
E. Beginning families

Student Name____

C. Match the family role in the numbered column with the type of role in the lettered column. Answers may be used more than once.

(57)	**1.**	__________ Harmonizer	A.	Informal role
			B.	Formal role
(57)	**2.**	__________ Encourager		
(57)	**3.**	__________ Wife-mother		
(57)	**4.**	__________ Family scapegoat		
(57)	**5.**	__________ Husband-father		
(57)	**6.**	__________ Son-brother		
(57)	**7.**	__________ Family caretaker		
(57)	**8.**	__________ Daughter-sister		

D. Match the characteristic of communication in the numbered column with the type of communication in the lettered column. Answers may be used more than once.

(58)	**1.**	__________ Dynamic, two-way process	A.	Functional communication
			B.	Dysfunctional communication
(58)	**2.**	__________ Acceptance of individual differences		
(58)	**3.**	__________ Unclear transmission of a message		
(58)	**4.**	__________ Verbal messages of caring		
(58)	**5.**	__________ Inability to focus on one issue		
(58)	**6.**	__________ Forbidden subjects for discussion		
(58)	**7.**	__________ Mutual respect for each other's feelings		

MULTIPLE-CHOICE QUESTIONS

E. Choose the most appropriate answer.

(57) **1.** The most consistent family developmental task that must be met throughout the family life cycle is:

1. defining the roles of the family members.
2. continuing education.
3. maintaining the marital relationship.
4. maintaining individual independence.

(57) **2.** One of the most important influences on family interaction is:

1. self-esteem of each member.
2. family income.
3. family size.
4. type of family configuration.

(59) **3.** A negative strategy for adapting to family stress is:

1. problem solving.
2. mastery.
3. coping behavior.
4. defense mechanism.

(59) **4.** Assessment of families and their coping strategies consists of all *except* which one of the following?

1. determine stressors being experienced
2. assess family communication patterns
3. find out what kinds of coping strategies are used
4. explore each family member's political views

(59) **5.** When assisting families to cope, it is most important to:

1. encourage all family members to be involved in the process.
2. work with the most influential member of the family.
3. make the family members use all new coping strategies.
4. tell the family they are dysfunctional and need help.

(59) **6.** When taking care of a patient in the hospital, it is important to:

1. keep the family members out of the room.
2. ignore the family members because the patient is the focus of care.
3. determine whether the family members are supportive or detrimental in the recovery process.
4. provide information only to the patient because of confidentiality.

(56) **7.** A developmental task of families with adolescents is to:

1. work out satisfactory relationships with the spouse's family.
2. refocus on the marital relationship.
3. expand the family circle to include new family members.
4. assist aging and ill parents.

(56) **8.** Maintaining ties between aging parents and growing children is a developmental task of:

1. beginning families.
2. families with young children.
3. launching children and moving on.
4. families in later life.

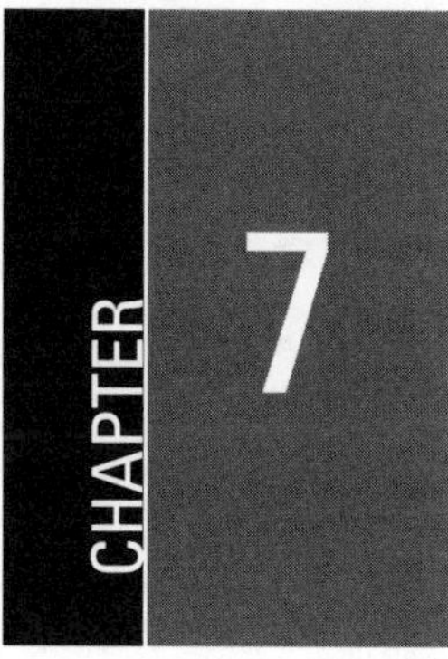

Student Name ______________________________

Health and Illness

Answer Key: Textbook page references are provided as a guide for answering these questions. A complete answer key was provided for your instructor.

OBJECTIVES

1. Describe the health-illness continuum.
2. Discuss traditional and current views of health and illness.
3. List Maslow's five basic human needs and explain why they constitute a hierarchy.
4. Explain the four levels of adaptability to stress.
5. Discuss concepts related to health promotion, disease prevention, and health maintenance.
6. Define acute and chronic illness.
7. Discuss illness behavior and the impact of illness on the family.
8. Describe nursing measures for health promotion, health maintenance, and illness.
9. Describe complementary and alternative therapies and the nurse's role in relation to both.

LEARNING ACTIVITIES

A. List the five levels of human needs in Maslow's hierarchy.

(63) **1.** ______________________________

(63) **2.** ______________________________

(63) **3.** ______________________________

(63) **4.** ______________________________

(63) **5.** ______________________________

B. Maslow's Hierarchy: Match the need in the numbered column with the correct level in the lettered column.

(63) **1.** ________ Oxygen, fluid, nutrition, temperature, elimination, shelter, rest, and sex

(63) **2.** ________ Security, protection from harm, freedom from anxiety and fear

(63) **3.** ________ Feeling loved by family and friends, and accepted by peers and community

(63) **4.** ________ Feeling good about oneself and feeling that others hold one in high regard

(63) **5.** ________ Self-fulfillment; able to problem-solve, accept criticism from others, and eager to acquire new knowledge; self-confidence; maturity

A. Self-esteem
B. Safety and security
C. Physiologic
D. Self-actualization
E. Love and belonging

C. List the three stages of the general adaptation syndrome.

(65) **1.** ______________________________

(65) **2.** ______________________________

(65) **3.** ______________________________

Student Name ____________________

D. Match Henderson's 14 components of basic nursing care in the numbered column with Maslow's hierarchy of human needs in the lettered column. Answers may be used more than once.

(68) **1.** __________ Learn, discover, or satisfy curiosity

(68) **2.** __________ Breathe normally

(68) **3.** __________ Worship according to one's faith

(68) **4.** __________ Eat and drink adequately

(68) **5.** __________ Eliminate body wastes

(68) **6.** __________ Play or participate in various forms of recreation

(68) **7.** __________ Move and maintain desirable posture

(68) **8.** __________ Sleep and rest

(68) **9.** __________ Select suitable clothing, dress and undress

(68) **10.** __________ Avoid dangers in the environment and avoid injuring others

(68) **11.** __________ Maintain body temperature within the normal range by adjusting clothing and modifying the environment

(68) **12.** __________ Communicate with others in expressing emotions, needs, fears, and opinions

(68) **13.** __________ Work in such a way that there is a sense of accomplishment

(68) **14.** __________ Keep the body clean and well-groomed and protect the integument

A. Physiologic needs
B. Safety and security needs
C. Love and belonging needs
D. Self-esteem and self-actualization needs

E. Match the statement in the numbered column with the correct method of increasing adaptability in the lettered column.

(68) **1.** ________ "What is your worst possible stressor, and how does this present stress compare with the worst?"

(68) **2.** ________ "What ways have you coped with stress in the past that have been successful for you?"

(68) **3.** ________ "What kinds of things do you do when you are stressed? Do you eat more or less?"

(68) **4.** ________ "Whom do you turn to when you are feeling stressed?"

A. Assess past methods of coping with stress
B. Assess internal coping strategies
C. Determine external coping strategies
D. Assess the degree of stress

F. Match the descriptions in the numbered column with traditional or current view in the lettered column.

(62) **1.** ________ Emphasis is on maintenance of health and prevention of disease.

(62) **2.** ________ Health and illness are separate entities.

(63) **3.** ________ Focus is on curing disease or injury.

(62) **4.** ________ Health and illness are relative and ever-changing.

A. Traditional view
B. Current view

Student Name____

G. Match the herbal-drug combination in the numbered column with the interaction in the lettered column. Answers may be used more than once.

(71) **1.** __________ Echinacea and immunosuppressants

(71) **2.** __________ Aloe and diuretics

(71) **3.** __________ Garlic and anticoagulants

(71) **4.** __________ Ephedra and antihypertensives

(71) **5.** __________ Kava-kava and CNS depressants

(71) **6.** __________ Goldenseal and antihypertensives

(71) **7.** __________ Ginseng and aspirin

(71) **8.** __________ Hawthorne and cardiac glycosides

A. Inhibit immunosuppression
B. Increased risk of bleeding
C. Increased blood pressure
D. Increased risk of digitalis toxicity
E. Increased risk of hypokalemia
F. Increased sedation

H. Match the examples of complementary therapies in the numbered column with the type of therapy in the lettered column. Answers may be used more than once.

(71) **1.** __________ Acupuncture

(71) **2.** __________ Meditation

(71) **3.** __________ Ginkgo biloba

(71) **4.** __________ Antioxidants

(71) **5.** __________ Herbal tea for a cold

(71) **6.** __________ Laser surgery

(71) **7.** __________ Chiropractic

(71) **8.** __________ High-dose vitamin therapy

(71) **9.** __________ St. John's wort

(71) **10.** __________ Prayer

A. Alternative systems of medical practice
B. Mind-body interventions
C. Manual healing methods
D. Bioelectromagnetic applications
E. Herbal medicine
F. Pharmacologic and biologic treatments
G. Diet and nutrition changes

I. Maslow's Hierarchy: Indicate for each finding in the numbered column the appropriate level of needs to which it relates in Maslow's hierarchy in the lettered column. Answers may be used more than once.

Your patient is a 45-year-old male who has been admitted to the hospital with pneumonia. As you are conducting your admission interview, you find out the following:

(63)	**1.**	________	He has recently separated from his wife and three children.	A.	Physiologic needs
				B.	Safety and security
				C.	Love and belonging
				D.	Self-esteem and self-actualization
(63)	**2.**	________	He is afraid to jog due to crime in neighborhood.		
(63)	**3.**	________	He states that he feels like he will never amount to anything.		
(63)	**4.**	________	He eats "fast foods," drinks a lot of coffee.		
(63)	**5.**	________	He states he does not feel very positive about himself right now.		
(63)	**6.**	________	His parents live 300 miles away; he has few close friends in town.		
(63)	**7.**	________	He states he fears he will lose his job if he is in the hospital too long.		
(63)	**8.**	________	He states he feels alone a lot.		
(63)	**9.**	________	He sleeps only 4–5 hours per night.		
(63)	**10.**	________	He lives in a poor section of town.		

Student Name____

MULTIPLE-CHOICE QUESTIONS

J. Choose the most appropriate answer.

(64) **1.** Which of the following is an internal stressor?

1. loss of relationship
2. economic inadequacies
3. sensory deprivation
4. feelings of powerlessness

(66) **2.** Which is an appropriate coping strategy for making plans?

1. problem solving
2. self-control
3. confrontation
4. faith

(64) **3.** Which type of stress occurs when you feel angry while fearing the consequences of expressing it?

1. internal, physical
2. internal, psychological
3. external, interpersonal relations
4. external, socioeconomic

(63) **4.** Oxygen, food, and safety are examples of:

1. psychological needs.
2. physiologic needs.
3. emotional needs.
4. affectional needs.

(66) **5.** A patient's refusal of treatment is an example of which coping strategy?

1. confrontation
2. denial
3. problem solving
4. event review

(67) **6.** What is one of the leading health indicators covered in the *Healthy People 2010* report?

1. physical activity
2. vision and hearing
3. medical product safety
4. oral health

(63) **7.** The highest level of Maslow's hierarchy is:

1. love and belonging.
2. self-esteem.
3. physiologic needs.
4. self-actualization.

(63) **8.** The most fundamental needs that sustain life are:

1. physiologic needs.
2. safety needs.
3. belonging needs.
4. self-esteem needs.

(64) **9.** Which is included as one of the top 10 major stressors?

1. death of a close family member
2. marriage of a child
3. celebration of 25th wedding anniversary
4. first employee evaluation

(64) **10.** Areas in which most people seek control even while they are sick include their:

1. work environment.
2. play environment.
3. treatments and procedures.
4. local adaptation syndrome.

(64) **11.** Wound healing and inflammation are examples of:

1. general adaptation syndrome.
2. local adaptation syndrome.
3. negative feedback response.
4. countercurrent response.

(65) **12.** A physiologic response of the body to stress is:

1. bronchoconstriction.
2. increased heart rate.
3. decreased respirations.
4. decreased blood pressure.

(65) **13.** Increased hormone levels, heart rate, and oxygen intake are components of the:

1. resistance stage.
2. exhaustion stage.
3. alarm reaction.
4. local adaptation stage.

(65) **14.** Adaptation to a stressor occurs in the:

1. resistance stage.
2. alarm stage.
3. exhaustion stage.
4. initial stage.

(65) **15.** With a long-term stressor such as a chronic physical or mental illness, the individual enters the third stage of adaptation, or the:

1. alarm stage.
2. exhaustion stage.
3. resistance stage.
4. local adaptation stage.

(65) **16.** Cold hands and feet and tensed muscles are signs or symptoms of:

1. withdrawal. 2. depression.
3. adaptation. 4. stress.

(65) **17.** Slowed speech, inability to concentrate, and hesitant speech may be signs of:

1. stress. 2. adaptation.
3. depression. 4. alarm.

(65) **18.** Behavioral or cognitive activities used to deal with stress are:

1. feedback behaviors.
2. coping behaviors.
3. depressive behaviors.
4. automatic behaviors.

(66) **19.** Maintaining stability of the internal environment is a definition of:

1. adaptation.
2. coping.
3. resistance.
4. homeostasis.

(67) **20.** An illness or disease that has a relatively rapid onset and short duration is said to be:

1. chronic.
2. acute.
3. disabling.
4. an emergency.

(67) **21.** Permanent impairments or disabilities, requiring long-term rehabilitation and treatment, are said to be:

1. disabling. 2. challenging.
3. chronic. 4. acute.

(67) **22.** Nursing interventions to increase adaptability in the elderly should be geared toward helping older clients to:

1. use past successful coping mechanisms to deal with new stressors.
2. assess their strengths and weaknesses in dealing with new stressors.
3. develop new coping mechanisms to deal with new stressors.
4. learn new methods of dealing with stressors.

(69) **23.** Biofeedback, meditation, and imagery are examples of measures that patients may use to help:

1. encourage exercise.
2. increase appetite.
3. relieve stress.
4. promote bowel regularity.

Student Name____

(69) **24.** Tasks for chronically ill individuals include:

1. ignoring disease.
2. preventing and managing crises.
3. curing disease.
4. promoting social isolation.

(66) **25.** Activities directed toward maintaining or enhancing well-being as a protection against illness are related to:

1. health adaptation.
2. health promotion.
3. prevention of illness.
4. homeostasis measures.

(62) **26.** Health and illness are:

1. absolute, unchanging states of being.
2. unconditional states of being.
3. relative, ever-changing states of being.
4. homeostasis measures.

(67) **27.** A leading health indicator for *Healthy People 2010* is:

1. infectious disease.
2. cardiovascular disease.
3. tobacco use.
4. nutrition.

(71) **28.** When garlic is taken by a patient who is also taking an anticoagulant, the patient is at risk for:

1. sedation.
2. hypotension.
3. bleeding.
4. infection.

(71) **29.** Immunosuppression may be inhibited when a patient who is taking immunosuppressant drugs also takes:

1. echinacea. 2. ginseng.
3. kava-kava. 4. garlic.

CHAPTER 8

Student Name ______________________

Nutrition

Answer Key: Textbook page references are provided as a guide for answering these questions. A complete answer key was provided for your instructor.

OBJECTIVES

1. Explain the role of the alimentary system in the digestion of food.
2. Describe how food is digested and absorbed.
3. List the functions of each of the six classes of essential nutrients.
4. List the functions of proteins, carbohydrates, and fats.
5. Identify the food sources of proteins, carbohydrates, and fats.
6. Identify the food sources of dietary fiber.
7. List the possible health benefits of dietary fiber.
8. Identify the food sources of each of the vitamins and minerals.
9. Describe the changes in nutrient needs as an individual ages.
10. Differentiate anorexia nervosa, bulimia, and binge eating disorder.
11. Discuss the different types of nutritional support.
12. Identify guidelines for the nutritional assessment.

LEARNING ACTIVITIES

A. Match the definition in the numbered column with the most appropriate term in the lettered column.

(78) **1.** ________ Lipid-wrapped proteins carried into the bloodstream; includes high-density and low-density lipoproteins, which carry cholesterol

(81) **2.** ________ Small amounts of metals (calcium, sodium, and potassium) and nonmetals (chloride, phosphate) that are essential to the body; can build up

(78) **3.** ________ Lipids composed of three fatty acid chains and a glycerol molecule

(80) **4.** ________ Combination of incomplete proteins that provide all nine essential amino acids when consumed together

(78) **5.** ________ Compounds that come chiefly from animal sources and are usually solid at room temperature; also coconut and palm oils

A. Saturated fatty acids
B. Incomplete protein
C. Triglycerides
D. Calorie
E. Vitamins
F. Lipids
G. Minerals
H. Basal metabolic rate
I. Amino acids
J. Complementary protein
K. Complete protein
L. Insoluble fiber
M. Lipoproteins
N. Resting metabolic rate
O. Proteins
P. Unsaturated fatty acids

Continued next page

Student Name ______________________________

(79) **6.** __________ Large organic compounds made of various combinations of amino acids; found in meat, milk, fish, and eggs

(81) **7.** __________ Organic compounds supplied by food that the body requires for normal growth and development

(79) **8.** __________ A group of 22 substances that can be bonded in different ways to make a variety of proteins; the body can manufacture sufficient amounts of these provided the nine essential amino acids are derived from the diet

(77) **9.** __________ Indigestible roughage found in plant cells; aids in stool formation and elimination

(78) **10.** __________ Compounds that come from plants or fish and are generally liquid at room temperature; can be monounsaturated (olive, peanut, canola, and avocado oils) or polyunsaturated (corn, safflower, and sesame oils)

(75) **11.** __________ Energy expended in the resting state; measured in the morning with the body at complete mental and physical rest, but not asleep

(79) **12.** __________ Plant protein lacking one or more essential amino acids

(78) **13.** __________ Fats in solid or liquid form; store energy, carry fat-soluble vitamins, and maintain healthy skin and hair; supply essential fatty acids and promote a feeling of fullness (satiety)

(76) **14.** __________ Standard unit for measuring energy; the amount of heat needed to raise the temperature of 1 kg of water at a standard temperature by 1° Celsius

(75) **15.** __________ Measurement of energy expenditure taken at any time of the day and 3–4 hours after the last meal

(79) **16.** __________ Protein containing all nine essential amino acids; usually of animal origin (e.g., meat, eggs)

B. List six nutrients.

(74) **1.** ______________________ (74) **4.** ______________________

(74) **2.** ______________________ (74) **5.** ______________________

(74) **3.** ______________________ (74) **6.** ______________________

C. List six hormones that affect the basal metabolic rate (BMR).

(75) **1.** ______________________ (75) **4.** ______________________

(75) **2.** ______________________ (75) **5.** ______________________

(75) **3.** ______________________ (75) **6.** ______________________

D. List two reasons why the BMR of a sleeping person is lower than that of an awake, alert person.

(75) **1.** ____

(75) **2.** ____

E. List the number of calories per gram provided by lipids, carbohydrates, and protein.

(79) **1.** Lipids ____

(77, 79) **2.** Carbohydrates ____

(79) **3.** Protein ____

F. List six sources of complete proteins in foods.

(79) **1.** ______________________ (79) **4.** ______________________

(79) **2.** ______________________ (79) **5.** ______________________

(79) **3.** ______________________ (79) **6.** ______________________

Student Name____

G. Label the food groups, including recommended amounts of servings (A–F) in the food guide pyramid (Fig. 8-1). *(86)*

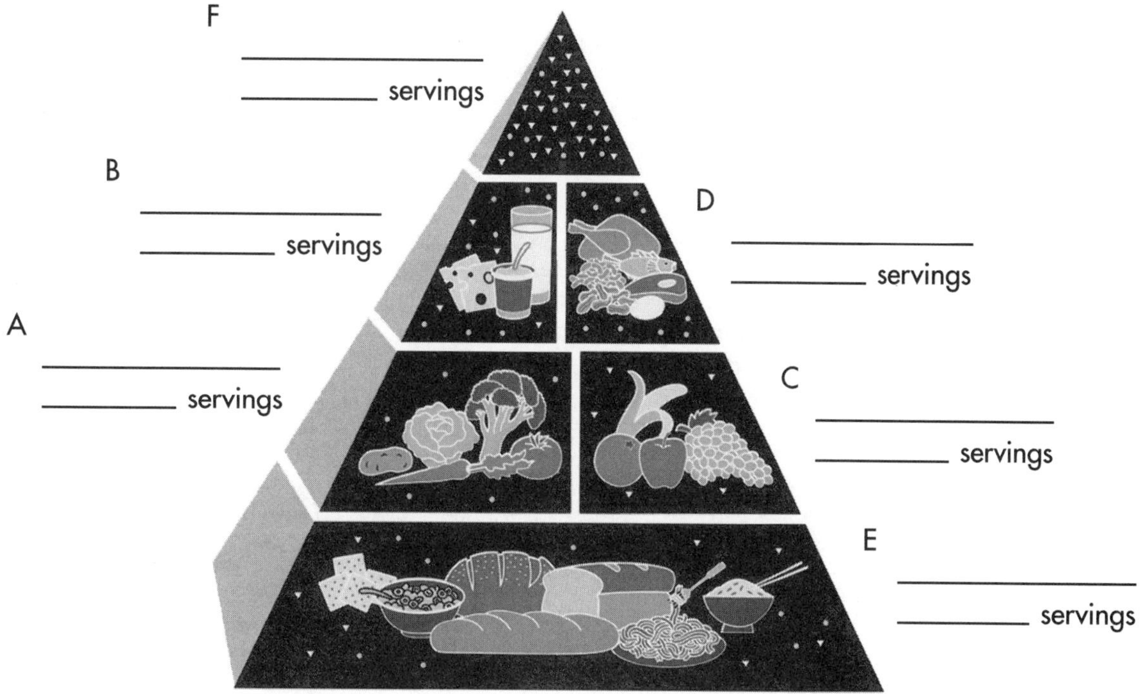

H. Label the feeding tubes in Figure 8-4 (A–D) using the following terms:

nasogastric
nasoduodenal
nasojejunal
PEG

(94) **A.** ____________________

(94) **B.** ____________________

(94) **C.** ____________________

(94) **D.** ____________________

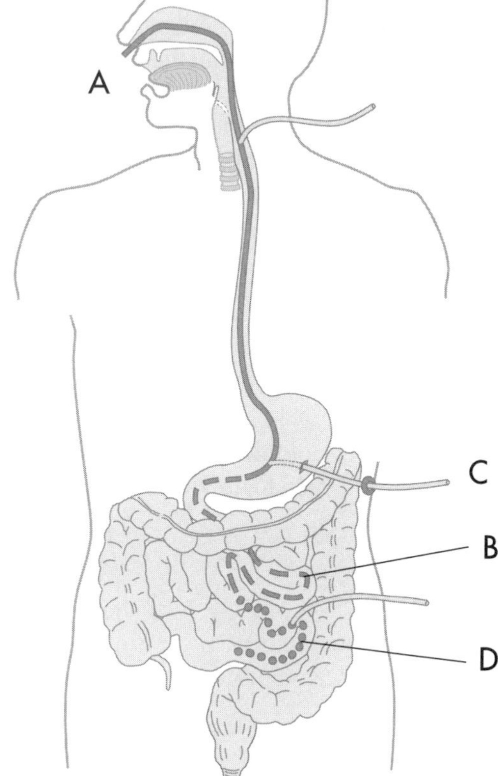

MULTIPLE-CHOICE QUESTIONS

I. Choose the most appropriate answer.

(74) **1.** The stomach is normally emptied in:

1. 30–60 minutes.
2. 1–4 hours.
3. 5–8 hours.
4. 10–12 hours.

(74) **2.** What is one type of carbohydrate that cannot be digested and is excreted unchanged in the feces?

1. fiber
2. glucose
3. glycogen
4. monosaccharide

(73) **3.** What is the parasympathetic effect in the stomach carried by the vagus nerve in response to the sight or smell of food ?

1. increases the appetite
2. increases gastric acid secretions
3. increases the feeling of fullness
4. speeds the movement of food through the intestines

(78) **4.** Which lipoprotein increases the risk of atherosclerosis by contributing to plaque buildup on the artery walls?

1. triglycerides
2. LDLs
3. HDLs
4. phospholipids

(75) **5.** Colonic bacteria are needed to help form vitamin:

1. C.
2. D.
3. K.
4. A.

(75) **6.** Which foods are the most easily digested?

1. raw foods
2. cooked foods
3. fried foods
4. foods with additives

(75) **7.** An endocrine hormone that regulates the metabolic rate is:

1. thyroxine.
2. melatonin.
3. aldosterone.
4. estrogen.

(79) **8.** For which body tissue are lipids NOT a source of energy?

1. bladder
2. stomach
3. heart
4. brain

(76) **9.** A calorie is the amount of heat energy required to raise the temperature of 1 gram of water at a standard initial temperature by:

1. 1° C.
2. 10° C.
3. 25° C.
4. 50° C.

(76) **10.** Carbohydrates are organic compounds that consist of carbon, hydrogen, and:

1. nitrogen.
2. oxygen.
3. iron.
4. calcium.

(76) **11.** For immediate use by the body's cells, carbohydrates are converted primarily to:

1. glycogen.
2. glucose.
3. sucrose.
4. fructose.

Student Name____

(77) **12.** What acts like a sponge to absorb many times its weight in water and helps provide a full feeling long after eating?

1. soluble fiber
2. monosaccharides
3. insoluble fiber
4. glycerols

(77) **13.** Diets without at least 50 to 100 grams of carbohydrates per day are likely to lead to:

1. ketosis.
2. alkalosis.
3. hyperglycemia.
4. hypernatremia.

(79) **14.** Which of the following nutrients releases the most energy?

1. fiber
2. carbohydrates
3. protein
4. lipid

(78) **15.** Which nutrient can be stored in the body compactly with little or no water?

1. carbohydrate
2. lipid
3. protein
4. glucose

(78) **16.** Neutral fats, the most common fats found in foods of both plant and animal origin, are called:

1. corticosteroids.
2. insoluble fibers.
3. soluble fibers.
4. triglycerides.

(79) **17.** Adipose cells can store up to 95% of their volume as:

1. glucose.
2. glycogen.
3. amino acids.
4. triglycerides.

(79) **18.** Most human adipose cells are in the form of white fat, which accumulates in:

1. subcutaneous tissue.
2. epidermis.
3. dermis.
4. muscles.

(79) **19.** Lipids are a major source of energy for:

1. subcutaneous tissue.
2. epidermis tissue.
3. muscle tissue.
4. mucous membrane.

(79) **20.** Where are most lipids carried to be converted to energy or used in the synthesis of new triglycerides?

1. gallbladder 2. liver
3. heart 4. kidney

(79) **21.** Most nutritionists recommend that the daily fat intake should be what percentage of the daily caloric intake?

1. 50% or less
2. 30% or less
3. 15% or less
4. 10% or less

(79) **22.** To minimize the risk of heart disease, people should eat more:

1. saturated fats.
2. polyunsaturated fats.
3. glycerol fats.
4. unsaturated fats.

(79) **23.** The main source of saturated fats in the American diet comes from:

1. vegetable oil.
2. cottonseed oil.
3. animal products.
4. safflower oil.

(80) **24.** When various incomplete proteins are consumed at the same time, the body can use them together to obtain a balance of the essential amino acids. Incomplete proteins consumed together are called:

1. plant proteins.
2. complementary proteins.
3. animal proteins.
4. enzyme proteins.

(79) **25.** The nine amino acids that must be obtained from the diet are called:

1. dietary amino acids.
2. essential amino acids.
3. incomplete amino acids.
4. complementary amino acids.

(80) **26.** Which of the following foods has the highest protein content?

1. cereals 2. beans
3. poultry 4. lentils

(81) **27.** Vitamins A, D, E, and K are:

1. fat soluble.
2. water soluble.
3. insoluble.
4. complementary.

(81) **28.** In addition to fat-soluble vitamins, which group of nutrients needs bile and pancreatic juices for absorption?

1. carbohydrates
2. proteins
3. amino acids
4. lipids

(83) **29.** The intake of water is controlled by:

1. exercise.
2. thirst.
3. metabolism.
4. stress.

(84) **30.** How much water should adults drink daily?

1. 500 ml 2. 1000 ml
3. 2500 ml 4. 5000 ml

(84) **31.** The diet for the elderly should include:

1. low-fat foods.
2. low-sodium foods.
3. all the food groups.
4. high-protein foods.

(84) **32.** Older adults with chronic diseases have an increased risk for negative nitrogen balance and:

1. protein deficiency.
2. vitamin deficiency.
3. mineral deficiency.
4. carbohydrate deficiency.

(86) **33.** Guidelines for the amounts of nutrients that healthy people should consume daily are called:

1. basic four food groups.
2. recommended daily allowances.
3. food pyramid.
4. minimum food requirements.

(91) **34.** Overweight individuals are considered obese if their weight is what percent above the ideal body weight?

1. 5% or more
2. 10% or more
3. 20% or more
4. 30% or more

(80) **35.** Which nutrient must be eaten daily, as it cannot be stored in the body?

1. carbohydrates
2. protein
3. lipids
4. minerals

Student Name ____________________

(92) **36.** A method of administering nutrients only if the gastrointestinal tract cannot be used is called:

1. enteral tube feedings.
2. nasogastric tube feedings.
3. duodenal tube feedings.
4. total parenteral nutrition.

(93) **37.** Total parenteral nutrition or TPN feedings are used for patients who are usually debilitated and malnourished with a weight loss of what percent of body weight?

1. 10% or more
2. 20% or more
3. 50% or more
4. 75% or more

(93) **38.** What type of solution is administered through a Hickman- or Broviac-type catheter?

1. hypotonic
2. hypertonic
3. isotonic
4. glucose and sterile water

(92) **39.** What is a complication of enteral tube feedings when viscous formulas and crushed medications are inadequately flushed?

1. dumping syndrome
2. diarrhea
3. GI bleeding
4. tube blockage

(94) **40.** If patients who have been without food for an extended period of time are given food too quickly, they may develop:

1. hypernatremia.
2. hypercalcemia.
3. hypophosphatemia.
4. hypoglycemia.

(94) **41.** When moving from enteral to oral feedings, the patient may experience:

1. breathing difficulties.
2. bleeding at the TPN site.
3. heart palpitations.
4. poor appetite.

CHAPTER 9

Student Name ______________________________

Developmental Processes

Answer Key: Textbook page references are provided as a guide for answering these questions. A complete answer key was provided for your instructor.

OBJECTIVES

1. List the developmental tasks for successful adulthood.
2. Identify the health problems specific to the adult age groups.
3. Discuss the health care needs of young, middle-aged, and older adults.

LEARNING ACTIVITIES

A. Match the definition in the numbered column with the most appropriate term in the lettered column.

(99) **1.** __________ The functional capabilities of various organ systems in the body

(99) **2.** __________ The behavioral capacity of a person to adapt to changing environmental demands

(99) **3.** __________ The roles and habits of a person in relation to other members of society

(99) **4.** __________ The number of years a person has lived

A. Chronologic age
B. Social age
C. Biologic age
D. Psychological age

B. Match the definition in the numbered column with the most appropriate developmental stage in the lettered column. Answers may be used more than once.

(96)	**1.**	________	Focus on marriage, childbearing, and work	A. Young adulthood B. Middle age C. Old age
(98)	**2.**	________	45–65 years of age	
(99)	**3.**	________	Over the age of 65	
(98)	**4.**	________	"Sandwich" generation	
(100)	**5.**	________	Redirection of energy and talents to new roles and activities	
(96)	**6.**	________	20–45 years of age	

C. Match the characteristic in the numbered column with the most appropriate developmental stage in the lettered column. Answers may be used more than once.

(98)	**1.**	________	Earn most of their money	A. Young adulthood B. Middle years C. Older adulthood
(99)	**2.**	________	Retirement	
(96)	**3.**	________	Marriage, childbearing, and work	
(96)	**4.**	________	Settling down to job and raising a family	
(99)	**5.**	________	Decreased short-term memory	
(98)	**6.**	________	Pay most of taxes	
(96)	**7.**	________	Establishing career goals	

Student Name____

D. Match the developmental task in the numbered column with the developmental stage in the lettered column. Answers may be used more than once.

(100)	**1.**	__________	Guidance of grown children	A.	Young adulthood
				B.	Middle age
(96)	**2.**	__________	Home and time management	C.	Older adulthood
(100)	**3.**	__________	Learn to combine new dependency needs with the continuing need for independence		
(98)	**4.**	__________	Help growing and grown children to become happy, responsible adults		
(99)	**5.**	__________	Adjust to decreasing physical strength and health changes		
(96)	**6.**	__________	Establish independence from parental home and financial aid		
(99)	**7.**	__________	Accept role reversal with aging parents		
(100)	**8.**	__________	Adjust to loss of physical strength, illness, and the approach of one's death		
(96)	**9.**	__________	Accept self and stabilize self-concept		
(96)	**10.**	__________	Become established in a vocation or profession		
(99)	**11.**	__________	Balance work and other roles, preparing for retirement		
(100)	**12.**	__________	Maintain emotional satisfaction in relationships with spouse, children, grandchildren, and other living relatives		

E. Match the health developmental task in the numbered column with the developmental stage in the lettered column.

(97) 1. ________ Generativity versus stagnation

(97) 2. ________ Intimacy versus isolation

(97) 3. ________ Ego integrity versus despair

A. Young adulthood
B. Middle years
C. Older adulthood

F. Match the health problem in the numbered column with the most appropriate developmental stage in the lettered column. Answers may be used more than once.

(100) 1. ________ Benign or malignant prostate enlargement

(99) 2. ________ Respiratory disease, causing absence from work among women

(99) 3. ________ Bone mass begins to decline

(97) 4. ________ Complications of pregnancy

(97) 5. ________ Smoking; alcohol and drug abuse

(99) 6. ________ Injuries, frequently causing absence from work among men

(100) 7. ________ Chronic illness a major cause of death

(97) 8. ________ Vehicular accidents and suicide

(100) 9. ________ Breast cancer common in women

(97) 10. ________ Stress related to managing a household

A. Young adulthood
B. Middle years
C. Older adulthood

Student Name____

G. Match the health problem in the numbered column with the most appropriate developmental age in the lettered column. Answers may be used more than once.

(99) **1.** __________ Development of presbyopia

(100) **2.** __________ Peptic ulcer

(97) **3.** __________ Homicide and accidents

(100) **4.** __________ Arthritis

(99) **5.** __________ Obesity

(100) **6.** __________ Childbearing complications

(100) **7.** __________ Accidental falls

(100) **8.** __________ Emphysema

(97) **9.** __________ HIV infection

(99) **10.** __________ Alcoholism

A. Young adulthood
B. Middle years
C. Older adulthood

MULTIPLE-CHOICE QUESTIONS

H. Choose the most appropriate answer.

(100) **1.** Establishing independence from parental home and financial aid is a developmental task of the:

1. middle-aged adult.
2. older adult.
3. young adult.
4. teenager.

(100) **2.** Guidance of grown children and care of aging parents are developmental tasks of the:

1. young adult.
2. middle-aged adult.
3. older adult.
4. retired adult.

(100) **3.** Learning to combine new dependency needs with the need for independence are developmental tasks of the:

1. teenager.
2. young adult.
3. middle-aged adult.
4. older adult.

(96) **4.** Developmental tasks that focus on marriage, parenthood, and career choice are related to:

1. teenagers.
2. young adults.
3. middle-aged adults.
4. older adults.

(98) **5.** Stress and conflict related to balancing caring for children as well as caring for aging parents are related to:

1. teenagers.
2. young adults.
3. middle-aged adults.
4. older adults.

(97) **6.** If older adults cannot adjust to the physical, psychological, and sociologic changes that occur as they age, they are at risk for:

1. isolation.
2. stagnation.
3. generativity.
4. despair.

(97) **7.** To assess the developmental tasks of young adulthood, you ask:

1. whether the patient has meaningful, intimate relationships.
2. what the patient does for leisure or recreation.
3. what the patient does each day.
4. what signs of depression the patient has.

(98) **8.** A baseline mammogram is recommended for women at age:

1. 20.
2. 25.
3. 35.
4. 45.

(98) **9.** Health promotion for persons in their thirties includes:

1. effective parenting, stress management.
2. yearly blood pressure screening.
3. influenza vaccinations.
4. yearly mammograms.

CHAPTER 10

Student Name ______________________________

The Older Patient

Answer Key: Textbook page references are provided as a guide for answering these questions. A complete answer key was provided for your instructor.

OBJECTIVES

1. Describe the roles of the gerontological nurse.
2. Compare the myths and stereotypes of the aging population with current statistical trends.
3. Describe biologic and physiologic factors associated with aging.
4. Explain psychosocial factors associated with aging.
5. Describe modifications needed for activities of daily living.

LEARNING ACTIVITIES

A. Match the drug in the numbered column with the adverse drug reaction in older persons in the lettered column. Answers may be used more than once.

(112) **1.** ________ Analgesics (aspirin)

(112) **2.** ________ Antibiotics (doxycycline)

(112) **3.** ________ Anticoagulants (warfarin)

(112) **4.** ________ Antidepressants (imipramine)

(112) **5.** ________ Antihypertensives (hydrochlorothiazide)

(112) **6.** ________ Antiparkinsonians (levodopa)

A. Hyponatremia
B. Drowsiness
C. Confusion
D. Hypotension
E. Bleeding or hemorrhage
F. Uremia
G. Arrhythmias

Continued next page

(112) **7.** ________ Antipsychotics (lithium)

(112) **8.** ________ Diuretics (chlorothiazide)

(112) **9.** ________ Sedative/hypnotics (flurazepam)

B. Match the change in the numbered column with the result described in the lettered column. Answers may be used more than once.

(105) **1.** ________ Pain, touch, and tactile sensation

(108) **2.** ________ Sense of smell

(105) **3.** ________ Conduction speed in CNS

(106) **4.** ________ Renal function

(105) **5.** ________ Pulmonary blood flow

(106) **6.** ________ Force of pulse

(105) **7.** ________ Intellectual capability

(105) **8.** ________ Sound judgment

(105) **9.** ________ Creativity

(105) **10.** ________ Exertional dyspnea

(106) **11.** ________ Cerebral blood flow

(105) **12.** ________ Loss of neurons (brain cells)

(105) **13.** ________ Functional ability of brain cells

(105) **14.** ________ Conduction speed associated with synaptic transmission

A. Decrease
B. Increase
C. No change

Continued next page

Student Name____

(104) **15.** __________ Intelligence

(106) **16.** __________ Heart size

(105) **17.** __________ Short-term memory

(105) **18.** __________ Vital capacity

(105) **19.** __________ Long-term memory

(105) **20.** __________ Chronic hypoxia of brain

C. Match the physiological assessment values in the numbered column with age-related causes in the lettered column.

(106) **1.** __________ By the age of 70, BP is 150/90

(106) **2.** __________ Resting cardiac output falls 30 to 40%

(105) **3.** __________ Difficulty remembering planned events for the day

(105) **4.** __________ Slow responses, impeded short-term memory

(106) **5.** __________ Problems with acid-base regulation

(106) **6.** __________ Increased residual urine and urinary tract infections

(106) **7.** __________ Increased BUN

(106) **8.** __________ Decreased ability to concentrate or dilute urine

(106) **9.** __________ Increased urge incontinence

(107) **10.** __________ Constipation

(106) **11.** __________ Heart murmurs

A. Decreased neurons and conduction speed at synapses
B. Decreased baroreceptor reflexes and inelasticity of vessel walls
C. Chronic hypoxic state of the brain
D. Decreased heart rate and stroke volume
E. Increasing valvular rigidity and incomplete closure of the aortic and pulmonic valves
F. Bladder capacity reduced by half; delayed response to stretch receptors in the bladder
G. Decreased intestinal motility
H. Decreased secretion of ADH by the pituitary
I. Lax muscle tone and incomplete emptying of bladder
J. Decreases in filtration rate, plasma flow rate, and tubular reabsorption and secretion
K. Renal tubules are less able to eliminate excess hydrogen ions

MULTIPLE-CHOICE QUESTIONS

D. Choose the most appropriate answer.

(102) **1.** The study of aging is called:

1. geriatrics.
2. ageism.
3. gerontology.
4. pulmonology.

(105) **2.** A stressor, such as illness, may impair the older person's ability to compensate, resulting in:

1. disorientation.
2. hypotension.
3. loss of brain neurons.
4. sedation.

(105) **3.** Which system shows only slight decline with age?

1. renal system
2. central nervous system
3. respiratory system
4. cardiovascular system

(105) **4.** A frequent concern of the aged is:

1. long-term memory loss.
2. creativity loss.
3. short-term memory loss.
4. judgment loss.

(105) **5.** Neurologic features that show age-related changes include:

1. size of the brain, oxygenation function, and emotions.
2. personality, cardiac output, and excretion of drugs.
3. elasticity of cells, vision changes, and gastric secretions.
4. temperature regulation, pain perception, and tactile sensation.

(105) **6.** To compensate for neurologic changes, the aged individual may:

1. avoid temperature extremes and accomplish tasks at a slower pace.
2. wear warm clothes and exert extra effort to get tasks accomplished.
3. wear hats and concentrate for longer periods of time.
4. check blood pressure frequently.

(105) **7.** Kyphosis, vertebral loss of calcium, and calcification of costal cartilage result in:

1. increased vital capacity.
2. decreased vital capacity.
3. decreased anteroposterior chest diameter.
4. contractures.

(105) **8.** A frequent respiratory complaint of the aged is:

1. orthostatic hypotension.
2. inability to breathe.
3. increased respirations.
4. exertional dyspnea.

(106) **9.** Standard components of respiratory care for the older adult include:

1. coughing and deep-breathing exercises and range-of-motion exercises to facilitate lung expansion.
2. frequent ambulation and auscultation of lungs.
3. intake and output and postural drainage exercises.
4. deep-breathing exercises and positioning to facilitate lung expansion and gas exchange.

Student Name ____________________

(106) **10.** In the absence of cardiovascular disease, heart size:

1. remains unchanged or slightly decreases.
2. increases markedly.
3. decreases markedly.
4. remains unchanged or slightly increases.

(106) **11.** With increasing age, a person's reduced tolerance for physical work may be due to the decreased:

1. size of the brain.
2. capacity of heart cells to utilize oxygen.
3. size of the heart.
4. resistance to blood flow in many organs.

(106) **12.** Which changes occur in aging kidneys?

1. decreased filtration rate
2. increased extracellular fluid
3. increased cell mass
4. increased renal function

(106) **13.** One of the first signs of aging of the skin is:

1. infection. 2. thickening.
3. elasticity. 4. wrinkles.

(107) **14.** An age change that occurs due to loss of oils in the skin is:

1. infection.
2. itching.
3. wrinkles.
4. brown spots.

(107) **15.** Which symptoms are suggestive of possible gastrointestinal system illness?

1. anorexia
2. dry mouth
3. constipation
4. unexplained weight loss

(107) **16.** The leading cause of disability in old age is:

1. urinary tract infection.
2. pelvic inflammatory disease.
3. pressure ulcers.
4. arthritis.

(107) **17.** The curvature of the thoracic spine that causes a bent over appearance in some older adults is:

1. kyphosis. 2. arthritis.
3. scoliosis. 4. lordosis.

(108) **18.** The term for hearing loss associated with age is:

1. tinnitus.
2. ototoxicity.
3. presbyopia.
4. presbycusis.

(108) **19.** What percentage of older adults are hearing impaired?

1. 10% 2. 50%
3. 25% 4. 75%

(108) **20.** The type of hearing loss most easily treated is:

1. sensorineural.
2. tinnitus.
3. conduction.
4. ototoxicity.

(108) **21.** The type of hearing loss that results from exposure to loud noises, disease, and certain drugs is:

1. conduction.
2. ototoxicity.
3. infection.
4. sensorineural.

(108) **22.** The leading cause of new cases of blindness in older people is age-related:

1. glaucoma.
2. cataracts.
3. corneal abrasion.
4. macular degeneration.

(107) **23.** Which of the following is a normal aging change?

1. decreased secretion of saliva
2. increased acidity of saliva
3. increased peristalsis
4. decreased gastric emptying

(108) **24.** Presbyopia is corrected by:

1. laser surgery.
2. reading eyeglasses.
3. treatment with antibiotics.
4. eye patches.

(108) **25.** The leading cause of blindness in this country is:

1. glaucoma.
2. presbyopia.
3. cataract.
4. conjunctivitis.

(109) **26.** What percentage of the aged are able to function independently and sustain a sense of well-being?

1. 15% 2. 25%
3. 50% 4. 85%

(109) **27.** The developmental challenge in old age is to:

1. develop close relations with other people; to learn and experience love.
2. find a vocation or hobby where the individual can help others or in some way contribute to society.
3. establish trusting relationships with other people.
4. review life and gain a feeling of accomplishment or fulfillment.

(110) **28.** Two-thirds of the suicides among older people are due to depression resulting from:

1. loneliness.
2. loss.
3. medication.
4. denial.

(110) **29.** For effective gerontological care, the crucial denominator in deciding care needs is:

1. medical diagnosis.
2. functional assessment.
3. activities of daily living.
4. community resources.

(111) **30.** With aging, there is decreased body size and increased:

1. serum albumin.
2. drug clearance.
3. lean body mass.
4. fat.

(111) **31.** A highly fat-soluble drug such as diazepam (Valium) may result in:

1. shorter storage of drug before excretion.
2. higher blood concentrations of the drug.
3. lower blood concentrations of the drug.
4. longer storage of drug before excretion.

(111) **32.** Age-related changes of decreased liver size, reduced blood flow through the liver, and reduced liver enzyme activity affect the:

1. storage of drugs.
2. tissue sensitivity of drugs.
3. inactivation of drugs.
4. absorption of drugs.

Student Name____________________

(112) **33.** Which drug may counteract the effects of diuretics in the older adult?

1. Tylenol
2. nasal decongestant
3. sodium bicarbonate
4. aspirin

(109) **34.** The developmental task associated with old age is:

1. generativity vs. stagnation.
2. intimacy vs. isolation.
3. autonomy vs. dependence.
4. ego-integrity vs. despair.

(105) **35.** Because older adults have a decreased number and sensitivity of sensory receptors and neurons, they should:

1. avoid temperature extremes and accomplish tasks at a slower pace.
2. do deep-breathing exercises and positioning to facilitate lung expansion.
3. use mnemonics and rehearsal memory training to improve memory performance.
4. use assistive devices for walking and preventing falls.

(107) **36.** Because of age-related changes in bone density in the spine, the thoracic spine curves, causing:

1. lordosis. 2. scoliosis.
3. kyphosis. 4. arthritis.

(105) **37.** Progressive slowing of responses and reflexes is due to:

1. decreased impulse conduction speed.
2. loss of neurons in the brain.
3. inadequate tissue oxygenation.
4. atherosclerosis and decreased cellular respiration.

Student Name ______________________________

The Nursing Process and Critical Thinking

Answer Key: Textbook page references are provided as a guide for answering these questions. A complete answer key was provided for your instructor.

OBJECTIVES

1. Describe the five components of the nursing process.
2. Describe the formats for North American Nursing Diagnosis Association (NANDA) diagnoses, Nursing Interventions Classification (NIC) interventions, and Nursing Outcome Classification (NOC) outcomes.
3. Explain the role of the licensed practical nurse in the nursing process.
4. Describe the proper documentation of the nursing process using a problem-oriented medical record format, nurses' notes, and flow sheets.
5. Explain the relationship between the nursing process and critical thinking.
6. Describe the characteristics of a critical thinker.
7. Describe how critical thinking skills are used in clinical practice.

LEARNING ACTIVITIES

A. Match the definition in the numbered column with the most appropriate term in the lettered column.

(117) **1.** __________ A systematic, thorough way of obtaining objective data

(127) **2.** __________ Method of record-keeping that focuses on patient problems rather than on medical diagnoses

A. Auscultation
B. Objective data
C. Clinical pathway
D. Nursing diagnosis
E. Problem-oriented medical record
F. Subjective data
G. Nursing process
H. Percussion
I. Inspection
J. Assessment
K. Palpation
L. Physical assessment

Continued next page

(114) **3.** ________ Systematic, problem-solving approach to providing nursing care in an organized, scientific manner

(117) **4.** ________ Tapping on the skin to assess the underlying tissues

(117) **5.** ________ Method of physical examination that uses the sense of touch to assess various parts of the body

(118) **6.** ________ Listening to sounds produced by the body, such as heart, lung, and intestinal sounds

(117) **7.** ________ Purposeful observation or scrutiny of the person as a whole and then of each body system

(119) **8.** ________ Actual or potential health problems derived from data gathered during the assessment of a patient or client

(115) **9.** ________ Information reported by patients or family members

(114) **10.** ________ Collection of data about the health status of a patient or client

(115) **11.** ________ Information about the patient collected by the nurse or other members of the health care team

(124) **12.** ________ Standard care plan with patient outcomes and timelines for specific interventions

B. Match the definition in the numbered column with the most appropriate component of the nursing process in the lettered column.

(122) **1.** ________ Putting the plan into action

(114) **2.** ________ Systematic collection of data relating to patients and their problems

(124) **3.** ________ Assessing the achievement of patient goals

(122) **4.** ________ Setting goals

A. Assessment
B. Nursing diagnosis
C. Planning
D. Intervention
E. Evaluation

Continued next page

Student Name____

(119) **5.** __________ Interpretation of the data for problem identification

(119) **6.** __________ Identify health problems or potential health problems

(122) **7.** __________ Determine priorities from the list of nursing diagnoses

(114) **8.** __________ Collect data, including height and weight and vital signs

(115) **9.** __________ Obtain information through a health history by direct questioning

(124) **10.** __________ Measure the patient's progress toward meeting goals

(122) **11.** __________ Actual performance of nursing interventions identified in the care plan

(122) **12.** __________ Set short-term and long-term goals to determine outcomes of care

C. Match the description in the numbered column (objective data) with the problem in the lettered column.

(116) **1.** __________ A patient's disheveled appearance based on sight

(116) **2.** __________ A patient's noisy and labored breathing based on hearing

(116) **3.** __________ A fruity mouth odor based on smell

(116) **4.** __________ Cold, clammy skin based on touch

A. Possible respiratory problems
B. Possible sign of diabetic acidosis
C. May indicate that patient is in shock
D. May indicate inability to carry out self-care activities at home

D. Match the description in the numbered column with the method of charting in the lettered column.

(127) **1.** _________ Charting by different health care team members on the same page

(127) **2.** _________ Charting narrative notes only when there is a change in the patient's condition

(127) **3.** _________ Nursing notes recorded on computers

(127) **4.** _________ Using key words to organize charting, such as action or response

(127) **5.** _________ Charting on separate sheets for different health care workers

(127) **6.** _________ Recordkeeping that focuses on patient problems rather than on medical diagnoses

(127) **7.** _________ Charting that includes the problem, intervention, and evaluation

A. POMR
B. Focus charting
C. Source-oriented charting
D. Multidisciplinary charting
E. CBE
F. CPR
G. PIE

Student Name____

E. Match the description of critical thinking tools in the numbered column with the corresponding critical thinking tool in the lettered column.

(129) **1.** __________ Deriving alternatives and drawing conclusions

(129) **2.** __________ Clarifying the meaning of events and data

(129) **3.** __________ Reconsidering conclusions and recognizing the need to make changes

(129) **4.** __________ Presenting arguments for decisions and justifying

(129) **5.** __________ Examining ideas and breaking down into components

(129) **6.** __________ Assessing possibilities, opinions, and usual practices

A. Interpretation
B. Analysis
C. Evaluation
D. Inference
E. Explanation
F. Self-regulation

F. Match the description in the numbered column with the correct component of SOAPE notes in the lettered column.

(127) **1.** __________ Turn from side to side q 2 hr. Get out of bed at least twice a day. Begin ambulating as tolerated.

(127) **2.** __________ Turned q 2 hr. OOB twice a day; taking 6 small steps to and from bed. Pressure ulcer healing; now 1.5 cm.

A. S
B. O
C. A
D. P
E. E

Continued next page

(127) **3.** ________ Feels weak; "does not have the energy" to move around

(127) **4.** ________ Pressure ulcer on sacrum related to immobility

(127) **5.** ________ Does not turn self in bed; 2 cm, stage 2 pressure ulcer on sacrum

G. Match the description of critical thinking characteristics in the numbered column with the critical thinking characteristic in the lettered column. Answers may be used more than once.

(129) **1.** ________ Willing to consider various alternatives

(129) **2.** ________ Examines parts and sees how they fit together

(129) **3.** ________ Recognizes that many variables are at work in patient situations

(129) **4.** ________ Seeks answers and reevaluates "common knowledge"

(129) **5.** ________ Uses an organized approach to problem solving

(129) **6.** ________ Sense of assurance that the problem-solving process produces a good plan

(129) **7.** ________ The desire, not just to know, but to understand how to apply the knowledge

(129) **8.** ________ Recognizes that sometimes the best plans do not work and goes back to the drawing board

(129) **9.** ________ Applies knowledge from various disciplines

A. Systematic thinking
B. Analytical
C. Open-minded
D. Self-confident
E. Maturity
F. Truth-seeking
G. Curiosity

Student Name ____________________

H. List five new nursing diagnoses included in the 2001 NANDA list.

(119) **1.** ____________________ *(119)* **4.** ____________________

(119) **2.** ____________________ *(119)* **5.** ____________________

(119) **3.** ____________________

I. Match the term in the numbered column with the type of diagnosis in the lettered column.

(121-122) **1.** __________ Peptic ulcer

(121-122) **2.** __________ Pneumonia

(122-123) **3.** __________ Ineffective airway clearance

(122-123) **4.** __________ Myocardial infarction

(122-123) **5.** __________ Hiatal hernia

(122-123) **6.** __________ Impaired mobility

(122-123) **7.** __________ Wandering

(122-123) **8.** __________ Powerlessness

(122-123) **9.** __________ Fatigue

(122-123) **10.** __________ Risk for falls

A. Nursing diagnosis
B. Medical diagnosis

J. Match the description in the numbered column with the type of data it represents in the lettered column.

(115) **1.** __________ A shooting pain in my arm

(115) **2.** __________ Noisy, labored breathing

(115) **3.** __________ Fruity mouth odor

(115) **4.** __________ Cold, clammy skin

(115) **5.** __________ Blood pressure 120/80

(115) **6.** __________ Headache

(115) **7.** __________ Fear of surgery

(115) **8.** __________ Disheveled appearance

A. Subjective data
B. Objective data

K. Match the condition to be assessed in the numbered column with the appropriate technique in the lettered column.

(117) **1.** __________ Bowel sounds

(117) **2.** __________ Pitting edema

(117) **3.** __________ Mucous membranes

(117) **4.** __________ Jaundice

(118) **5.** __________ Blood pressure

(117) **6.** __________ Radial pulse

(118) **7.** __________ Lung sounds

(117) **8.** __________ Cyanosis

A. Inspection
B. Percussion
C. Palpation
D. Auscultation

MULTIPLE-CHOICE QUESTIONS

L. Choose the most appropriate answer.

(114) **1.** The goal of the nursing process is to:
1. obtain information through observation, physical examination, or diagnostic testing.
2. interview the patient or family in a goal-directed, orderly, and systematic way.
3. record objective data, writing exactly what is observed.
4. alleviate, minimize, or prevent real or potential health problems.

(122) **2.** In the planning phase of the nursing process, which of the following actions occurs first?
1. Set short-term goals to determine outcomes of care.
2. Set long-term goals to determine outcomes of care.
3. Develop objectives to meet goals.
4. Determine priorities from the list of nursing diagnoses.

(122) **3.** The role of the LPN in relation to the planning phase of the nursing process is to:
1. perform a physical assessment.
2. perform therapeutic nursing measures.
3. assist with the development of nursing care plans.
4. evaluate the nursing care given.

(124) **4.** The role of the LPN in relation to the evaluation phase of the nursing process is to:
1. report observed outcomes and make necessary changes.
2. carry out the established plan of care.
3. collect data and take objective measurements of body functions.
4. develop nursing care plans.

Student Name____

(114) **5.** When admitting a patient with pneumonia, which step of the nursing process is done first?
1. implementation
2. determine outcome criteria
3. set short-term goals
4. collect data

(124) **6.** Which step of the nursing process do you use to determine whether outcome criteria have been met?
1. assessment
2. planning
3. implementation
4. evaluation

(124) **7.** An organization that requires systematic review of hospitals and other health care organizations is:
1. Joint Commission on Accreditation of Healthcare Organizations (JCAHO)
2. Medicare
3. Medicaid
4. ANA Standards of Care

(117-118) **8.** Why is auscultation done before percussion and palpation when doing a physical assessment of the abdomen?
1. Auscultation aids in the palpation process.
2. Palpation can alter auscultation findings.
3. Auscultation can alter palpation findings.
4. Auscultation findings determine where to perform percussion.

(127) **9.** The POMR is a method of recordkeeping that focuses on:
1. medical diagnoses.
2. patient problems.
3. medical treatments.
4. diagnostic tests.

(126) **10.** If an error in charting is made, the entry should be:
1. erased, new entry entered, and initialed.
2. erased, "error" or "mistaken entry" written in, and initialed.
3. crossed out, "error" or "mistaken entry" written above, initialed.
4. crossed out, new entry written above, and initialed.

(127) **11.** Which of the following describes critical thinking?
1. thinking based on learning many facts.
2. reasonable thinking focused on deciding what to do.
3. thinking based on the utilization of the nursing process.
4. reflective thinking related to reading and gathering information.

(127) **12.** The statement, "Does not turn self in bed; 2 cm, stage 2 pressure ulcer on sacrum," refers to which component of SOAPIER charting?
1. subjective information
2. assessment
3. plan
4. objective information

(127) **13.** The statement, "Turn from side to side every 2 hours. Get out of bed at least twice a day. Begin ambulating as tolerated," refers to which component of SOAPE charting?
1. plan
2. assessment
3. evaluation
4. objective information

(115) **14.** Which would you chart under objective data?
1. lumbar back pain
2. nausea
3. no shortness of breath
4. pupils equal and reactive

(115) **15.** Which is a correct recording of observational data?
1. The skin is cool and clammy.
2. The skin looks good.
3. The patient states, "My skin is cool and clammy."
4. The patient's skin has improved.

(119) **16.** Which is a nursing diagnosis?
1. Pneumonia
2. Wandering
3. Diabetes mellitus
4. Urinary tract infection

(119) **17.** Which is a medical diagnosis?
1. Altered tissue perfusion
2. Impaired skin integrity
3. Diabetes mellitus
4. Fatigue

(121) **18.** Which is a nursing diagnosis?
1. Fear
2. Asthma
3. Bronchitis
4. Manic-depressive disorder

(118) **19.** Auscultation is used to assess the:
1. skin.
2. joints.
3. lungs.
4. head.

(115) **20.** Which of the following observations about the patient is documented as subjective data?
1. Patient is 6' 3" tall and weighs 180 pounds.
2. Patient's skin is jaundiced.
3. Patient has pain associated with taking deep breaths.
4. Patient's blood pressure is 130/80.

(116) **21.** Which of the following is the best method for obtaining objective data?
1. asking the patient about his pain
2. observing the patient to see if he is afraid
3. watching the patient for signs of fatigue
4. inspecting the color of the patient's skin

(122) **22.** A new patient is admitted to the hospital with the following nursing diagnoses: Fatigue, Nausea, Ineffective individual coping, and Ineffective breathing pattern. Which diagnosis requires immediate attention?
1. Fatigue
2. Nausea
3. Ineffective individual coping
4. Ineffective breathing pattern

(122) **23.** Which of the following short-term goals is incomplete?
1. The patient will drink 1500 mL by 8:00 AM on 3/22.
2. The patient will ambulate in the hall twice a day on 3/22.
3. The patient will have less pain by 8:00 AM on 3/22.
4. The patient will cough and deep breathe every 4 hours on 3/22.

(122) **24.** A patient states, "I hope I can leave the hospital soon and return to my neighborhood association meetings. I am the president." According to Maslow's hierarchy of needs, which level does this indicate?
1. physiological need
2. safety and security
3. love and belonging
4. self-esteem

CHAPTER 12

Student Name ______________________________

Inflammation, Infection, and Immunity

Answer Key: Textbook page references are provided as a guide for answering these questions. A complete answer key was provided for your instructor.

OBJECTIVES

1. Describe physical and chemical barriers.
2. Describe how inflammatory changes act as bodily defense mechanisms.
3. Identify the signs and symptoms of inflammation.
4. Discuss the process of repair and healing.
5. Differentiate infection from inflammation.
6. Discuss the actions of commonly found infectious agents.
7. Describe the ways that infections are transmitted.
8. Identify the signs and symptoms of infection.
9. Compare community-acquired and nosocomial infections.
10. Discuss the nursing care of patients with infections.
11. Describe the Centers for Disease Control standard precautions guidelines for infection control.
12. Describe the Centers for Disease Control isolation guidelines for airborne, droplet, and contact (transmission-based) precautions.
13. Describe the immune response.
14. Identify organs involved in immunity.
15. Compare natural and acquired immunity.
16. Differentiate between humoral (antibody-mediated) and cell-mediated immunity.
17. Describe the nursing care of patients with immunodeficiency and of those with allergies.
18. Describe the process of autoimmunity.

LEARNING ACTIVITIES

A. Match the definition in the numbered column with the most appropriate term in the lettered column. Some terms may be used more than once and some terms may not be used.

(145) **1.** _________ An antigen that causes a hypersensitive reaction

(143) **2.** _________ A protein that is created in response to a specific antigen

(138) **3.** _________ Limiting the spread of microorganisms; often called *clean technique*

(138) **4.** _________ Elimination of microorganisms from any object that comes in contact with the patient; often called *sterile technique*

(132) **5.** _________ Nonspecific immune response that occurs in response to bodily injury; condition in which the body is invaded by infectious organisms that multiply, causing injury and inflammatory response

(137) **6.** _________ Hospital-acquired infections (infections that were not present at the time of admission)

(136) **7.** _________ Presence of an infectious organism on a body surface or an object

A. Allergen
B. Antibody
C. Antigen
D. Autoimmunity
E. Bacteria
F. Communicable disease
G. Contamination
H. Fungi
I. Immunity
J. Immunodeficiency
K. Infection
L. Inflammation
M. Medical asepsis
N. Nosocomial infections
O. Surgical asepsis
P. Viruses

Continued next page

Student Name ____________________

(135) **8.** ________ Vegetable-like organisms that feed on organic matter and are capable of producing disease

(143) **9.** ________ A substance, usually a protein, that is capable of stimulating a response from the immune system

(132) **10.** ________ A condition in which the body is invaded by infectious organisms that multiply, causing injury

(134) **11.** ________ One-celled organisms capable of multiplying rapidly and causing illness

(147) **12.** ________ A condition in which the body is unable to distinguish self from nonself, causing the immune system to react and destroy its own tissues

(137) **13.** ________ Illness, caused by infectious organisms or their toxins, that can be transmitted, either directly or indirectly, from one person to another

(144) **14.** ________ Condition in which the immune system is unable to defend the body against organisms

(135) **15.** ________ Infectious microorganisms that can live and reproduce only within living cells; capable of causing illness, inflammation, and cell destruction

(143) **16.** ________ Resistance to or protection from a disease

B. Match the definition in the numbered column with the most appropriate term in the lettered column. Some answers may be used more than once, and some may not be used

(135) **1.** ________ One-celled organisms capable of producing disease, which is usually spread by contaminated food and water

(135) **2.** ________ Vegetable-like organisms that exist by feeding on organic matter and that are capable of producing disease

A. Helminths
B. Rickettsiae
C. Protozoa
D. Fungi
E. Mycoplasmas
F. Viruses

Continued next page

(135) **3.** ______ Worms that are parasites found in the soil and water and are transmitted to humans from hand to mouth

(135) **4.** ______ Microorganisms that cause illness by stimulating an antigen-antibody response in the tissues, producing inflammation and cell destruction

(135) **5.** ______ Microorganisms that are usually transmitted to humans through flea and tick bites

(135) **6.** ______ Gram-negative organisms usually causing infections in the respiratory tract

C. List four observable signs (objective data) of infection.

(136) **1.** ____________________

(136) **2.** ____________________

(136) **3.** ____________________

(136) **4.** ____________________

D. Match the definition in the numbered column with the most appropriate term in the lettered column.

(132) **1.** ______ Tumor

(132) **2.** ______ Dolor

(132) **3.** ______ Calor

(132) **4.** ______ Rubor

A. Heat
B. Swelling
C. Redness
D. Pain

E. List two reasons why the healing process can be delayed in the elderly.

(134) **1.** ____________________

(134) **2.** ____________________

Student Name ____________________

F. Match the definition or description in the numbered column with the most appropriate term in the lettered column.

(134) **1.** ________ Round bacteria that cluster in groups of two

(134) **2.** ________ Rod-shaped organisms that form spirals

(134) **3.** ________ Chains of round bacteria

(134) **4.** ________ One-celled microorganisms that retain a violet-colored stain

(134) **5.** ________ Bacteria that do not grow in the presence of oxygen

(134) **6.** ________ Clusters of round bacteria

(134) **7.** ________ Rod-shaped organisms

(134) **8.** ________ Bacteria that grow in the presence of oxygen

(134) **9.** ________ Round bacteria

(134) **10.** ________ Rod-shaped organisms with tapered ends

(135) **11.** ________ One-celled microorganisms that can be decolorized and counterstained pink

(134) **12.** ________ One-celled microorganisms capable of multiplying rapidly within a susceptible host

A. Anaerobes
B. Gram-positive bacteria
C. Bacilli
D. Aerobes
E. Spirochetes
F. Diplococci
G. Streptococci
H. Bacteria
I. Staphylococci
J. Fusiform bacilli
K. Gram-negative bacteria
L. Cocci

G. Match each disease or infection in the numbered column with the most appropriate causative agent in the lettered column. Some agents may be used more than once and some agents may not be used.

(135)	**1.** ________ Malaria	A.	Fungi
		B.	Protozoa
(135)	**2.** ________ Hookworm infection	C.	Mycoplasmas
		D.	Viruses
		E.	Helminths
(135)	**3.** ________ Pneumocystis pneumonia	F.	Rickettsiae
(135)	**4.** ________ Primary atypical pneumonia		
(135)	**5.** ________ Measles		
(135)	**6.** ________ Typhus		
(135)	**7.** ________ Common cold		
(135)	**8.** ________ Rocky Mountain spotted fever		
(135)	**9.** ________ Tapeworm infection		
(135)	**10.** ________ Ringworm		

H. List six factors, in sequence, that must happen for human infectious disease to occur, known as the "chain of infection."

(135) **1.** ______________________________

(135) **2.** ______________________________

(135) **3.** ______________________________

(135) **4.** ______________________________

(135) **5.** ______________________________

(135) **6.** ______________________________

I. List three common portals of entry.

(136) **1.** ______________________________

(136) **2.** ______________________________

(136) **3.** ______________________________

Student Name____

J. Indicate which of the diseases below are (A) community-acquired and which are (B) hospital-acquired.

A. Community-acquired
B. Hospital-acquired

(138) **1.** __________ Urinary tract infections

(137) **2.** __________ Food-borne illness

(138) **3.** __________ Hepatitis B

(137) **4.** __________ Nosocomial infection

(138) **5.** __________ Superinfection

(137) **6.** __________ Syphilis

(137) **7.** __________ Gonorrhea

(138) **8.** __________ Iatrogenic infection

(136) **9.** __________ Tuberculosis

(137) **10.** __________ Hepatitis A

(138) **11.** __________ VRE

(137) **12.** __________ AIDS

(137) **13.** __________ Anthrax

K. List three barriers to providing immunizations to everyone.

(137) **1.** ____

(137) **2.** ____

(137) **3.** ____

L. List seven CDC-recommended guidelines for limiting patient-to-patient transmission of VRE infection.

(138) **1.** ____

(138) **2.** ____

(138) **3.** ____

(138) **4.** ____

(138) **5.** ____

(138) **6.** ____

(138) **7.** ____

M. List four reasons why resistant bacterial strains develop.

(138) **1.** ______________________

(138) **2.** ______________________

(138) **3.** ______________________

(138) **4.** ______________________

N. List three common sites for nosocomial infections in hospitalized patients.

(138) **1.** ______________________

(138) **2.** ______________________

(138) **3.** ______________________

O. List four examples of clean technique (medical asepsis) that help prevent infection in hospitalized patients.

(138) **1.** ______________________

(138) **2.** ______________________

(138) **3.** ______________________

(138) **4.** ______________________

P. When you perform procedures, list six contacts of substances that require the use of standard precautions.

(139) **1.** ______________________

(139) **2.** ______________________

(139) **3.** ______________________

(139) **4.** ______________________

(139) **5.** ______________________

(139) **6.** ______________________

Q. List three new types of transmission-based precautions.

(139) **1.** ______________________

(140) **2.** ______________________

(140) **3.** ______________________

Student Name ______________________

R. For each disease or condition in the numbered column, indicate all of the types of precautions in the lettered column that are appropriate.

A. Airborne precautions
B. Droplet precautions
C. Contact precautions

(140) **1.** ________ Mumps

(140) **2.** ________ Scabies

(140) **3.** ________ Influenza

(140) **4.** ________ Impetigo

(140) **5.** ________ Rubeola (measles)

(140) **6.** ________ Respiratory syncytial virus (RSV)

(140, 142) **7.** ________ Varicella (chickenpox)

(140) **8.** ________ Rubella

(140) **9.** ________ Tuberculosis

(140) **10.** ________ Diphtheria (pharyngeal)

S. List five laboratory tests used to screen patients for infection.

(142) **1.** ______________________

(142) **2.** ______________________

(142) **3.** ______________________

(142) **4.** ______________________

(142) **5.** ______________________

T. List four complications for which you monitor the patient during hyperbaric oxygen therapy.

(142) **1.** ______________________

(142) **2.** ______________________

(142) **3.** ______________________

(142) **4.** ______________________

U. Fill in the blanks.

(143) **1.** The body's resistance to invading organisms and its ability to fight off invaders once they have gained access to the body is called ______________________.

V. List five factors that can compromise the immune system.

(143) **1.** ______________ *(143)* **4.** ______________

(143) **2.** ______________ *(143)* **5.** ______________

(143) **3.** ______________

W. List five examples of antigens.

(143) **1.** ______________ *(143)* **4.** ______________

(143) **2.** ______________ *(143)* **5.** ______________

(143) **3.** ______________

X. List five body organs that are involved in immunity.

(143) **1.** ______________ *(143)* **4.** ______________

(143) **2.** ______________ *(143)* **5.** ______________

(143) **3.** ______________

Y. List four classifications of medications that often place patients at risk for infection.

(145) **1.** ______________ *(145)* **3.** ______________

(145) **2.** ______________ *(145)* **4.** ______________

Z. List the primary nursing responsibility in cases of patients with immunodeficiencies.

(145) ______________________________

Student Name____

AA. Match the example of antigen in the numbered column with the appropriate classification in the lettered column. Some classifications may be used more than once and classifications may not be used.

(143) **1.** __________ Food

(143) **2.** __________ Fungi

(143) **3.** __________ Parasites

(143) **4.** __________ Organ transplant cells

(143) **5.** __________ Penicillin

(143) **6.** __________ Bacteria

(143) **7.** __________ Insect venoms

(143) **8.** __________ Pollens

(143) **9.** __________ Viruses

(143) **10.** __________ Blood transfusion cells

A. Environmental substances
B. Drugs
C. Microorganisms
D. Transplanted cells

BB. List nine common allergens.

(145) **1.** ____________________

(145) **2.** ____________________

(145) **3.** ____________________

(145) **4.** ____________________

(145) **5.** ____________________

(145) **6.** ____________________

(145) **7.** ____________________

(145) **8.** ____________________

(145) **9.** ____________________

CC. List five effects of histamine on the body when it is released during anaphylaxis.

(146) **1.** ____

(146) **2.** ____

(146) **3.** ____

(146) **4.** ____

(146) **5.** ____

DD. Indicate the stages of the inflammatory response outlined in Figure 12-1 using the letters A–D.

(133)	**1.**	________	Release of chemical mediators	A. Normal tissue
(133)	**2.**	________	Ingestion and destruction of foreign agents	B. Stage I
(133)	**3.**	________	Repair and regeneration	C. Stage 2
(133)	**4.**	________	Cellular injury	D. Stage 3
(133)	**5.**	________	Movement of proteins, water, and white blood cells out of capillaries into injured tissues	
(133)	**6.**	________	Exudate formation	
(133)	**7.**	________	Normal tissue	
(133)	**8.**	________	Phagocytic lymphocytes enter area of injury	
(133)	**9.**	________	Dilated blood vessels and increased capillary permeability	

A

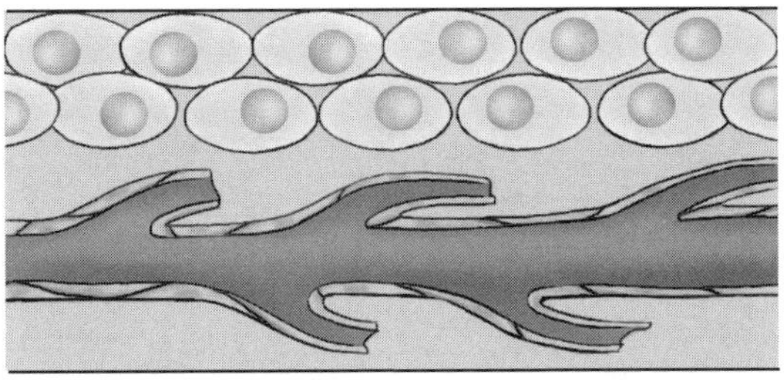

B

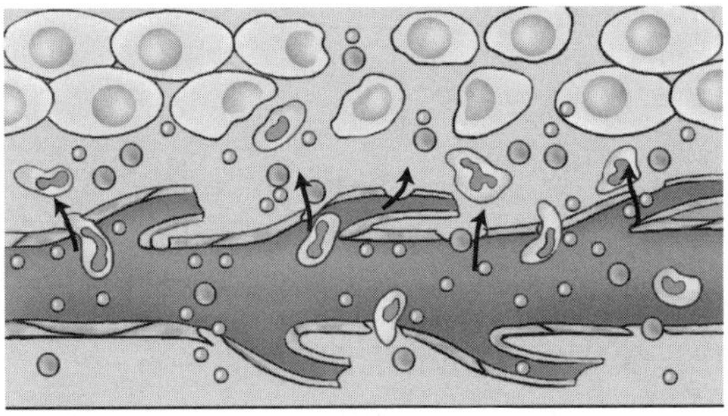

C

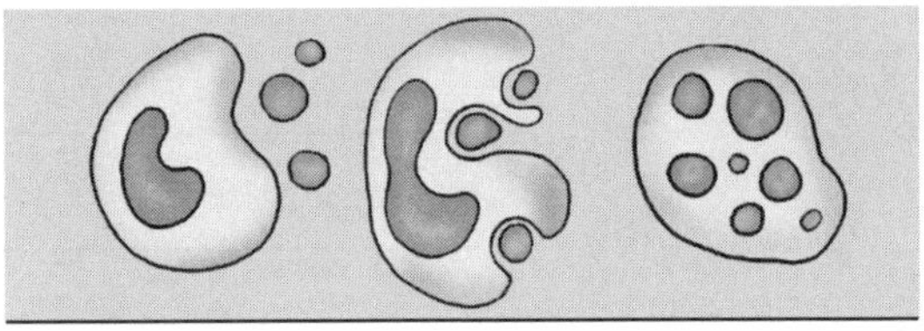

D

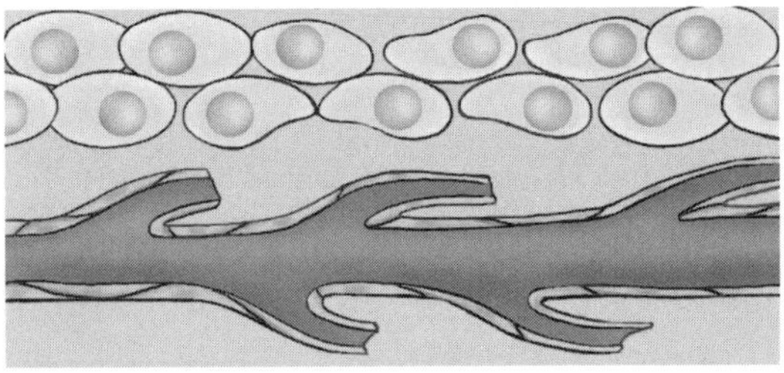

Student Name____

EE. Using Figure 12-4, label organs involved in immunity (A–G).

(144)	**A.**	________________	*(144)*	**E.**	________________
(144)	**B.**	________________	*(144)*	**F.**	________________
(144)	**C.**	________________	*(144)*	**G.**	________________
(144)	**D.**	________________			

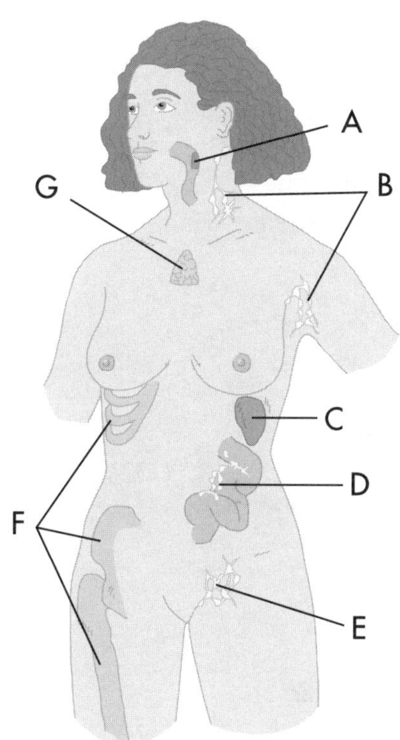

FF. Match the allergic reaction in the numbered column with the most appropriate stimuli in the lettered column. Some stimuli may be used more than once and some stimuli may not be used.

(146) **1.** __________ Gastrointestinal allergy

(146) **2.** __________ Atopic dermatitis (eczema)

(146) **3.** __________ Asthma

(146) **4.** __________ Urticaria (hives)

(146) **5.** __________ Allergic contact dermatitis

(146) **6.** __________ Allergic rhinitis

(146) **7.** __________ Anaphylaxis

A. Pollens, dust, molds, animal dander
B. Antibiotics (penicillin), blood transfusions, insect venom
C. Soaps, cosmetics, chemicals, fabrics
D. Food, drugs
E. Pollens, dust, molds, cigarette smoke, air pollutants, animal dander
F. Plants (poison ivy), metals (nickel), chemicals, cosmetics, latex gloves

MULTIPLE-CHOICE QUESTIONS

GG. Choose the most appropriate answer.

(132) **1.** Which types of leukocytes are especially involved with fighting infection?

1. erythrocytes and neutrophils
2. neutrophils and monocytes
3. monocytes and thrombocytes
4. eosinophils and neutrophils

(134) **2.** Which gram-positive bacteria clusters cause pneumonia, cellulitis, peritonitis, and toxic shock?

1. Staphylococcus
2. Streptococcus
3. Pneumococcus
4. Enterococcus

(132) **3.** The literal meaning of inflammation is:

1. red flame.
2. great fire.
3. inner infection.
4. fire within.

(135) **4.** What are small intracellular parasites that only live inside cells?

1. gram-negative bacteria
2. gram-positive bacteria
3. viruses
4. fungi

(132) **5.** The increase in blood flow to an inflamed area is due to:

1. increased permeability.
2. chemical mediators.
3. hemodynamic changes.
4. hormonal factors.

(132) **6.** The process by which the increased blood flow brings leukocytes to line the small blood vessel walls near the inflamed site is called:

1. phagocytosis.
2. leukocytosis.
3. pavementing.
4. vasodilation.

(132) **7.** The hemodynamic changes and vascular permeability in inflammation occur with the help of:

1. hormonal factors.
2. chemical mediators.
3. erythrocytes.
4. thrombocytes.

(132) **8.** Prostaglandins, histamine and leukotrienes are examples of:

1. hormonal factors.
2. chemical mediators.
3. erythrocytes.
4. thrombocytes.

(132) **9.** A hormone produced by the adrenal cortex that is anti-inflammatory is:

1. epinephrine.
2. cortisol.
3. aldosterone.
4. thyroxine.

(132) **10.** Cells that are produced to clean up inflammatory debris are called:

1. fibroblasts.
2. platelets.
3. neutrophils.
4. macrophages.

Student Name____

(132) **11.** Which of the following is a sign of local infection?

1. fever 2. chills
3. warm skin 4. pale skin

(134) **12.** One-celled microorganisms capable of multiplying rapidly within a susceptible host are called:

1. fungi.
2. protozoa.
3. bacteria.
4. mycoplasmas.

(135) **13.** Many childhood illnesses such as measles and chickenpox, and some forms of hepatitis are caused by:

1. viruses. 2. bacteria.
3. protozoa. 4. fungi.

(135) **14.** The best way to fight viral illness is:

1. antibiotics.
2. prevention.
3. drug therapy.
4. vitamin therapy.

(135) **15.** It is seldom possible to kill viruses because:

1. replication of the virus occurs within the host cell.
2. the cell wall can be destroyed with drugs.
3. the cell wall requires oxygen for functions.
4. the host cell is separate from the virus.

(135) **16.** Vegetable-like organisms that exist by feeding on organic matter are called:

1. bacteria. 2. viruses.
3. protozoa. 4. fungi.

(135) **17.** Ringworm (tinea corporis) and athlete's foot (tinea pedis) are examples of disease caused by:

1. bacteria. 2. viruses.
3. fungi. 4. protozoa.

(135) **18.** One-celled organisms that produce diseases such as malaria and amoebic dysentery are called:

1. fungi. 2. protozoa.
3. viruses. 4. helminths.

(135) **19.** Microorganisms between the size of bacteria and viruses that are transmitted to humans through the bites of fleas and ticks are called:

1. rickettsiae.
2. protozoa.
3. helminths.
4. mycoplasmas.

(135) **20.** Parasites that are found in soil and water and are generally transmitted from hand to mouth are called:

1. rickettsiae.
2. protozoa.
3. helminths.
4. mycoplasmas.

(135) **21.** Gram-negative multishaped organisms without cell walls, also known as *pleuropneumonia-like organisms*, are called:

1. helminths.
2. protozoa.
3. mycoplasmas.
4. viruses.

(135) **22.** Microorganisms present in sufficient number and virulence to damage human tissue are called:

1. reservoirs.
2. causative agents.
3. portals of exit.
4. portals of entrance.

(136) **23.** The route by which the infectious agent leaves one host and travels to another is called:

1. portal of entry.
2. mode of transfer.
3. host.
4. portal of exit.

(138) **24.** Two groups of patients who are most susceptible to hospital-acquired infections include patients with:

1. pneumonia and patients requiring insulin.
2. myocardial infarction and patients with tachycardia.
3. AIDS and cancer patients receiving chemotherapy.
4. emphysema and patients with bronchitis.

(138) **25.** The type of infection resulting from giving immunosuppressive drugs to prevent rejection of a transplanted organ is:

1. sexually transmitted infection.
2. superinfection.
3. iatrogenic infection.
4. fungal infection.

(138) **26.** The overgrowth of a second microorganism that can cause illness following antibiotic therapy for one microorganism is called:

1. thrombophlebitis.
2. superinfection.
3. sexually transmitted infection.
4. septicemia.

(138) **27.** The most basic and most effective method of preventing cross-contamination is:

1. hand washing.
2. antibiotics.
3. isolation.
4. use of gown and gloves.

(138) **28.** The primary cause of nosocomial infections is:

1. soiled hands.
2. faulty equipment.
3. airborne droplets.
4. open wounds.

(139) **29.** The elimination of microorganisms from any object that comes in contact with the patient is called:

1. medical asepsis.
2. clean technique.
3. isolation technique.
4. surgical asepsis.

(141) **30.** How much fluid is required by patients with infection?

1. 1 liter/day
2. 2 liters/day
3. 5 liters/day
4. 10 liters/day

(142) **31.** Patient teaching for persons undergoing hyperbaric oxygen therapy includes:

1. do not take aspirin one week before.
2. do not wear watches.
3. swallow first to prevent pressure buildup.
4. wear everyday clothes.

(142) **32.** A CNS complication of oxygen toxicity that my occur during hyperbaric oxygen therapy is:

1. respiratory problems.
2. sinus pain.
3. bradycardia.
4. seizures.

Student Name____

(142) **33.** An advantage of home health care for infected patients is that the patient is:

1. exposed to fewer nosocomial infections.
2. capable of spreading infections to others.
3. susceptible to poorly prepared food.
4. vulnerable to poor hygiene.

(141) **34.** Which type of precaution is used to treat methicillin-resistant *Staphylococcus aureus* infections?

1. airborne
2. droplet
3. respiratory
4. contact

(139) **35.** Precautions developed to reduce the risk of airborne, droplet, and contact transmission in hospitals are known as:

1. reverse isolation.
2. compromised host precautions.
3. enteric precautions.
4. transmission-based precautions.

(141) **36.** Which precautions are used with patients who have MRSA?

1. contact precautions
2. airborne precautions
3. droplet precautions
4. compromised host precautions

(141) **37.** People with generalized infections become dehydrated because of:

1. poor skin turgor and dry mouth.
2. dry mucous membranes and decreased metabolism.
3. inflammation and pain.
4. fever and anorexia.

(141) **38.** A diet recommended for patients with infection is:

1. low sodium.
2. high fiber.
3. high protein.
4. low potassium.

(138) **39.** Which guidelines are used for limiting patient-to-patient transmission in order to prevent VRE infection?

1. check air conditioning system for infected water
2. use separate thermometers and stethoscopes for VRE patients
3. change bed linen frequently
4. use sterile technique when caring for VRE patients

(138) **40.** Decreased bone mass due to the administration of cortisone is an example of a(n):

1. VRE infection.
2. MRSA infection.
3. nosocomial infection.
4. iatrogenic infection.

(138) **41.** A common side effect of broad-spectrum antibiotics is:

1. superinfection.
2. hemorrhage.
3. hypotension.
4. hypokalemia.

(139) **42.** Isolation precautions and disease-specific precautions are now classified under Standard Precautions as:

1. universal precautions.
2. enteric precautions.
3. transmission-based precautions.
4. compromised host precautions.

(137) **43.** Food-borne illness is a common community-acquired infectious disease often caused by:

1. pseudomonas.
2. diphtheria.
3. tuberculosis.
4. *Salmonella.*

(144) **44.** Antibody-mediated immunity is:

1. immediate.
2. delayed.
3. cell-mediated.
4. altered.

(144) **45.** A delayed response to injury or infection is called:

1. humoral immunity.
2. interferon immunity.
3. cell-mediated immunity.
4. pyrogen immunity.

(145) **46.** What percentage of the U.S. population suffers from allergies of some sort?

1. 20–25%
2. under 5%
3. 40–45%
4. 50–75%

(145) **47.** Someone who is prone to allergies may be referred to as:

1. infectious.
2. immunocompromised.
3. atopic.
4. symptomatic.

(145) **48.** Antigens that cause hypersensitivity reactions are called:

1. antibodies.
2. complement.
3. allergens.
4. interferon.

(146) **49.** Allergy testing is performed by injecting small amounts of allergen:

1. intradermally.
2. intramuscularly.
3. intravenously.
4. interstitially.

(146) **50.** In anaphylaxis, what causes bronchospasm, vasodilation, and increased vascular permeability?

1. interferon
2. pyrogen
3. phagocytosis
4. histamine

(146) **51.** Drugs used in the treatment of anaphylaxis include diphenhydramine, corticosteroids, epinephrine, and:

1. atropine.
2. morphine.
3. propranolol.
4. aminophylline.

(147) **52.** The body's ability to determine self from nonself is called:

1. tolerance.
2. phagocytosis.
3. immunity.
4. inflammation.

(147) **53.** Autoimmunity can involve any tissue or organ system. In multiple sclerosis, what is (are) affected?

1. heart and kidney tissue
2. white matter of brain and spinal cord
3. lung tissue and liver cells
4. spleen tissue and thymus gland

(147) **54.** Two central nervous system autoimmune disorders are:

1. ulcerative colitis and Crohn's disease.
2. rheumatoid arthritis and SLE.
3. hyperthyroidism and Addison's disease.
4. multiple sclerosis and myasthenia gravis.

Student Name____

(137) **55.** Barriers to providing immunizations to large groups of the population include:

1. using fixed sites such as health departments.
2. sliding fee schedules.
3. educating persons on benefits.
4. increased infectious diseases caused by new organisms.

(137) **56.** Control of vectors aimed at interrupting the transmission of infectious agents is:

1. spraying for mosquitos.
2. using antibiotics to prevent traveler's diarrhea.
3. prompt treatment of strep throat.
4. cooking meat, egg, and poultry until well-done.

(137) **57.** Two measures to prevent the spread of VRE are:

1. careful use of antibiotics and infection control.
2. proper hygiene and cooking meats until well-done.
3. sanitation of water and antidiarrheal agents.
4. screening and education of blood handlers.

(136) **58.** Flu and cold viruses often enter the body through the mucous membranes of the nose and mouth; the nose and mouth areas are:

1. susceptible hosts.
2. portals of exit.
3. portals of entry.
4. causative agents.

(137) **59.** Malaise, anorexia, and prostration are symptoms of:

1. generalized infection.
2. localized infection.
3. community-acquired infection.
4. nosocomial infection.

(136) **60.** It is now necessary to give two or more drugs to tuberculosis patients because:

1. they prolong the effects of each drug.
2. they potentiate the effect of each drug.
3. strains of bacteria resistant to drugs have developed.
4. more people are susceptible to tuberculosis.

(135) **61.** A common protozoal infection that occurs as an opportunistic infection in HIV-positive persons is:

1. *Pneumocystis carinii.*
2. Rocky Mountain spotted fever.
3. hookworms.
4. conjunctivitis.

(135) **62.** Gram-negative organisms without cell walls that are responsible for primary atypical pneumonia are:

1. viruses.
2. rickettsia.
3. helminths.
4. mycoplasmas.

(146) **63.** A life-threatening allergic reaction that can quickly deteriorate into shock, coma, and death is called:

1. resistance.
2. septicemia.
3. anaphylaxis.
4. pneumonia.

(136) **64.** Any items that have been touched or cross-contaminated by the host, such as bed linens or side rails, are:

1. vectors.
2. common vehicles.
3. pathogens.
4. fomites.

(144) **65.** The condition when the body's self defenses against foreign invasion fail to function normally is:

1. infection.
2. inflammation.
3. immunodeficiency.
4. allergy.

CHAPTER 13

Student Name ______________________________

Fluid and Electrolytes

Answer Key: Textbook page references are provided as a guide for answering these questions. A complete answer key was provided for your instructor.

OBJECTIVES

1. Describe the extracellular and intracellular fluid compartments.
2. Describe the composition of the extracellular and intracellular body fluid compartments.
3. Discuss the mechanisms of fluid transport and fluid balance.
4. Identify the causes, signs and symptoms, and treatment of fluid imbalances.
5. Describe the major functions of the major electrolytes—sodium, potassium, calcium, and magnesium.
6. Identify the causes, signs and symptoms, and treatment of electrolyte imbalances.
7. List data to be collected in assessing the fluid and electrolyte status.
8. Discuss the medical treatment and nursing management of persons with fluid and electrolyte imbalances.
9. Explain why the elderly are at increased risk for fluid and electrolyte imbalances.
10. List the four types of acid-base imbalances.
11. Identify the major causes of each acid-base imbalance.
12. Explain the management of acid-base imbalances.

LEARNING ACTIVITIES

A. Select the correct word to complete each sentence.

(150) **1.** With increasing age, body water (increases/decreases).

(151) **2.** Fat cells contain (more/less) water than other cells.

(150) **3.** Females have (higher/lower) body water percentages than males.

(151) **4.** An obese person has a (higher/lower) percentage of body water than a thin person.

B. Indicate for each substance whether it is an electrolyte (A) or a nonelectrolyte (B).

(152) **1.** ________ Bilirubin

(152) **2.** ________ Urea

(151) **3.** ________ Magnesium

(151) **4.** ________ Phosphate

(152) **5.** ________ Creatinine

(151) **6.** ________ Bicarbonate

(151) **7.** ________ Potassium

(152) **8.** ________ Protein

(151) **9.** ________ Chloride

(151) **10.** ________ Calcium

(151) **11.** ________ Sodium

C. List 10 conditions that have great potential for altering fluid balance.

(155) **1.** ____________________

(155) **2.** ____________________

(155) **3.** ____________________

(155) **4.** ____________________

(155) **5.** ____________________

(155) **6.** ____________________

(155) **7.** ____________________

(155) **8.** ____________________

(155) **9.** ____________________

(155) **10.** ____________________

D. List three locations where skin turgor is best measured.

(156) **1.** ____________________

(156) **2.** ____________________

(156) **3.** ____________________

E. List four parts of the body against which skin is pressed to test for edema.

(156) **1.** ____________________

(156) **2.** ____________________

(156) **3.** ____________________

(156) **4.** ____________________

Student Name ______________________

F. List three reasons older people are at high risk for fluid and electrolyte imbalance.

(154) **1.** ______________________

(154) **2.** ______________________

(154) **3.** ______________________

G. What is the most serious effect of hyperkalemia? *(162)*

____

H. Indicate whether the statements are related to fluid volume excess (hypervolemia) (A) or fluid volume deficit (hypovolemia) (B).

(154) **1.** ________ Stimulates thirst

(154) **2.** ________ Dilute urine

(154) **3.** ________ Decreased urination

(154) **4.** ________ Stimulates aldosterone

(154) **5.** ________ Inhibits ADH

A. Hypervolemia
B. Hypovolemia

I. Regulation of body fluid volume: Match the condition in the numbered column with the most appropriate effect in the lettered column. Answers may be used more than once.

(153, 154) **1.** ________ Hyperkalemia

(153, 154) **2.** ________ Increased plasma osmolality

(153, 154) **3.** ________ Hyponatremia

(153, 154) **4.** ________ Decreased plasma osmolality

A. Stimulates ADH release
B. Inhibits ADH release
C. Stimulates aldosterone release
D. Inhibits aldosterone release

J. Match the vital sign change (assessment) finding in the numbered column with the most appropriate condition in the lettered column. More than one condition may be appropriate for each vital sign change.

(155) **1.** ________ Bounding pulse

(155) **2.** ________ Weak, irregular, and rapid pulse

(155) **3.** ________ Increased pulse

(155) **4.** ________ Decreased pulse

(155) **5.** ________ Increased blood pressure

(155) **6.** ________ Deep, fast respirations

(155) **7.** ________ Slow, shallow respirations with intermittent periods of apnea

(155) **8.** ________ Fall in systolic blood pressure >20 mm Hg from lying to standing

(155) **9.** ________ Fever

(155) **10.** ________ Increased respiratory rate

(155) **11.** ________ Subnormal body temperature

(155) **12.** ________ Hypotension

A. Hyponatremia
B. Increased metabolism, with fluid loss
C. Metabolic acidosis
D. Hypernatremia
E. Hyperkalemia
F. Hypermagnesemia
G. Metabolic alkalosis
H. Hypomagnesemia
I. Fluid volume excess
J. Fluid volume deficit

Student Name____

K. Add the arrows (↑ , ↓) or Normal in the table below. *(164)*

Arterial Blood Gas Values with Uncompensated Respiratory and Metabolic Acidosis and Alkalosis

CONDITION	CAUSE	pH	HCO_3	$PaCO_2$
Respiratory acidosis	Hypoventilation			
Respiratory alkalosis	Hyperventilation			
Metabolic acidosis	Diabetic ketoacidosis			
	Lactic acidosis			
	Diarrhea			
	Renal insufficiency			
Metabolic alkalosis	Vomiting			
	HCO_3 retention			
	Volume depletion			
	K^+ depletion			

MULTIPLE-CHOICE QUESTIONS

L. Choose the most appropriate answer.

(151) **1.** The major electrolytes in extracellular fluid are:

1. sodium and chloride.
2. potassium and phosphate.
3. calcium and bicarbonate.
4. magnesium and phosphate.

(151) **2.** Sodium, potassium, calcium, and magnesium are examples of:

1. anions. 2. cations.
3. filtrates. 4. enzymes.

(151) **3.** Chloride, bicarbonate, and phosphate are examples of:

1. cations. 2. anions.
3. filtrates. 4. enzymes.

(151) **4.** The concentration of electrolytes in a solution or body fluid compartment is measured in:

1. milligrams (mg).
2. grams (g).
3. milliliters (ml).
4. milliequivalents (mEq).

(153) **5.** What stimulates osmoreceptors in the hypothalamus to give the sensation of thirst?

1. increased plasma osmolality
2. decreased plasma osmolality
3. less concentrated urine
4. decreased urine volume

(153) **6.** Water loss via the skin and lungs increases in a:

1. hot, moist environment.
2. hot, dry environment.
3. cool, dry environment.
4. cool, moist environment.

(152) **7.** A measurement of the concentration of electrolytes in body water is called:

1. osmosis. 2. diffusion.
3. osmolality. 4. filtration.

(153) **8.** What percentage of the plasma is filtered by the glomerulus?

1. 5% 2. 20%
3. 50% 4. 80%

(153) **9.** Because the retention of sodium causes water retention, aldosterone acts as a regulator of:

1. acid balance.
2. base balance.
3. blood pH.
4. blood volume.

(158) **10.** One way the body tries to compensate for fluid volume deficits is to:

1. increase heart rate.
2. decrease heart rate.
3. increase blood pressure.
4. decrease ADH.

(154) **11.** ADH is decreased in response to:

1. fluid volume deficit.
2. fluid volume excess.
3. decreased urination.
4. concentrated urine.

(154) **12.** The body tries to compensate for fluid volume excess by:

1. inhibiting aldosterone.
2. stimulating ADH.
3. inhibiting epinephrine.
4. stimulating thirst.

(160) **13.** The two electrolytes that cause a majority of health problems when there is an imbalance are sodium and:

1. potassium. 2. chloride.
3. magnesium. 4. bicarbonate.

(151) **14.** The major cation involved in the structure of bones and teeth is:

1. sodium. 2. chloride.
3. calcium. 4. potassium.

(153) **15.** When your body goes without fluid intake, which hormone increases water reabsorption?

1. thyroxine 2. epinephrine
3. ADH 4. aldosterone

(162) **16.** Low levels of serum potassium can result in serious disturbances of neuromuscular function and:

1. metabolic function.
2. cardiac function.
3. bone structure.
4. acid-base balance.

(151) **17.** An extracellular anion that is usually bound with other ions, especially sodium or potassium, is:

1. chloride. 2. magnesium.
3. calcium. 4. iron.

(162) **18.** Which of the following drugs cause hypokalemia?

1. narcotics and salicylates
2. anticholinergics and antihistamines
3. calcium channel blockers and beta blockers
4. diuretics and corticosteroids

Student Name____

(151) **19.** Ninety-nine percent of the body's calcium is concentrated in the:

1. blood and muscles.
2. liver and brain.
3. bones and teeth.
4. kidneys and adrenal glands.

(151) **20.** If more calcium is needed in the bones, it is taken from the blood as well as reabsorbed through the:

1. lungs.
2. kidneys.
3. heart.
4. liver.

(151) **21.** Next to potassium, the most abundant cation in the intracellular fluid is:

1. calcium.
2. sodium.
3. chloride.
4. magnesium.

(156) **22.** Hard, edematous tissue, called *brawny edema*, occurs commonly after:

1. hysterectomy.
2. appendectomy.
3. tonsillectomy.
4. radical mastectomy.

(155) **23.** One liter of fluid retention equals a weight gain of:

1. 1 pound.
2. 2.2 pounds.
3. 5.4 pounds.
4. 10 pounds.

(156) **24.** Puffy eyelids and fuller cheeks suggest:

1. fluid volume excess.
2. fluid volume deficit.
3. potassium excess.
4. potassium deficit.

(154) **25.** Which assessment finding is the *least* reliable indicator of fluid status in an 80-year-old person?

1. pitting peripheral edema
2. poor tissue turgor
3. intake and output
4. mucous membrane moisture

(156) **26.** If a depression remains in the tissue after pressure is applied with a fingertip, the edema is described as:

1. excessive.
2. pitting.
3. depressed.
4. minimal.

(156) **27.** A deep and persistent pit that is approximately 1 inch deep is described as:

1. 1+.
2. 2+.
3. 3+.
4. 4+.

(156) **28.** When the edema is so severe that pitting is not possible and the tissue feels hard, the edema is described as:

1. 10+.
2. 5+.
3. tenacious.
4. brawny.

(156) **29.** A red, swollen tongue suggests an excess of:

1. potassium.
2. calcium.
3. sodium.
4. magnesium.

(156) **30.** A dry mouth may be the result of:

1. fluid volume excess.
2. fluid volume deficit.
3. hypochloremia.
4. hyperchloremia.

(156) **31.** Distention of the jugular neck vein can indicate:

1. fluid volume excess.
2. fluid volume deficit.
3. hypocalcemia.
4. hypercalcemia.

(156) **32.** If the veins take longer than 3 to 5 seconds to fill when placed in a dependent position, the patient may have:

1. hypokalemia.
2. hyperkalemia.
3. hypovolemia.
4. hypervolemia.

(162) **33.** Weakness and muscle cramps are symptoms of:

1. hyponatremia.
2. hypokalemia.
3. fluid volume deficit.
4. respiratory acidosis.

(157) **34.** The normal range for urine pH is:

1. 2.0–7.0. 2. 4.0–12.0.
3. 4.6–8.0. 4. 7.8–12.0.

(157) **35.** A urine specimen that is not tested within 4 hours of collection may become:

1. alkaline.
2. acidic.
3. more concentrated.
4. less concentrated.

(157) **36.** A measure of the kidneys' ability to dilute or concentrate urine is called:

1. pH.
2. urine potassium.
3. creatinine clearance.
4. specific gravity.

(157) **37.** In most instances, normal urine specific gravity is between:

1. 1.010 and 1.025.
2. 2.001 and 4.035.
3. 4.001 and 6.035.
4. 5.0 and 7.0.

(157) **38.** A good indicator of fluid balance is urine:

1. sodium.
2. creatinine clearance.
3. specific gravity.
4. potassium.

(157) **39.** A more precise measurement of the kidneys' ability to concentrate urine than the specific gravity is:

1. urine sodium.
2. urine pH.
3. urine osmolality.
4. urine potassium.

(158) **40.** A 24-hour urine specimen is required for:

1. creatinine clearance.
2. pH.
3. specific gravity.
4. osmolality.

(158) **41.** When the blood is more concentrated in a patient with fluid volume deficit, which blood study result is expected?

1. increased blood urea nitrogen (BUN)
2. increased creatine
3. increased hematocrit
4. decreased hemoglobin

(158) **42.** BUN provides a measure of:

1. blood volume.
2. renal function.
3. cardiac function.
4. liver function.

(158) **43.** In a patient with fluid volume excess, which blood study result would you expect?

1. increased albumin
2. decreased osmolality
3. decreased magnesium
4. increased potassium

Student Name____

(161) **44.** What one of the following is a symptom of hyponatremia?

1. palpitations 2. hypertension
3. confusion 4. insomnia

(153, 154) **45.** What amount of fluid per day is needed by the average person for adequate hydration?

1. 500–700 ml/day
2. 800–1000 ml/day
3. 1500–2000 ml/day
4. 3500–5000 ml/day

(160) **46.** When breathing problems occur in a patient with fluid volume excess, the patient should:

1. lie flat in bed.
2. have head of bed elevated 30 degrees.
3. ambulate frequently.
4. be in side-lying position.

(160) **47.** If pitting edema is present in patients with fluid volume excess, patients should:

1. be turned every 2 hours.
2. cough every 2 hours.
3. ambulate every 2 hours.
4. have blood pressure checked every 2 hours.

(161) **48.** To prevent hyponatremia in patients with feeding tubes, what should be used for irrigation?

1. sterile water
2. normal glucose
3. normal saline
4. sterile dextrose

(162) **49.** The heart rate of patients on digitalis should be closely watched because hypokalemia can contribute to:

1. congestive heart failure.
2. pericarditis.
3. digitalis toxicity.
4. diuresis.

(162) **50.** In order to prevent gastrointestinal irritation, oral potassium supplements should be given with:

1. meals.
2. a full glass of water or fruit juice.
3. a full glass of milk.
4. a teaspoon of water.

(162) **51.** Which must be checked before starting an intravenous infusion of potassium?

1. blood pressure
2. temperature
3. weight
4. urine output

(162) **52.** Decreased renal function can cause:

1. hyperkalemia.
2. hypokalemia.
3. hypercalcemia.
4. hypocalcemia.

(163) **53.** The homeostasis of the hydrogen ion concentration in the body fluids is:

1. acid-base balance.
2. active transport.
3. adaptation.
4. osmosis.

(163) **54.** The respiratory system regulates the pH by:

1. removing oxygen from the blood.
2. removing carbon dioxide from the blood.
3. removing sodium from the blood.
4. removing chloride from the blood.

(164) **55.** When the respiratory system fails to eliminate the appropriate amount of carbon dioxide to maintain the normal acid-base balance, what occurs?

1. respiratory alkalosis
2. respiratory acidosis
3. metabolic acidosis
4. metabolic alkalosis

(162) **56.** Nursing care for patients with hypokalemia includes monitoring serum potassium levels and:

1. EKG.
2. EEG.
3. arterial blood gas results.
4. intake and output.

(165) **57.** The most common cause of respiratory alkalosis is:

1. hypoventilation.
2. hyperventilation.
3. drowning.
4. obesity.

(163) **58.** Patients may develop high levels of magnesium in their blood if they are taking:

1. diuretics.
2. antihypertensives.
3. antacids.
4. salicylates.

(165) **59.** Hyperventilation is treated by having the patient:

1. breathe slowly.
2. increase fluid intake.
3. receive oxygen.
4. elevate legs.

(165) **60.** When patients with respiratory alkalosis are hyperventilating, they should be encouraged to breathe:

1. rapidly into a paper bag.
2. shallow breaths.
3. panting breaths.
4. slowly into a paper bag.

(165) **61.** When the body retains too many hydrogen ions or loses too many bicarbonate ions, what occurs?

1. respiratory acidosis
2. respiratory alkalosis
3. metabolic acidosis
4. metabolic alkalosis

(165) **62.** With too many acids and too few bases present in metabolic acidosis, the blood:

1. $PaCO_2$ increases.
2. pH remains the same.
3. pH rises.
4. pH drops.

(162) **63.** When cells are damaged because of an injury, which cation is released?

1. calcium 2. chloride
3. potassium 4. sodium

(165) **64.** Metabolic acidosis may be treated with intravenous infusion of:

1. potassium chloride.
2. normal saline.
3. calcium salts.
4. sodium bicarbonate.

(165) **65.** An increase in bicarbonate levels or a loss of hydrogen ions results in:

1. metabolic acidosis.
2. metabolic alkalosis.
3. respiratory alkalosis.
4. respiratory acidosis.

(151) **66.** Potassium is a critical factor for the transmission of nerve impulses, because it is necessary for:

1. muscular activity.
2. acid-base balance.
3. fluid balance.
4. membrane excitability.

Student Name____

(151) **67.** In addition to its role in regulating fluid balance, sodium is also necessary for:

1. nerve impulse conduction.
2. bone structure.
3. protein structure.
4. breakdown of glycogen.

(161) **68.** Symptoms of hyponatremia include:

1. headache, rapid breathing, nervousness.
2. confusion, abdominal cramps.
3. vomiting, diarrhea, shallow respirations.
4. irritability, edema, convulsions.

(163) **69.** The most common cause of hypocalcemia is related to problems with which hormone?

1. ADH
2. aldosterone
3. thyroxine
4. PTH

CHAPTER 14

Student Name ______________________________

Pain Management

Answer Key: Textbook page references are provided as a guide for answering these questions. A complete answer key was provided for your instructor.

OBJECTIVES

1. Define pain.
2. Explain the physiologic basis for pain.
3. Identify situations in which patients are likely to experience pain.
4. Explain the relationships between past pain experiences, anticipation, culture, anxiety, or activity and a patient's response to pain.
5. Identify differences in the duration of pain and patient responses to acute and chronic pain.
6. Explain the special needs of the elderly patient with pain.
7. List the data to be collected in assessing pain.
8. Describe interventions used in the management of pain.
9. Describe the nursing care of patients receiving opioid and nonopioid analgesics for pain.
10. List the factors that should be considered when pain is not relieved with analgesic medications.

LEARNING ACTIVITIES

A. Match the definition in the numbered column with the most appropriate term in the lettered column.

(168) **1.** __________ Process of pain transmission

(168) **2.** __________ Unpleasant sensory and emotional experience associated with actual or potential tissue damage, existing whenever the person says it does

A. Pain
B. Addiction
C. Acute pain
D. Pain tolerance
E. Nociception
F. Physical dependence
G. Tolerance
H. Chronic pain
I. Pain threshold
J. Analgesic

Continued next page

(168) **3.** __________ Drug that acts on the nervous system to relieve or reduce the suffering or intensity of pain

(182) **4.** __________ A physiologic result of repeated doses of an opioid where the same dose is no longer effective in achieving the same analgesic effect

(182) **5.** __________ Behavioral pattern of compulsive drug use characterized by craving for an opioid and obtaining and using the drug for effects other than pain relief

(182) **6.** __________ Physiologic adaptation of the body to an opioid so that a person exhibits withdrawal symptoms when the opioid is stopped abruptly after repeated administration

(170) **7.** __________ Amount of pain a person is willing to endure before taking action to relieve pain

(171) **8.** __________ Pain that lasts longer than 6 months

(170) **9.** __________ Point at which a stimulus causes the sensation of pain

(171) **10.** __________ Pain that occurs after injury to tissues from surgery, trauma, or disease

Student Name____

B. Indicate for each statement in the numbered column whether it (A) opens the gate or (B) closes the gate according to gate-control theory. Answers may be used more than once.

(169) **1.** __________ Distraction

(169) **2.** __________ Tissue damage

(169) **3.** __________ Massage

(169) **4.** __________ Heat application

(169) **5.** __________ Position change

(169) **6.** __________ Fear of pain

(169) **7.** __________ Guided imagery

(169) **8.** __________ Monotonous environment

(169) **9.** __________ Cold application

(169) **10.** __________ Preparatory information

A. Opens the gate
B. Closes the gate

C. Match the description in the numbered column with the most appropriate factor affecting pain response in the lettered column.

(170) **1.** __________ A patient who has received nitrous oxide during surgery and who says he does not have pain postoperatively

(170) **2.** __________ An older person who is stoic and does not want to bother the nurse

(171) **3.** __________ Pain associated with childbirth is usually short-lived, whereas cancer pain may be chronic

(170) **4.** __________ Anger, fatigue, insomnia, depression

(170) **5.** __________ A patient who prays and believes that divine intervention will help him to endure pain

A. Situational factors
B. Pain threshold
C. Religious beliefs
D. Age, culture
E. Anesthetic

D. A 42-year-old male with multiple fractures in the right arm used the numeric scale from 1 to 10 for rating pain. The patient complained of throbbing in his right arm and a backache. He rated the intensity of both pains at 7 on the scale at 8:00 PM. The nurse applied heat to the lower back as ordered, massaged his back, and administered 10 mg of morphine intramuscularly. At 9:00 PM, the patient rated intensity of both pains at 2 and stated that the pain was slowly going away.

(174) Were the interventions effective in relieving the pain?

(174) What evidence do you have that the pain was or was not relieved?

E. List seven possible nursing diagnoses for patients who have pain.

(176) **1.** ____________________

(176) **2.** ____________________

(176) **3.** ____________________

(176) **4.** ____________________

(176) **5.** ____________________

(176) **6.** ____________________

(176) **7.** ____________________

Student Name ______________________________

F. Match the characteristic in the numbered column with the most appropriate term in the lettered column. Answers may be used more than once.

A. Addiction
B. Tolerance
C. Physical dependence

(182) **1.** ________ Physiologic changes that occur from repeated doses of opioids

(182) **2.** ________ Compulsive obtaining and use of drug for psychic effects

(182) **3.** ________ Withdrawal symptoms may occur if the opioid is stopped abruptly (e.g., irritability, chills, sweating, nausea)

(182) **4.** ________ Psychological dependence characterized by continued craving for opioid for other than pain relief

(182) **5.** ________ The need for higher doses to achieve pain relief

G. List seven physical factors that influence response to pain.

(170) **1.** ______________________________

(170) **2.** ______________________________

(170) **3.** ______________________________

(170) **4.** ______________________________

(170) **5.** ______________________________

(170) **6.** ______________________________

(170) **7.** ______________________________

MULTIPLE-CHOICE QUESTIONS

H. Choose the most appropriate answer.

(171) **1.** One difference between acute and chronic pain is that a patient with acute pain:

1. often becomes depressed.
2. shows little facial expression.
3. feels isolated.
4. has a fast heart rate.

(169) **2.** Pathways that carry messages to the brain where the messages are interpreted are:

1. internal. 2. external.
3. afferent. 4. efferent.

(170) **3.** Factors influencing the response to pain include pain threshold, pain tolerance, age, physical activity, and the type of surgery. These factors are examples of:

1. psychosocial factors.
2. emotional factors.
3. sociological factors.
4. physical factors.

(170) **4.** The point at which a stimulus causes the sensation or feeling of pain is the pain:

1. duration. 2. peak.
3. threshold. 4. tolerance.

(170) **5.** When the pain threshold is lowered, the person experiences pain:

1. less easily.
2. more easily.
3. as excruciating.
4. as mild.

(170) **6.** Which age group tends to report their pain as much less severe than it really is?

1. older patients
2. middle-aged patients
3. adolescent patients
4. children

(170) **7.** Surgery in which area is reported to be the most painful for patients?

1. skull region
2. thoracic region
3. upper abdominal region
4. lower abdominal region

(171) **8.** Dilated pupils, perspiration, and pallor are results of which nervous system response to pain?

1. voluntary
2. somatic
3. parasympathetic
4. sympathetic

(171) **9.** Postoperative pain and pain in childbirth are examples of:

1. chronic pain.
2. permanent pain.
3. acute pain.
4. nonmalignant pain.

(172) **10.** An example of acute pain with recurrent episodes is pain associated with:

1. low back pain.
2. migraine headaches.
3. rheumatoid arthritis.
4. cancer pain.

Student Name____

(172) **11.** A pain that cannot be explained or that persists after healing has taken place is:

1. acute benign pain.
2. acute metastatic pain.
3. chronic benign pain.
4. chronic metastatic pain.

(172) **12.** The first step in pain management is:

1. assessment.
2. planning.
3. intervention.
4. evaluation.

(172) **13.** When possible, the information about pain should obtained from the:

1. nurse.
2. patient.
3. doctor.
4. patient's family.

(174) **14.** Factors that make the pain worse are called:

1. benign factors.
2. stoic factors.
3. psychological factors.
4. aggravating factors.

(177) **15.** The application of heat or cold, massage, and TENS are examples of:

1. physical comfort measures.
2. cutaneous stimulation.
3. environmental control.
4. psychological comfort measures.

(177) **16.** The longest time a cold application can be used without tissue injury would be:

1. 3 minutes.
2. 15 minutes.
3. 30 minutes.
4. 60 minutes.

(177) **17.** The application of cold is contraindicated in patients with:

1. hip fracture.
2. muscle sprain.
3. allergic reaction.
4. peripheral vascular disease.

(183) **18.** Duragesic or fentanyl transdermal patches are used to treat chronic pain by delivering:

1. NSAIDs.
2. salicylates.
3. opioids.
4. steroids.

(177) **19.** Which is the most expensive and least available pain treatment?

1. cold
2. heat
3. massage
4. TENS

(178) **20.** Focusing on stimuli other than pain is called:

1. massage.
2. stimulation.
3. distraction.
4. acupuncture.

(179) **21.** Relaxation is most effective for:

1. delusional pain.
2. mild to moderate pain.
3. moderate to severe pain.
4. severe pain.

(179) **22.** Using a person's imagination to help control pain is called:

1. environmental control.
2. stimulation.
3. imagery.
4. relaxation.

(179) **23.** When pain is unpredictable, analgesics are more effective when given:

1. once a day.
2. twice a day.
3. around the clock.
4. prn.

(179) **24.** The initial treatment choice for mild pain is:

1. opioid analgesics.
2. nonopioid analgesics.
3. narcotics.
4. anesthetics.

(179) **25.** Aspirin, acetaminophen, and NSAIDs are examples of:

1. opioid analgesics.
2. nonopioid analgesics.
3. narcotics.
4. anesthetics.

(180) **26.** Ketorolac tromethamine (Toradol) is generally used for the short-term management of:

1. cancer pain.
2. congestive heart failure.
3. urinary tract infection.
4. postoperative pain.

(180) **27.** Drugs, such as nonopioids, that do not improve analgesia beyond a certain dosage are said to have a:

1. peak effect.
2. duration effect.
3. ceiling effect.
4. onset effect.

(180) **28.** Some nonopioids should be used cautiously in patients with congestive heart failure or hypertension because of the side effect of:

1. decreased circulation.
2. depressed respirations.
3. tachycardia.
4. fluid retention.

(180) **29.** Nonopioids tend to block pain transmission:

1. at the central nervous system.
2. during cell wall synthesis.
3. at the myocardium.
4. on the peripheral nervous system.

(180) **30.** Nalbuphine (Nubain), butorphanol (Stadol), and pentazocine (Talwin) are examples of:

1. nonopioid analgesics.
2. anticholinergics.
3. opioid agonist-antagonists.
4. opioid agonists.

(181) **31.** A patient receiving 10 mg morphine IM for pain will be given what dose PO to receive an equianalgesic dose?

1. 10 mg
2. 30 mg
3. 60 mg
4. 80 mg

(182) **32.** If the patient is nauseated or has difficulty swallowing, which route is useful for administering opioids?

1. oral
2. rectal
3. topical
4. intradermal

(183) **33.** To evaluate the patient for constipation, the nurse must assess the patient for:

1. black, tarry stools and anorexia.
2. decreased blood pressure, itching, and respiratory distress.
3. abdominal distention, cramping, and abdominal pain.
4. intake and output, nausea and vomiting.

Student Name ______________________________

(183) **34.** Which effect of opioids is not potentiated by the use of promethazine (Phenergan)?

1. sedation
2. respiratory depression
3. hypotension
4. analgesia

(184) **35.** A drug classification that is effective in treating neuropathic pain is:

1. muscle relaxants.
2. benzodiazepines.
3. antidepressants.
4. corticosteroids.

(184) **36.** A patient who has had back surgery complains of muscle spasms. Which drug may be most effective in relieving his pain?

1. muscle relaxant
2. opioid
3. NSAID
4. aspirin

CHAPTER 15

Student Name ____________________

First Aid and Emergency Care

Answer Key: Textbook page references are provided as a guide for answering these questions. A complete answer key was provided for your instructor.

OBJECTIVES

1. List the principles of emergency and first aid care.
2. List the steps of the initial assessment and interventions for the person requiring emergency care.
3. Describe the components of the nursing assessment of the person requiring emergency care.
4. Outline the steps of the nursing process for emergency or first aid treatment of victims of cardiopulmonary arrest, choking, shock, hemorrhage, traumatic injury, burns, heat or cold exposure, poisoning, bites, and stings.
5. Explain the legal implications of administering first aid in emergency situations.

LEARNING ACTIVITIES

A. Match the definition in the numbered column with the most appropriate term in the lettered column.

(196) **1.** __________ Tearing away of tissue

(197) **2.** __________ Presence of air in the pleural cavity that causes the lung on the affected side to collapse

(193) **3.** __________ Loss of a large amount of blood

(194) **4.** __________ An injury to muscle tissue or the tendons that attach them to bones, or both

A. Shock
B. Hypothermia
C. Cardiopulmonary arrest
D. Hemothorax
E. Flail chest
F. Sprain
G. Evisceration
H. Avulsion
I. Hemorrhage
J. Hyperthermia
K. Strain
L. Poison
M. Respiratory arrest
N. Pneumothorax
O. Anaphylactic shock
P. Cardiac tamponade
Q. Epistaxis

Continued next page

(202) **5.** __________ A severe, potentially fatal, allergic reaction characterized by hypotension and bronchial constriction

(197) **6.** __________ Presence of blood in the pleural cavity causing the lung on the affected side to collapse

(198) **7.** __________ Elevation of body core temperature above 99° F

(197) **8.** __________ Blood in the pericardial sac that causes decreased cardiac output

(193) **9.** __________ Nosebleed

(198) **10.** __________ Decrease in body core temperature below 95° F

(194) **11.** __________ An injury to a ligament

(200) **12.** __________ Any substance that, in small quantities, is capable of causing illness or harm following ingestion, inhalation, injection, or contact with the skin

(189) **13.** __________ Absence of breathing

(196) **14.** __________ Protrusion of internal organs through a wound

(189) **15.** __________ Absence of heartbeat and breathing

(197) **16.** __________ Loss of support of chest wall where several adjacent ribs are broken in more than one place

(192) **17.** __________ Acute circulatory failure that can lead to death

B. List five steps in the initial assessment and immediate intervention in emergency care.

(188) **1.** ______________________________

(188) **2.** ______________________________

(188) **3.** ______________________________

(188) **4.** ______________________________

(188) **5.** ______________________________

C. List five general guidelines for first aid treatment of emergency patients.

(188-189) **1.** ______________________________

(188-189) **2.** ______________________________

Student Name____________________

(188-189) **3.** ____________________

(188-189) **4.** ____________________

(188-189) **5.** ____________________

D. List three nursing diagnoses for patients in cardiopulmonary arrest.

(190) **1.** ____________________

(190) **2.** ____________________

(190) **3.** ____________________

E. List two nursing diagnoses for the patient who is choking.

(192) **1.** ____________________

(192) **2.** ____________________

MULTIPLE-CHOICE QUESTIONS

F. Choose the most appropriate answer.

(188) **1.** General guidelines for first aid treatment of emergency patients include:

1. cover with wool blanket to prevent chills.
2. remove penetrating objects.
3. splint injured parts in the position they are found.
4. give orange juice with sugar if unconscious.

(188, 189) **2.** The first assessment priorities must be:

1. observation of uncontrolled bleeding or shock.
2. systematic head-to-toe assessment.
3. airway, breathing, and circulation.
4. palpation of carotid and peripheral pulses.

(189) **3.** The systematic assessment begins with inspection of the:

1. head. 2. chest.
3. abdomen. 4. lungs.

(189) **4.** When the heart stops beating, a person is in:

1. pulmonary arrest.
2. anaphylactic shock.
3. cardiac arrest.
4. cardiopulmonary arrest.

(189) **5.** When respirations cease, the person is in:

1. cardiac arrest.
2. anaphylactic shock.
3. cardiopulmonary arrest.
4. pulmonary arrest.

(190) **6.** In most cases, the brain begins to die after 4 minutes without oxygen due to susceptibility to hypoxia of:

1. heart tissue.
2. nerve tissue.
3. lung tissue.
4. blood vessels.

(190) **7.** Prompt recognition and treatment of cardiopulmonary arrest are so important due to the need to maintain the oxygen supply to the:

1. heart.
2. brain.
3. lungs.
4. blood vessels.

(189) **8.** The goal of CPR is to maintain:

1. the heartbeat until respirations are restored.
2. respirations until the heartbeat is restored.
3. circulation until the heartbeat and respirations are restored.
4. oxygenation until the heartbeat and respirations are restored.

(190) **9.** When cardiopulmonary arrest is suspected, the first step is to:

1. tap the victim urgently and ask "Are you okay?".
2. place the victim supine on a firm, flat surface.
3. put your ear near the victim's nose and mouth to listen for breathing.
4. give two full breaths.

(191) **10.** Check for cardiac arrest in the adult by palpating the:

1. brachial artery.
2. femoral artery.
3. carotid artery.
4. coronary artery.

(191) **11.** Airway obstruction caused by a foreign body that enters the airway is:

1. cardiac arrest.
2. respiratory arrest.
3. choking.
4. cardiopulmonary arrest.

(191) **12.** Grabbing the throat with one or both hands is the universal sign for:

1. heart attack.
2. choking.
3. danger.
4. loss of consciousness.

(192) **13.** If the choking victim is conscious, the rescuer performs:

1. the Heimlich maneuver.
2. CPR.
3. 15 chest compressions.
4. assessment of breathing.

(192) **14.** If a choking victim loses consciousness, the rescuer does a finger sweep, attempts to ventilate, straddles the victim's thighs, and gives:

1. 5 chest compressions.
2. 15 chest compressions.
3. 5 abdominal thrusts.
4. 10 abdominal thrusts.

(192) **15.** Choking deaths can be prevented by:

1. not talking while chewing.
2. lowering blood pressure.
3. decreasing weight.
4. increasing exercise.

(193) **16.** In an adult, what amount of blood loss may result in hypovolemic shock?

1. 30 ml or more
2. 1 pint or more
3. 1 liter or more
4. 10 liters or more

Student Name____

(193) **17.** Immediate treatment for external bleeding is:

1. application of ice.
2. elevate the site of bleeding.
3. direct, continuous pressure.
4. check vital signs.

(193) **18.** If direct wound pressure and elevation fail to control bleeding, pressure is applied to the:

1. coronary heart vessels.
2. cerebral blood vessels.
3. main artery that supplies the area.
4. main vein that supplies the area.

(194) **19.** A fracture that does not break the skin is:

1. compound. 2. open.
3. simple. 4. complete.

(194) **20.** A fracture in which the ends of the broken bone protrude through the skin is:

1. compound. 2. simple.
3. closed. 4. incomplete.

(194) **21.** A fracture in which the broken ends are separated is:

1. compound. 2. simple.
3. complete. 4. incomplete.

(194) **22.** A fracture in which the bone ends are not separated is:

1. complete. 2. incomplete.
3. compound. 4. simple.

(194) **23.** The primary symptom of fracture is:

1. numbness. 2. tingling.
3. pain. 4 hemorrhage.

(194) **24.** The key to emergency management of fractures is:

1. application of cold.
2. elevation of injury.
3. immobilization.
4. application of heat.

(194) **25.** Injuries to muscles and/or the tendons are called:

1. dislocations.
2. strains.
3. sprains.
4. fractures.

(194) **26.** Emergency treatment for sprains and strains include:

1. direct wound pressure.
2. immobilization.
3. application of heat.
4. application of splint.

(194) **27.** Nursing diagnoses that might apply to the patient with a head injury during the emergency phase of treatment include:

1. Decreased cardiac output related to hypovolemia and fear related to possible impending death.
2. Altered cerebral tissue perfusion related to hypovolemia and anxiety related to panic.
3. Ineffective breathing pattern related to neurologic trauma and risk for injury related to increasing intracranial pressure.
4. Risk for trauma related to improper movements of the spine.

(194) **28.** Altered mental function and unequal pupils are signs of:

1. anaphylactic shock.
2. altered breathing.
3. increased intracranial pressure.
4. spinal cord injury.

(195) **29.** When there is a neck or spinal injury, you first assess:

1. blood loss and level of consciousness.
2. breathing and circulation.
3. movement of extremities.
4. sensation in extremities.

(195) **30.** After a diving injury, while removing the victim from the water, efforts are made to:

1. immobilize the extremities.
2. immobilize the neck and back.
3. turn the victim in a prone position.
4. turn the victim in a supine position.

(195) **31.** The priority goal for the patient with a neck or spinal injury is to:

1. provide adequate ventilation.
2. increase cardiac output.
3. reduce fear.
4. decrease risk of additional injury.

(195) **32.** Outcome criteria for the patient with a neck or spinal injury is based on:

1. continuous monitoring for signs of increased intracranial pressure and oxygenation.
2. continuous immobilization of the back and spine and transport for medical care.
3. prevention of aspiration and maintenance of circulation.
4. prevention of skin breakdown and shock.

(195) **33.** The primary nursing diagnosis for the patient with an eye injury is:

1. Impaired self-image related to change in physical capacity.
2. Impaired coping related to change in vision.
3. Risk for impaired skin integrity related to immobility.
4. Risk for injury related to foreign body in eye.

(196) **34.** When chemicals come in contact with the eye, the nurse should:

1. cover the eye with a loose dressing.
2. flush with water to irrigate the eye for 30 minutes.
3. apply pressure with a sterile cloth.
4. place patient in shower under cold water.

(196) **35.** If bleeding is under control, the priority nursing diagnosis for a traumatic injury to the auricle is:

1. Impaired body image related to injury.
2. Anemia related to blood loss.
3. Impaired tissue integrity related to trauma.
4. Decreased cardiac output related to blood loss.

(196) **36.** The most critical chest injuries include:

1. tension pneumothorax, ulcer, and abdominal injuries.
2. pericarditis, lung contusion, and flail chest.
3. open pneumothorax, flail chest, and cardiac tamponade.
4. lung concussion and closed pneumothorax.

Student Name____

(196) **37.** Any chest injury at or below the nipple may cause both chest injuries and:

1. head injuries.
2. neck injuries.
3. shoulder injuries.
4. abdominal injuries.

(196) **38.** Signs and symptoms of chest injuries that impair respirations are:

1. unequal pupils and hypotension.
2. dyspnea and tachycardia.
3. shallow respirations and lethargy.
4. bradycardia and cyanosis.

(197) **39.** Open chest wounds that penetrate the pleural cavity allowing air to enter are referred to as:

1. pneumothorax.
2. cardiac tamponade.
3. flail chest.
4. hemothorax.

(197) **40.** The pneumothorax wound should be covered with which type of dressing?

1. saline 2. occlusive
3. vented 4. porous

(197) **41.** The term used when several adjacent ribs are broken in more than one place is:

1. pneumothorax.
2. cardiac tamponade.
3. flail chest.
4. hemothorax.

(197) **42.** The abnormal chest wall movement in flail chest would be described as what sort of motion?

1. sawing 2. paradoxical
3. pulsating 4. sucking

(197) **43.** The abnormal chest wall action in flail chest causes:

1. altered tissue perfusion.
2. increased cardiac output.
3. increased pulse strength.
4. impaired gas exchange.

(197) **44.** The accumulation of blood in the pleural cavity that causes the lung to collapse is:

1. pneumothorax.
2. cardiac tamponade.
3. flail chest.
4. hemothorax.

(196) **45.** Outcome criteria for evaluating emergency nursing care of the patient with an abdominal wound includes:

1. protection of injured tissue.
2. control of bleeding.
3. restoration of a strong pulse.
4. reduction in fear.

(198) **46.** First aid for minor superficial burns is to:

1. apply butter to the burn.
2. apply petroleum jelly to the burn.
3. cover the burn with a cloth.
4. immerse the injured body part in cool water.

(198) **47.** When a large body surface area is burned or any area is severely burned, the nurse should:

1. apply medications to the burn.
2. cover the burn with a clean dry dressing or cloth.
3. cover the burn with a cool wet dressing or cloth.
4. apply ice to the burn.

(198) **48.** Outcome criteria for emergency care of the burn victim are based on finding:

1. immobility, as well as circulatory and respiratory status maintained.
2. absence of symptoms of shock, burned areas covered, and coping supported.
3. improved gas exchange, skin surfaces free from burning materials, and pain reduced.
4. no symptoms of ileus and monitoring in place for signs of gastrointestinal bleeding and circulation.

(199) **49.** Heat exhaustion is treated by:

1. pushing fluids with caffeine.
2. ambulating the victim.
3. cooling and hydrating the victim.
4. placing victim in ice.

(199) **50.** Patients with heat exhaustion would be considered stable when they exhibit:

1. urine output of at least 10 ml/hr and pulse rate of 100 bpm or more.
2. ability to take a regular diet without nausea.
3. below-normal body temperature and tachycardia.
4. lowered body temperature and intake and retention of fluids.

(199) **51.** The skin is red, hot, and dry and perspiration is absent in:

1. heatstroke
2. heat exhaustion
3. hyperthermia
4. hypothermia

(199) **52.** Mild tissue damage caused by cold is called:

1. frostbite.
2. frostnip.
3. hypothermia.
4. cyanosis.

(199) **53.** The priority nursing diagnosis for the victim of frostbite is:

1. Sensory/perceptual alterations related to decreased circulation.
2. Risk for impaired skin integrity related to vascular changes caused by extreme cold exposure.
3. Risk for infection related to tissue damage.
4. Risk for disuse syndrome related to vascular changes.

(199) **54.** The immediate treatment of mild cold injury is:

1. rapid rewarming.
2. massaging to increase circulation.
3. covering with dressing.
4. immersing in tepid water.

(200) **55.** Any substance that in small quantities is capable of causing illness or harm following ingestion is a(n):

1. antitoxin.
2. emetic.
3. poison.
4. antiemetic.

(200) **56.** Carbon monoxide poisoning occurs because carbon monoxide:

1. is blown off too rapidly during exhalation.
2. binds to hemoglobin and occupies sites needed to transport oxygen to the cells.
3. binds to white blood cells and causes infection.
4. is retained and prevents oxygen from being inhaled in adequate amounts.

Student Name____

(200) **57.** The primary nursing diagnosis for the victim of carbon monoxide poisoning is:

1. Impaired gas exchange.
2. Ineffective breathing pattern.
3. Risk for aspiration.
4. Anxiety related to ineffective breathing pattern.

(200) **58.** The primary nursing diagnosis for the victim of drug or chemical poisoning is:

1. Altered thought processes.
2. Risk for infection.
3. Risk for injury.
4. Risk for suffocation.

(202) **59.** Flulike symptoms following a tick bite may be symptoms of:

1. poisoning.
2. Lyme disease.
3. Staph infection.
4. hypersensitivity.

(200) **60.** Which drugs increase the risk of heat stroke by affecting the body's heat-reducing mechanisms?

1. adrenergics and bronchodilators.
2. diuretics and anticholinergics.
3. steroids and salicylates.
4. anticoagulants and antihistamines.

(203) **61.** Local effects of venom on blood and blood vessels include:

1. skin breakdown, petechiae, and clubbing of nails.
2. coolness of extremities, shiny skin, and blood clots.
3. discoloration, pain, and edema.
4. brittle nails, hair loss, and cellulitis.

(203) **62.** After a bite, epinephrine may be given to prevent:

1. hypotension.
2. aspiration.
3. blood clots.
4. anaphylaxis.

(202) **63.** A victim of a bite would be considered improved when:

1. wound has only clear or white drainage, pulse is 100 bpm or less, and respiratory rate is increased.
2. patient is sleepy but able to be aroused, wound has only slight drainage, and only slight toxic effects are noted.
3. patient is alert, respiratory rate is 30 or more, and blood pressure is normal.
4. wound is free from debris, patient is alert without dyspnea, and specific toxic effects are absent.

Student Name ________________________________

Surgical Care

Answer Key: Textbook page references are provided as a guide for answering these questions. A complete answer key was provided for your instructor.

OBJECTIVES

1. State the purpose of each type of surgery: diagnostic, exploratory, curative, palliative, and cosmetic.
2. List data to be included in the nursing assessment of the preoperative patient.
3. Assist in identifying the nursing diagnoses, goals and outcome criteria, and interventions during the preoperative phase of the surgical experience.
4. Outline a preoperative teaching plan.
5. List the responsibilities of each member of the surgical team.
6. Explain the nursing implications of each type of anesthesia.
7. Explain how the nurse can help prevent postoperative complications.
8. List data to be included in the nursing assessment of the postoperative patient.
9. Identify nursing diagnoses, goals and outcome criteria, and interventions for the postoperative patient.
10. Explain patient needs to be considered in discharge planning.

LEARNING ACTIVITIES

A. List three reasons why older persons are often at greater risk for surgical complications.

(208) **1.** ________________________________

(208) **2.** ________________________________

(208) **3.** ________________________________

B. List three reasons why smoking increases the risk of pulmonary complications.

(209) **1.** ________________________________

(209) **2.** ________________________________

(209) **3.** ________________________________

C. List four diagnostic tests that are done preoperatively.

(210) **1.** ____________ *(210)* **3.** ____________

(210) **2.** ____________ *(210)* **4.** ____________

D. List the four components of a consent form for surgery.

(212) **1.** ____________ *(212)* **3.** ____________

(212) **2.** ____________ *(212)* **4.** ____________

E. Explain why each of the following classifications of drugs is given preoperatively.

(215) **1.** Opioid: ____________

(215) **2.** Antiemetic: ____________

(215) **3.** Anticholinergic: ____________

F. List three nursing interventions following administration of the preoperative medication.

(217) **1.** ____________

(217) **2.** ____________

(217) **3.** ____________

G. List 3 complications of local anesthesia.

(220) **1.** ____________

(220) **2.** ____________

(220) **3.** ____________

H. List four methods by which general anesthetic agents can be given.

(220) **1.** ____________ *(220)* **3.** ____________

(220) **2.** ____________ *(220)* **4.** ____________

I. List two reasons why there is a risk of shock in the immediate postoperative period.

(221) **1.** ____________

(221) **2.** ____________

Student Name____

J. List four reasons why hypoxia may occur in the immediate postoperative period.

(221) **1.** ______________________________________

(221) **2.** ______________________________________

(221) **3.** ______________________________________

(221) **4.** ______________________________________

K. Match the condition in the numbered column with the effect in the lettered column.

(221) **1.** __________ Spasm of larynx or bronchi

(221) **2.** __________ General anesthesia

(221) **3.** __________ Patient is unconscious

A. Depresses respirations, cough, and swallowing reflex
B. Narrows airway and obstructs air flow
C. Tongue falls back and blocks airway

L. List three classifications of drugs that depress respiratory function and cause pulmonary secretions to be drier and thicker during the postoperative phase.

(223) **1.** ______________________________________

(223) **2.** ______________________________________

(223) **3.** ______________________________________

M. List three complications of wound healing.

(223) **1.** ______________________________________

(223) **2.** ______________________________________

(223) **3.** ______________________________________

N. Match the description in the numbered column with the most appropriate term in the lettered column. Answers may be used more than once.

(223) **1.** __________ Most likely to occur between the 5th and 12th postoperative days

(223) **2.** __________ Protrusion of body organs through the open wound

(223) **3.** __________ Reopening of the surgical wound

(223) **4.** __________ Likely to happen when there is excessive strain on the suture line

A. Dehiscence
B. Evisceration

O. List four factors that may cause peristalsis to be impaired after surgery.

(223) **1.** ______________________________

(223) **2.** ______________________________

(223) **3.** ______________________________

(223) **4.** ______________________________

P. List three causes of urinary retention following surgery.

(224) **1.** ______________________________

(224) **2.** ______________________________

(224) **3.** ______________________________

Q. List three nursing measures to improve oxygenation during the immediate postoperative period.

(224) **1.** ______________________________

(224) **2.** ______________________________

(224) **3.** ______________________________

R. List six criteria that determine when the patient can be moved from the recovery room to the nursing unit.

(225) **1.** ______________________________

(225) **2.** ______________________________

(225) **3.** ______________________________

(225) **4.** ______________________________

(225) **5.** ______________________________

(225) **6.** ______________________________

S. List four safety precautions that should be taken when patients are transferred to their own bed on the nursing unit.

(225) **1.** ______________________________

(225) **2.** ______________________________

(225) **3.** ______________________________

(225) **4.** ______________________________

Student Name ______________________________

T. List three types of surgeries in which coughing is contraindicated.

(232) **1.** ______________________________

(232) **2.** ______________________________

(232) **3.** ______________________________

U. List four measures to prevent thrombophlebitis and related pulmonary emboli.

(232) **1.** ______________________________

(232) **2.** ______________________________

(232) **3.** ______________________________

(232) **4.** ______________________________

V. List four signs and symptoms that would alert the nurse to possible pulmonary emboli.

(232) **1.** ______________________________

(232) **2.** ______________________________

(232) **3.** ______________________________

(232) **4.** ______________________________

W. List four characteristics of paralytic ileus.

(233) **1.** ______________________________

(233) **2.** ______________________________

(233) **3.** ______________________________

(233) **4.** ______________________________

X. List criteria for evaluating the outcomes of nursing goals for the following nursing diagnoses.

(227) **1.** Pain: ______________________________

(227) **2.** Impaired tissue integrity: ______________________________

(227) **3.** Risk for infection: ______________________________

(227) **4.** Impaired gas exchange: ______________________________

(227) **5.** Urinary retention: ______________________________

(227) **6.** Constipation: ______________________________

(227) **7.** Risk for deficient fluid volume: ____________________

(227) **8.** Impaired physical mobility: ____________________

(227) **9.** Disturbed body image: ____________________

Y. Using Figure 16-10, label each method of wound closure (A–F).

(229) **A.** ____________________ *(229)* **D.** ____________________

(229) **B.** ____________________ *(229)* **E.** ____________________

(229) **C.** ____________________ *(229)* **F.** ____________________

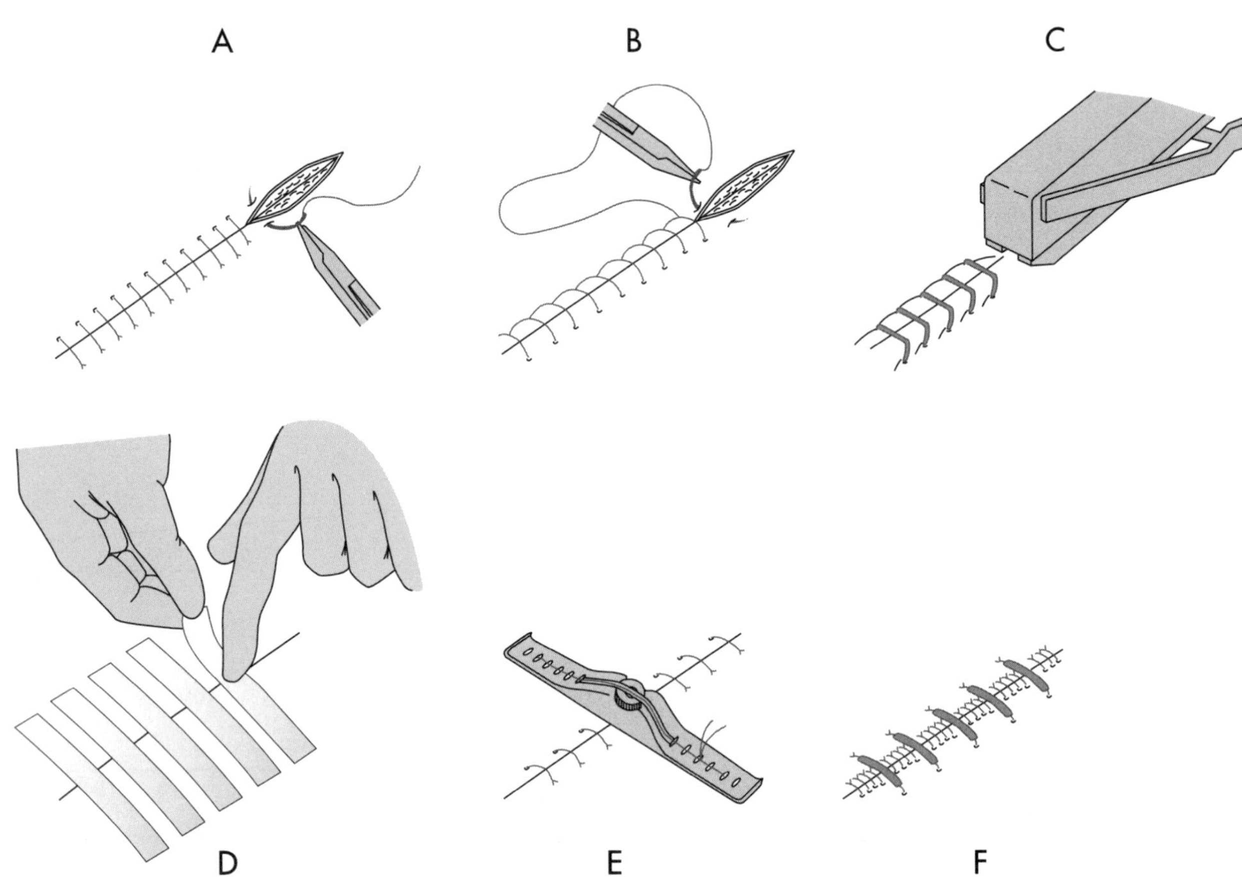

Student Name____

Z. Using Figure 16-9, label each complication of wound healing (A and B).

(223) **A.** ________________________________

(223) **B.** ________________________________

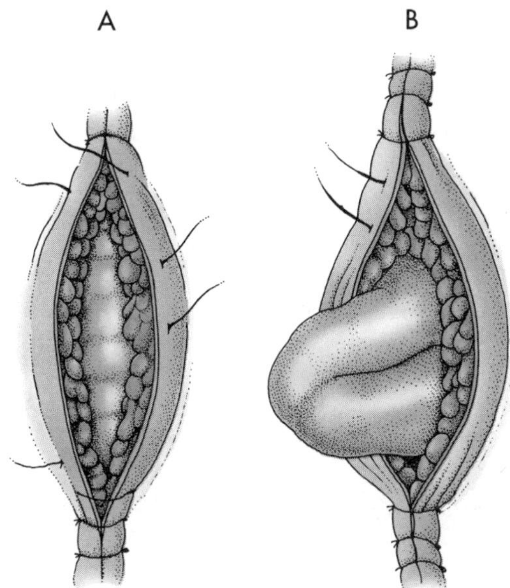

AA. Using Figure 16-8, label each part of the drawing representing inhalation anesthesia given through an endotracheal tube.

(220) **A.** ____________________ *(220)* **E.** ____________________

(220) **B.** ____________________ *(220)* **F.** ____________________

(220) **C.** ____________________ *(220)* **G.** ____________________

(220) **D.** ____________________ *(220)* **H.** ____________________

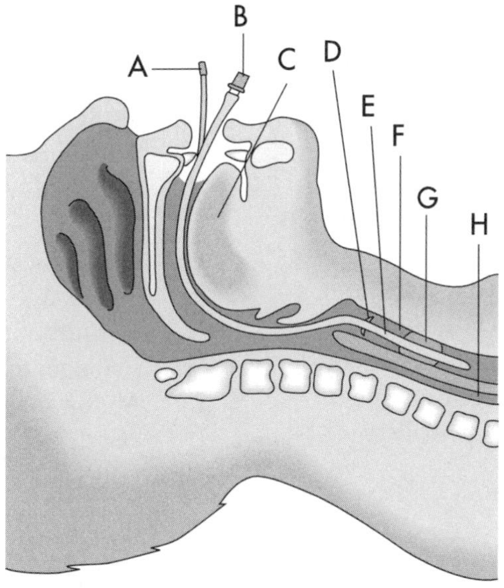

BB. Match the preoperative drug in the numbered column with the most appropriate classification for use with preoperative surgical patients in the lettered column. Some answers may be used more than once.

(215) **1.** __________ Glycopyrrolate (Robinul)

(215) **2.** __________ Chloral hydrate (Noctec)

(215) **3.** __________ Promethazine hydrochloride (Phenergan)

(215) **4.** __________ Pentobarbital sodium (Nembutal Sodium)

(215) **5.** __________ Diazepam (Valium)

(215) **6.** __________ Atropine sulfate

(215) **7.** __________ Meperidine hydrochloride (Demerol HCl)

(215) **8.** __________ Secobarbital sodium (Seconal Sodium)

(215) **9.** __________ Morphine sulfate (MS Contin, Duramorph)

A. Tranquilizer
B. Analgesic
C. Anticholinergic
D. Sedative or hypnotic
E. Antiemetic
F. Skeletal muscle relaxant

CC. Match the treatment in the numbered column with the complication it is used for in the lettered column. Some complications may be used more than once, and some treatments may match more than one complication.

(222) **1.** __________ Administer oxygen

(222) **2.** __________ Pour warm water over perineum

(222) **3.** __________ Give intravenous (IV) fluids as ordered; encourage oral intake when allowed

A. Fluid and electrolyte imbalances
B. Altered elimination
C. Impaired wound healing
D. Shock
E. Nausea and vomiting
F. Hypoxia
G. Thrombophlebitis
H. Inadequate oxygenation
I. Abdominal distention
J. “Gas” pains/constipation

Continued next page

Student Name ____

(222) **4.** __________ Ambulate frequently when permitted; laxatives or enemas, or both, as ordered

(222) **5.** __________ Vasopressors (drugs to raise blood pressure) as ordered

(222) **6.** __________ Position to promote effective ventilation

(222) **7.** __________ Cover the open wound with a sterile dressing; if organs protrude, saturate the dressing with normal saline, notify physician, and keep patient still and quiet

(222) **8.** __________ Antiemetic drugs as ordered

(222) **9.** __________ Encourage deep breathing and coughing

(222) **10.** __________ Bed rest; anticoagulant therapy as ordered

(222) **11.** __________ Rectal tube, heat to abdomen, bisacodyl suppositories as ordered; position on right side; nasogastric intubation with suction as ordered

(222) **12.** __________ Fluid or blood replacement

(222) **13.** __________ Rest; oxygen and antibiotics as ordered

(222) **14.** __________ Additional surgery to control bleeding

(222) **15.** __________ Suction as necessary

MULTIPLE-CHOICE QUESTIONS

DD. Choose the most appropriate answer.

(208) **1.** The surgical patient who is malnourished is at risk for:

1. excessive bleeding and hemorrhage.
2. drug toxicity and ineffective metabolism.
3. cardiac complications and dyspnea.
4. poor wound healing and infection.

(208) **2.** Obese surgical patients are more likely to have postoperative:

1. infection and increased temperature.
2. excessive bleeding and hemorrhage.
3. headache and bradycardia.
4. respiratory and wound healing complications.

(208) **3.** Excess body fluid in the surgical patient can overload the:

1. brain.
2. heart.
3. muscles.
4. lungs.

(208) **4.** Electrolyte imbalances may predispose the surgical patient to:

1. cardiac arrhythmias.
2. lung complications.
3. liver malfunction.
4. bone tissue loss.

(212) **5.** Before surgery, a patient must sign a legal document called a(n):

1. bill of rights.
2. consent form.
3. advance directive.
4. living will.

(212) **6.** If the patient is a minor, who signs the surgical consent form?

1. physician
2. registered nurse
3. parent or guardian
4. close relative

(215) **7.** Shaving the skin in preparation for surgery is often delayed until shortly before surgery in order to:

1. improve wound healing.
2. control bleeding.
3. allow less time for organisms to multiply.
4. prevent postoperative edema.

(217) **8.** The use of local anesthetics that block the conduction of nerve impulses in a specific area is called:

1. general anesthesia.
2. sedative anesthesia.
3. anticonvulsant anesthesia.
4. regional anesthesia.

(219) **9.** The injection of an anesthetic agent into and under the skin around the area of treatment is called:

1. local infiltration.
2. topical administration.
3. nerve block technique.
4. intravenous infusion.

(219) **10.** One complication of spinal anesthesia is:

1. tachycardia.
2. hemorrhage.
3. headache.
4. shock.

(219) **11.** Postspinal headache can be relieved by:

1. elevating the head of the bed.
2. lying flat.
3. early ambulation.
4. coughing and deep breathing.

(219) **12.** A "blood patch" may help treat:

1. hemorrhage.
2. postspinal headache.
3. shock.
4. tachycardia.

(220) **13.** Which of the following adverse effects of anesthetic agents may be reduced by giving preanesthetic medications?

1. tachycardia
2. dry mouth
3. urinary retention
4. vomiting

(220) **14.** Inhalation anesthetic agents and the endotracheal tube can cause irritation of the:

1. lungs.
2. heart.
3. kidney.
4. larynx.

Student Name ________________

(220) **15.** A life-threatening complication of inhalation anesthesia characterized by increasing body temperature and metabolic rate, tachycardia, hypotension, cyanosis, and muscle rigidity is called:

1. anaphylactic shock.
2. malignant hyperthermia.
3. hypotensive shock.
4. hyperglycemia.

(229) **16.** The patient develops rupture of the suture line and states: "My incision is breaking open." Which of the following actions should the nurse take to prevent complications in this patient?

1. Keep the patient in bed.
2. Administer opioid analgesics as ordered.
3. Have the patient cough and deep-breathe every 2 hours.
4. Auscultate breath sounds.

(231) **17.** An infection of the lungs due to immobility is called:

1. hypovolemic pleurisy.
2. atelectasis.
3. hypostatic pneumonia.
4. emphysema.

(233) **18.** When peristalsis is slow, gas builds up, causing:

1. abdominal cramping and distention.
2. diarrhea and tachycardia.
3. fever and infection.
4. nausea and vomiting.

(223) **19.** "Gas pains" typically occur:

1. during surgery.
2. immediately after surgery.
3. 6 hours after surgery.
4. on second or third day after surgery.

(223) **20.** With urinary retention, the kidneys:

1. produce no urine and the patient is unable to empty the bladder.
2. produce urine and the patient is able to empty the bladder.
3. produce no urine and the patient is able to empty the bladder.
4. produce urine but the patient is unable to empty the bladder.

(224) **21.** The inflammation of veins with the formation of blood clots is:

1. hemorrhage.
2. shock.
3. thrombophlebitis.
4. pericarditis.

(224) **22.** Clots that cling to the walls of blood vessels are called:

1. emboli.
2. platelets.
3. thrombi.
4. anticoagulants.

(227) **23.** An outcome criterion related to absence of thrombophlebitis is:

1. adequate oxygenation.
2. normal arterial blood gases.
3. negative Homans' sign.
4. normal wound healing.

(224) **24.** If intravenous fluids are given too rapidly postoperatively, they can overload the circulatory system, causing:

1. lung failure.
2. heart failure.
3. brain failure.
4. kidney failure.

(224) **25.** What is used to monitor the oxygenation of the blood?

1. sphygmomanometer
2. incentive spirometer
3. oximeter
4. stethoscope

(225) **26.** When regional block anesthesia is used during surgery, the nurse must remember that after surgery:

1. sensation in the area is impaired.
2. circulation in the area is impaired.
3. infection is likely to occur.
4. fever may make the patient drowsy.

(224) **27.** Once the immediate postoperative phase has passed, which risks lessen?

1. fever and infection
2. pneumonia and atelectasis
3. shock and hemorrhage
4. thrombophlebitis and decubitus ulcer

(228) **28.** Two common narcotic analgesics that are given postoperatively are:

1. acetaminophen and aspirin.
2. meperidine and morphine.
3. codeine and tincture of opium.
4. alprazolam and diazepam.

(228) **29.** Clean sutured incisions heal by:

1. first intention.
2. second intention.
3. third intention.
4. fourth intention.

(229) **30.** After the first 24 hours following surgery, which finding should be reported to the physician if it is observed?

1. respirations of 20 bpm
2. temperature of 98.8° F
3. blood pressure of 110/70 mm Hg
4. continued or excessive bleeding

(229) **31.** A soft tube that permits passive movement of fluids from the wound is called a(n):

1. active drain
2. Hemovac
3. Penrose drain
4. Jackson-Pratt drain

(229) **32.** In the immediate postoperative phase, wound drainage is often bright red; as the amount of blood in the drainage decreases, the fluid becomes:

1. straw-colored and then clear and pink.
2. clear and then pink and straw-colored.
3. pink and then clear and straw-colored.
4. pink and then straw-colored and clear.

(229) **33.** What may precede wound dehiscence? A sudden:

1. decrease in wound drainage.
2. increase in wound drainage.
3. increase in temperature.
4. increase of purulent drainage.

(229) **34.** If evisceration occurs, the usual practice is to cover the wound with:

1. dry sterile dressings.
2. saline-soaked gauze with a dry dressing over it.
3. antibiotic ointment and dry dressings.
4. steroid ointment and dry dressings.

Student Name____

(230) **35.** Signs and symptoms of wound infection usually do not develop until:

1. the first hour after surgery.
2. 12 hours after surgery.
3. the first and second days after surgery.
4. the third to fifth day after surgery.

(230) **36.** A postoperative patient complains of pain, fever, swelling, and purulent drainage. These signs and symptoms are indications of:

1. thrombophlebitis.
2. evisceration.
3. dehiscence.
4. wound infection.

(230) **37.** Which finding in a postoperative patient should be reported to the physician?

1. redness that spreads to the surrounding area
2. redness at the wound suture site
3. low-grade fever
4. serosanguineous drainage

(230) **38.** To prevent pneumonia, the patient must be assisted to turn initially every:

1. 5 minutes. 2. 15 minutes.
3. 2 hours. 4. 6 hours.

(231) **39.** A device used to promote lung expansion postoperatively is the:

1. Penrose drain.
2. sphygmomanometer.
3. inhaler.
4. incentive spirometer.

(232) **40.** Pulmonary emboli usually originate from thrombi that develop in veins of the:

1. chest.
2. arms and shoulders.
3. legs and pelvis.
4. abdomen.

(232) **41.** Emboli may be treated with:

1. phenytoin (Dilantin) and anticonvulsants.
2. morphine and analgesics.
3. heparin and thrombolytic agents.
4. furosemide (Lasix) and diuretics.

(232) **42.** Catheterization is usually done postoperatively if the patient does not void in:

1. 2 hours. 2. 4 hours.
3. 8 hours. 4. 10 hours.

(232) **43.** When a patient passes small amounts of urine frequently without feeling relief of fullness, this indicates:

1. retention with overflow.
2. stress incontinence.
3. urge incontinence.
4. kidney failure.

(232) **44.** Some agencies have policies that limit the amount of urine that can be drained from a full bladder at one time; these limits are usually:

1. 5–10 ml.
2. 50–100 ml.
3. 400–500 ml.
4. 750–1000 ml.

(233) **45.** Most patients pass flatus:

1. 15 minutes after surgery.
2. 1 hour after surgery.
3. 48 hours after surgery.
4. 1 week after surgery.

(233) **46.** The best way to prevent gastrointestinal discomfort postoperatively is:

1. administration of antacids.
2. early, frequent ambulation.
3. administration of laxatives.
4. early, frequent meals.

(229) **47.** Which surgical drain works by creating negative pressure when the receptacle is compressed?

1. Penrose
2. urinary
3. Hemovac
4. passive

(220) **48.** Which drug supplements the effects of local anesthetics?

1. propranolol (Inderal)
2. atropine
3. morphine
4. epinephrine

(230) **49.** A week after surgery, the patient develops pain, fever, swelling, and purulent drainage around the wound site. Which of the following actions should the nurse take to prevent complications?

1. keeping the patient in bed
2. early, frequent ambulation
3. monitoring intake and output
4. good hand washing

(229) **50.** A patient states that his wound feels as if it is "pulling apart." This is an indication of:

1. healing by first intention.
2. dehiscence.
3. evisceration.
4. singultus.

(222) **51.** One way to prevent shock as a surgical complication is to:

1. keep airway in place until patient is alert.
2. splint incision during activity.
3. keep IV fluid rate on schedule.
4. change patient's position at least every 3 hours.

(216) **52.** Which of the following postoperative drugs causes urinary retention?

1. antibiotics
2. thrombolytics
3. opioid analgesics
4. anticoagulants

(221) **53.** The use of IV drugs to reduce pain intensity or awareness without loss of reflexes is called:

1. regional anesthesia.
2. conscious sedation.
3. general anesthesia.
4. balanced anesthesia.

(220, 221) **54.** Which is a commonly used IV drug for conscious sedation?

1. succinylcholine
2. isoflurane
3. nitrous oxide
4. midazolam (Versed)

(220) **55.** Which drug is often given along with a general anesthetic agent to prevent movement of muscles?

1. midazolam (Versed)
2. succinylcholine
3. ketamine hydrochloride (Ketalar)
4. thiopental sodium (Pentothal)

(220) **56.** Enflurane (Ethrane) and nitrous oxide are administered by:

1. inhalation.
2. IV infusion.
3. intramuscular (IM) injection.
4. rectal insertion.

CHAPTER 17

Student Name ___________________________________

Intravenous Therapy

Answer Key: Textbook page references are provided as a guide for answering these questions. A complete answer key was provided for your instructor.

OBJECTIVES

1. List the indications for intravenous fluid therapy.
2. Describe the types of fluids used for intravenous fluid therapy.
3. Describe the types of venous access devices and other equipment used for intravenous therapy.
4. Given the prescribed hourly flow rate, calculate the correct drop rate for an intravenous fluid.
5. Explain the causes, signs and symptoms, and nursing implications of the complications of intravenous fluid or drug therapy.
6. Explain the nursing responsibilities when a patient is receiving intravenous therapy.

LEARNING ACTIVITIES

A. Match the definition in the numbered column with the most appropriate term in the lettered column.

(237) **1.** __________ A liquid containing one or more dissolved substances

(237) **2.** __________ A term used to describe a solution that has a higher concentration of electrolytes than normal body fluids

A. Hypotonic
B. Cannula
C. Solution
D. Hypertonic
E. Extravasation
F. Isotonic
G. Tonicity

Continued next page

(237) **3.** __________ A term used to describe a solution that has the same concentration of electrolytes as normal body fluids

(237) **4.** __________ A term used to describe a solution that has a lower concentration of electrolytes than normal body fluids

(237) **5.** __________ A measure of the concentration of electrolytes in a fluid

(246) **6.** __________ Escape of fluid or blood from a blood vessel into body tissue

B. Match the definition or description in the numbered column with the most appropriate term in the lettered column.

(239) **1.** __________ Used for single-dose therapy, therapy of short duration, for infants and for adults with poor veins

(238) **2.** __________ Hickman-Broviac catheters inserted by physicians

(239) **3.** __________ Small plastic tubes that fit over or inside needles

(238) **4.** __________ Needles and catheters

(240) **5.** __________ Inserted in antecubital space and advanced into the axillary subclavian vein or superior vena cava

A. Catheters
B. Winged infusion needle
C. Central venous tunneled catheters
D. Cannulas
E. Peripherally inserted central catheters

Student Name______________________________

C. Match the definition or description in the numbered column with the most appropriate term in the lettered column.

(243, 244)	**1.**	________	Maintain infusion rate set by nurses; saves time and prevents accidental delivery of large amounts of fluid	A.	Piggyback infusion
				B.	Electronic infusion pump
				C.	Heparin lock (saline lock)
				D.	Infusion port
(240)	**2.**	________	Implanted under skin; allows immediate access to vein without repeated venipunctures		
(241)	**3.**	________	Short cannula with attached injection port; usually flushed with dilute heparin or saline solution		
(241)	**4.**	________	Catheter and a chamber into which fluids are directly injected into vein or artery		

D. Match the definition or description in the numbered column with the most appropriate term in the lettered column.

(246)	**1.**	________	Leakage of fluid from a blood vessel	A.	Thrombus
				B.	Embolism
				C.	Infiltration
				D.	Catheter embolus
(247)	**2.**	________	Piece of catheter breaks off in vein	E.	Embolus
				F.	Trauma
				G.	Phlebitis
(246)	**3.**	________	Skin torn or irritated by tape or insertion of cannula	H.	Extravasation
(247)	**4.**	________	Attached blood clot		
(247)	**5.**	________	Obstruction caused by trapped embolus		

Continued next page

(246) **6.** __________ Collection of infused fluid in tissue surrounding the cannula

(247) **7.** __________ Unattached blood clot

(246) **8.** __________ Inflammation of the vein

E. Match the outcome criteria in the numbered column with the nursing diagnoses in the lettered column.

(246) **1.** __________ Pulse and blood pressure within normal limits

(246) **2.** __________ Patient activities completed without disruption of intravenous therapy

(246) **3.** __________ Normal body temperature; no purulent drainage or redness at venipuncture site

(246) **4.** __________ Fluid output equal to intake; no dyspnea or edema

A. Decreased cardiac output related to blood loss through disrupted intravenous line
B. Self-care deficit related to restricted movement of infusion site
C. Fluid volume excess related to rapid fluid infusion
D. Risk for infection related to disruption of skin integrity

MULTIPLE-CHOICE QUESTIONS

F. Choose the most appropriate answer.

(237) **1.** Tonicity of IV fluid is important because it affects:

1. acid-base balance.
2. blood volume.
3. buffer action.
4. electrolytes.

(247) **2.** Irrigation of an occluded IV cannula is not recommended because:

1. the IV cannula may become infiltrated.
2. clots may be forced into the bloodstream.
3. the IV cannula may become dislodged.
4. thrombophlebitis may occur.

Student Name____

(237) **3.** Normal saline is:

1. 0.25% sodium chloride.
2. 0.45% sodium chloride.
3. 0.9% sodium chloride.
4. 1.5% sodium chloride.

(237) **4.** An IV solution of 0.45% sodium chloride is:

1. hypertonic. 2. isotonic.
3. hypotonic. 4. equivalent.

(237) **5.** An IV solution of 0.45% sodium chloride is given if the patient has experienced:

1. excessive water loss.
2. cerebral edema.
3. excessive sodium loss.
4. burns.

(247) **6.** In which position should you place a patient if air accidentally enters a central line?

1. on the right side
2. on the left side
3. semi-Fowler's
4. Fowler's

(240) **7.** Advantages of peripherally inserted central catheters (PICCs) over other central catheters include:

1. smaller needle, cost savings, and reduced risk of pneumothorax or air embolism.
2. easier insertion, less expense, and reduced risk of infection.
3. remaining in place longer, fewer dressing changes, and no risk of dislodgment.
4. easier insertion, cost savings, and reduced risk of pneumothorax or air embolism.

(244) **8.** Short peripheral cannulas and tubing are usually changed every:

1. 1–2 hours.
2. 4–8 hours.
3. 12–24 hours.
4. 48–72 hours.

(242) **9.** You notice that the IV on your patient is running in too fast. To slow the rate down, you:

1. vent the IV container.
2. splint the arm with an armboard.
3. turn the arm so that the IV site is free.
4. lower the fluid container.

(242) **10.** In order to calculate the IV infusion rate, you must know the:

1. ordered fluid volume per hour and number of drops equal to 1 ml in the tubing set.
2. number of milliliters of fluid in a solution container.
3. ordered fluid volume minus the urine output.
4. ordered fluid volume and the prior 24 hours' IV intake.

(247) **11.** Symptoms of an air embolus include:

1. pulmonary edema; frothy, pink sputum; and a feeling of doom.
2. chest pain, diminished respirations, and lethargy.
3. shortness of breath, hypotension, and possibly shock and cardiac arrest.
4. nausea, vomiting and diarrhea, hepatomegaly, and pink sputum.

(246) **12.** Edema, coolness, and pain at the IV insertion site are indications of:

1. thrombophlebitis.
2. infection.
3. air embolus.
4. infiltration.

(246) **13.** Which IV complication is characterized by redness, swelling, and warmth?

1. phlebitis
2. infiltration
3. hemorrhage
4. catheter embolus

(247) **14.** Signs of fluid volume excess include:

1. confusion.
2. bounding pulse.
3. inflammation.
4. redness.

(247) **15.** If signs of fluid volume excess occur, you should:

1. turn the patient to the right side.
2. elevate the head of the bed.
3. check the vital signs.
4. lower the head of the bed.

(247) **16.** The patient with an air embolus is placed on the left side to trap air:

1. in the left atrium so that it can be gradually absorbed.
2. in the right ventricle so that it is not transferred to the lungs.
3. in the left ventricle so that it is not transferred to the lungs.
4. in the right atrium so that it can be gradually absorbed.

(247) **17.** When a central catheter is inserted or removed, the patient is instructed to:

1. take a deep breath and hold it for 30 seconds.
2. take a deep breath and bear down.
3. breathe normally.
4. take a normal breath and hold it for 30 seconds.

(247) **18.** When a central catheter is inserted or removed, the patient is asked to take a deep breath and bear down in order to help:

1. prevent air from entering the lungs.
2. prevent air from entering the bloodstream.
3. air enter the bloodstream.
4. air enter the lungs.

(246) **19.** Outcome criteria for evaluating the nursing care of a patient with an IV include the *absence* of:

1. palpitations and pain and redness at the infusion site.
2. blood return and swelling and pain at the infusion site.
3. edema, pallor, redness, and drainage at the infusion site.
4. movement, erythema, and firmness at the infusion site.

(247) **20.** As you are making your morning rounds at 7:00 AM, you note that your patient's IV has 900 ml and is running at 75 ml/hour as ordered. When you check the IV on your 10:00 AM rounds, you note that there is only 100 ml remaining. Which signs and symptoms do you need to be alert for with this patient?

1. flushing of the face
2. nausea and vomiting
3. puffy eyelids
4. diarrhea

Student Name____

(247) **21.** Which nursing intervention may prevent fluid volume excess during IV therapy?

1. Encourage the patient to ambulate.
2. Encourage the patient to cough.
3. Time-tape the IV bag and monitor closely.
4. Keep an accurate intake and output record.

(247) **22.** Your patient complains of crushing chest pain and difficulty breathing and has a rapid, thready pulse. You suspect that he is experiencing an air embolism. Which interventions are appropriate?

1. Turn the patient onto his left side, raise the head of the bed, and notify the charge nurse or physician.
2. Turn the patient onto his left side, lower the head of the bed, and notify the charge nurse or physician.
3. Place the patient on his back, lower the head of the bed, and notify the charge nurse.
4. Ambulate the patient for 15 minutes and notify the charge nurse.

(246) **23.** The hand in which an IV is infusing is puffy and cool. This is a sign of:

1. phlebitis.
2. infection.
3. infiltration.
4. air embolus.

(246) **24.** When the IV line has infiltrated, nursing interventions are as follows.

1. Discontinue IV, apply ice, and place area lower than the heart.
2. Slow down the IV rate, apply ice, and elevate affected arm.
3. Discontinue IV and restart in a different vein; elevate affected arm.
4. Slow down the IV rate, apply warm compresses, and place the area lower than the heart.

(246) **25.** You check your patient's IV site and find that her vein is cordlike. The IV is running well, but the site is red; the patient tells you that the site is "sore when touched." These are signs of:

1. infiltration.
2. catheter embolus.
3. air embolus.
4. phlebitis.

(243) **26.** What does a "drop factor of 15" mean?

1. The infusion set will deliver 15 ml of fluid for every drop.
2. The infusion set will deliver 1 ml of fluid for every 15 drops.
3. The infusion set will deliver 1 ml of fluid in 15 minutes.
4. The infusion set will deliver 15 ml of fluid in 1 minute.

(242) **27.** You checked the patient's IV 1 hour ago, and it was running at the correct rate of 50 ml/hour. Now you find that the IV is running at 100 ml/hour. What may be the cause of this increased rate?

1. The tubing has a kink in it.
2. The clamp has slipped.
3. The fluid container is too low.
4. The filter is blocked.

(247) **28.** How much air does it take to cause an air embolism in an adult?

1. 5 cc
2. 10 cc
3. 15 cc
4. 25 cc

(244) **29.** An IV fluid container should not be used for more than:

1. 12 hours.
2. 24 hours.
3. 48 hours.
4. 72 hours.

(245) **30.** Because older people often have less efficient cardiac function, you should monitor an older person with an IV for:

1. fluid volume excess.
2. bleeding.
3. infection.
4. infiltration.

(247) **31.** A cannula with a clot in it should not be irrigated because it could cause:

1. extravasation.
2. infiltration.
3. air embolism.
4. pulmonary embolism.

(237) **32.** Administering a hypertonic IV solution causes fluid to be pulled from:

1. blood into the cells.
2. cells into the blood.
3. cells into interstitial tissue.
4. blood into interstitial tissue.

(246) **33.** An elderly patient is receiving IV fluids to treat dehydration. When he complains of pain and a burning sensation at the IV site, your assessment reveals that the IV site is pale, puffy, and cool. Which complication do you suspect?

1. phlebitis
2. infiltration
3. fluid volume excess
4. embolism

(238) **34.** Which vein is usually used for administering solutions through a central vein?

1. subclavian vein
2. brachial vein
3. femoral vein
4. pulmonary vein

(247) **35.** Your patient is an 80-year-old male with a history of high blood pressure. When you come in to give him a bath, you notice that his IV of 5% D/W, which was hung 1 hour before you came into his room, contains 500 ml. 1000 ml was ordered to run in over 8 hours. You should observe him for signs of:

1. infection.
2. shock.
3. hemorrhage.
4. heart failure.

(237) **36.** Hypertonic IV solutions should be used cautiously in patients with:

1. renal disease.
2. burns.
3. cancer.
4. GI disease.

CHAPTER 18

Student Name ____________________

Shock

Answer Key: Textbook page references are provided as a guide for answering these questions. A complete answer key was provided for your instructor.

OBJECTIVES

1. List the types of shock.
2. Describe the pathophysiology of each type of shock.
3. List the signs and symptoms of each stage of shock.
4. Explain the first aid emergency treatment of shock outside the medical facility.
5. Identify general medical and nursing interventions for shock.
6. Explain the rationale for medical/surgical treatment of shock.
7. Assist in developing care plans for patients in each type of shock.

LEARNING ACTIVITIES

A. Match the definition in the numbered column with the correct term in the lettered column.

(257) **1.** ________ Presence of SIRS with a confirmed infection

(257) **2.** ________ Generalized inflammatory condition that follows serious physiologic threat; characterized by damage to vascular endothelium and hypermetabolic state

(251) **3.** ________ Deficiency of blood flow

A. Ischemia
B. Metabolic acidosis
C. Multiple organ dysfunction syndrome (MODS)
D. Sepsis
E. Shock
F. Systemic inflammatory response syndrome (SIRS)

Continued next page

(257) **4.** __________ Failure of more than one organ as a result of SIRS

(249) **5.** __________ A state of acute circulatory failure and impaired tissue perfusion

(250, 253) **6.** __________ A pathologic condition associated with an increase in acid relative to bicarbonate content; increased hydrogen ion concentration

B. Match the description in the numbered column with the type of shock in the lettered column.

A. Hypovolemic
B. Cardiogenic
C. Distributive

(249) **1.** __________ Caused by hemorrhage, severe diarrhea or vomiting, and excessive perspiration

(249) **2.** __________ Complicated by increased capillary permeability

(249) **3.** __________ Includes classification of obstructive shock

(249) **4.** __________ Associated with pulmonary embolism and tension pneumothorax

(249) **5.** __________ Occurs when the circulating blood volume is inadequate to maintain the supply of oxygen and nutrients to tissue

(249) **6.** __________ Fluid pools in dependent areas of the body

(249) **7.** __________ Related to excessive blood or fluid loss, inadequate fluid intake, or a shift of plasma from blood into body tissues

Continued next page

Student Name ______________________

(249) **8.** __________ Occurs when heart fails as a pump

(249) **9.** __________ Problem is with excessive dilation of blood vessels

(249) **10.** __________ Related to burns, peritonitis, and intestinal obstruction

(249) **11.** __________ Associated with congestive heart failure (CHF), acute myocardial infarction (MI), and heart rhythm disturbances

C. Match the classification of drugs in the numbered column with the type of shock treated by the drugs in the lettered column.

(254) **1.** __________ Bronchodilators

(254) **2.** __________ Low-dose inotropics

(254) **3.** __________ Thrombolytics

(254) **4.** __________ Antidysrhythmics

(254) **5.** __________ Corticosteroids

(254) **6.** __________ H_1 blockers

(254) **7.** __________ Inotropics

(254) **8.** __________ Vasopressors

(254) **9.** __________ Epinephrine and theophylline

(254) **10.** __________ Anticoagulants

A. Cardiogenic shock
B. Hypovolemic shock
C. Anaphylactic shock

MULTIPLE-CHOICE QUESTIONS

D. Choose the most appropriate answer.

(249) **1.** Anaphylactic, septic, and neurogenic are examples of which types of shock?

1. hypovolemic
2. cardiogenic
3. obstructive
4. distributive

(249) **2.** Following an automobile accident, a 35-year-old man experienced severe hemorrhage. This type of shock is classified as:

1. hypovolemic.
2. cardiogenic.
3. obstructive.
4. distributive.

(249) **3.** A woman experiences burns over 80% of her body. You suspect she has:

1. hypovolemic shock.
2. cardiogenic shock.
3. obstructive shock.
4. distributive shock.

(249) **4.** Inadequate tissue perfusion deprives cells of essential oxygen, forcing cells to rely on:

1. anabolic metabolism.
2. catabolic metabolism.
3. aerobic metabolism.
4. anaerobic metabolism.

(250) **5.** A person has a severe allergic reaction that results in bronchoconstriction and increased capillary permeability. This type of shock is:

1. anaphylactic.
2. cardiogenic.
3. hypovolemic.
4. septic.

(250) **6.** Which type of shock occurs suddenly, following exposure to a substance for which the patient had already developed antibodies?

1. neurogenic
2. septic
3. anaphylactic
4. cardiogenic

(250) **7.** Following a spinal cord injury, a 24-year-old man develops hypotension and bradycardia. This type of shock is:

1. hypovolemic.
2. septic.
3. anaphylactic.
4. neurogenic.

(250) **8.** The body of a patient with neurogenic shock is unable to compensate with vasoconstriction because:

1. the vasomotor center is incapacitated.
2. chemicals released as a result of tissue ischemia depress the myocardium.
3. bronchoconstriction and airway obstruction occur.
4. systemic inflammatory response syndrome occurs.

(250) **9.** One of the effects of shock on the neuroendocrine system is:

1. release of catecholamines.
2. decreased ADH.
3. increased cerebral blood flow.
4. decreased aldosterone.

(250) **10.** One of the effects of shock on the respiratory system is:

1. metabolic alkalosis.
2. tissue hypoxia.
3. depressed immune system.
4. bronchodilation.

(250) **11.** Assessment findings in the compensatory stage are likely to include:

1. drowsiness.
2. slightly increased blood pressure.
3. increased blood glucose.
4. increased bowel sounds.

(250) **12.** The stage of shock during which cells resort to anaerobic metabolism producing lactic acid is called:

1. compensatory.
2. progressive.
3. irreversible.
4. refractory.

Student Name ____________________

(251) **13.** Which assessment data would you expect to find in a patient in the progressive stage of shock?

1. increased pulse pressure
2. weak, thready pulse
3. warm, flushed skin
4. increased blood pressure

(251) **14.** The stage of shock in which death is imminent is known as:

1. compensatory.
2. refractory.
3. progressive.
4. hypovolemic.

(251) **15.** Assessment data in the irreversible stage of shock include:

1. loss of consciousness.
2. a drop in diastolic blood pressure to 50.
3. rapid, shallow respirations.
4. warm, flushed skin.

(251) **16.** A priority in shock treatment is to:

1. correct acid-base balances.
2. manage cardiac dysrhythmias.
3. administer antishock drugs.
4. improve blood flow and oxygen supply to vital organs.

(252) **17.** Which position is best to maintain blood flow to vital organs for a patient with hypovolemic shock?

1. supine with head lowered.
2. Fowler's.
3. supine with legs elevated 45 degrees.
4. left side-lying.

(252) **18.** The purpose of giving blood and fluids to improve cardiac output in a patient with cardiogenic shock is to:

1. promote delivery of oxygen to cells.
2. correct acid-base imbalances.
3. improve fluid and electrolyte imbalances.
4. decrease the incidence of infection.

(252) **19.** Which type of shock does *not* have replacement of fluid as a priority?

1. distributive
2. neurogenic
3. hypovolemic
4. cardiogenic

(253) **20.** Sodium bicarbonate and mechanical ventilation are used to promote:

1. acid-base imbalances.
2. fluid replacement.
3. oxygen perfusion.
4. cardiac output.

(249) **21.** Which patient condition is likely to have a history of severe vomiting and diarrhea?

1. hypovolemic shock
2. cardiogenic shock
3. distributive shock
4. progressive shock

(254) **22.** For which type of shock are antimicrobials prescribed?

1. hypovolemic
2. cardiogenic
3. distributive
4. septic

(254) **23.** Why is atropine prescribed for neurogenic shock?

1. raise heart rate
2. raise blood pressure
3. treat pain
4. dilate blood vessels

(251) **24.** Why is improving blood flow and oxygen supply to the vital organs a priority in shock treatment?

1. Brain cells begin to die after 4 minutes without oxygen.
2. Cells resort to anaerobic metabolism, producing lactic acid immediately.
3. Acidosis has a depressant effect on myocardial cells.
4. If compensatory mechanisms are effective, the blood pressure will remain normal.

(252) **25.** Why is Trendelenburg's (head down) position *not* recommended for shock treatment?

1. It can stimulate respirations and filling of coronary arteries.
2. It can impair cerebral blood flow and increase intracranial pressure.
3. It can cause fluid overload.
4. It can lead to metabolic acidosis.

(254) **26.** For which type of shock are inotropic and antidysrhythmic agents ordered?

1. neurogenic
2. distributive
3. cardiogenic
4. anaphylactic

(256) **27.** A patient in shock has a pulse of 120, BP of 80/40, and respirations 28. These signs represent:

1. deficient fluid volume.
2. ineffective tissue perfusion.
3. decreased cardiac output.
4. electrolyte imbalance.

(257) **28.** Hypermetabolism in shock causes which type of malnutrition?

1. decreased carbohydrate
2. decreased glucose
3. decreased protein
4. increased nitrogen

(251) **29.** Which assessment finding would you expect to see in a patient with septic shock that would not be present in a patient with hypovolemic shock?

1. cool skin
2. fever
3. low blood pressure
4. dizziness

(250) **30.** A patient with a wound infection is likely to develop which type of shock?

1. hypovolemic
2. cardiogenic
3. septic
4. neurogenic

CHAPTER 19

Student Name ______________________________

Falls

Answer Key: Textbook page references are provided as a guide for answering these questions. A complete answer key was provided for your instructor.

OBJECTIVES

1. Define falls.
2. Give the incidence of falls.
3. Describe factors that increase the risk of falls.
4. Discuss the relationship between restraint use and falls, types of restraints, and regulations for restraint use.
5. Describe fall prevention techniques.
6. Describe nursing interventions to use when a fall occurs.

LEARNING ACTIVITIES

A. Match the definition in the numbered column with the most appropriate term in the lettered column.

(261) **1.** __________ Anything that restricts movement

(260) **2.** __________ Circumstance in which one unintentionally falls to the ground or hits an object such as a chair or stair

(260) **3.** __________ Factors related to the internal functioning of an individual, such as the aging process or physical illness, that can cause falls

A. Chemical restraints
B. Extrinsic factors
C. Fall
D. Omnibus Reconciliation Act (OBRA)
E. Physical restraint
F. Intrinsic factors

Continued next page

(260) **4.** ______ Psychotropic medication given to subdue agitated or confused patients

(262) **5.** ______ Law enacted in 1987 to protect patients from unnecessary restraints in nursing homes

(260) **6.** ______ Factors in the environment that can cause falls

B. List seven factors associated with people at greatest risk for injury from falls.

(261) **1.** ______

(261) **2.** ______

(261) **3.** ______

(261) **4.** ______

(261) **5.** ______

(261) **6.** ______

(261) **7.** ______

C. List nine damaging psychological effects of restraints on older patients.

(262) **1.** ______

(262) **2.** ______

(262) **3.** ______

(262) **4.** ______

(262) **5.** ______

(262) **6.** ______

(262) **7.** ______

(262) **8.** ______

(262) **9.** ______

Student Name____

D. Match each risk factor in the numbered column with the most appropriate intervention in the lettered column.

(263) **1.** __________ Musculoskeletal disorders

(263) **2.** __________ Impaired adaptation to the dark

(263) **3.** __________ Balance disorders

(263) **4.** __________ Stroke

(263) **5.** __________ Reduced visual acuity

(263) **6.** __________ Postural hypotension

(263) **7.** __________ Impacted cerumen (earwax)

(263) **8.** __________ Peripheral neuropathy

(263) **9.** __________ Impaired color perception

(263) **10.** __________ Foot disorders

(263) **11.** __________ Presbycusis

A. Maintain adequate lighting; reduce glare from shiny floors and allow time for eyes to adjust to light levels (e.g., from a dark room to outside); use night-light in bedroom and bathroom

B. Trim toenails; use appropriate footwear

C. Speak slowly; use low voice; decrease background noise; encourage use of hearing aid

D. Remove earwax

E. Use bright colors as markers, especially orange, yellow, and red

F. Be sure that individual wears glasses, if appropriate; keep glasses clean; encourage regular eye examinations

G. Use correctly sized footwear with firm soles

H. Encourage balance, gait training, and muscle-strengthening exercises

I. Encourage dorsiflexion exercises; use pressure-graded stockings (TEDs); elevate head of bed; teach individual to get up from chair or bed slowly to avoid tipping head backward

J. Encourage balance exercises

K. Place call bell in visual field and within reach of arm that has use; anticipate needs for toileting, dressing, eating, and bathing; assist with transfer; provide passive range of motion exercises to improve functional ability

E. List four basic strategies for reducing all types of falls.

(263) **1.** ____

(263) **2.** ____

(263) **3.** ____

(263) **4.** ____

F. List three important factors to document when a fall occurs.

(264) **1.** ____

(264) **2.** ____

(264) **3.** ____

MULTIPLE-CHOICE QUESTIONS

G. Choose the most appropriate answer.

(260) **1.** What is the estimated ratio of persons aged 65 or older who fall in a given year?

1. 1 in 3
2. 1 in 10
3. 1 in 20
4. 1 in 100

(260) **2.** After what age does there appear to be a steady increase in the number of falls?

1. 40
2. 65
3. 75
4. 85

(260) **3.** Of the total number of deaths due to falls, which percentage of the victims are elderly?

1. 10%
2. 20%
3. 50%
4. 72%

(260) **4.** Which percentage of deaths due to falls does the U.S. Public Health Service state are preventable?

1. one fifth
2. one third
3. one half
4. two thirds

(260) **5.** Factors such as the aging process and physical illness that increase the possibility of falling are called:

1. extrinsic factors.
2. environmental factors.
3. intrinsic factors.
4. physical factors.

(260) **6.** Factors that increase the opportunity to fall are called:

1. extrinsic factors.
2. aging process factors.
3. intrinsic factors.
4. physical illness factors.

(261) **7.** Of all reported falls, what percentage do not result in injury?

1. 10–20%
2. 25–35%
3. 40–50%
4. 65–75%

(261) **8.** What is the most frequent type of injury from falls, occurring in 25–30% of all falls?

1. deep tissue damage
2. contusions, cuts, or lacerations
3. concussion
4. fractures

(261) **9.** Geriatric chairs and side rails are examples of:

1. environmental restraints.
2. social restraints.
3. physical restraints.
4. chemical restraints.

(261) **10.** Older patients are more likely than younger patients to be physically restrained because of their greater likelihood of:

1. mental decline and weight loss.
2. chronic illness and physical decline.
3. heart disease and insomnia.
4. falling and confusion.

Student Name ______________________________

(262) **11.** The major complications from using physical restraints include:

1. sedation from medications administered and accidental aspiration.
2. falls from wheelchairs and beds (when patients are able to untie restraints or wriggle out of them) and accidental strangulation.
3. fatigue from fighting the restraints and confusion resulting from fatigue.
4. skin breakdown from friction and wound development.

(262) **12.** The Omnibus Reconciliation Act of 1987 (OBRA) states that nursing home residents have the right to be free from any physical restraints imposed or psychoactive drug administered for the purposes of:

1. discipline or convenience.
2. safety or public health.
3. exercise or physical therapy.
4. strict confinement.

(262) **13.** Physical restraints should be removed and released every:

1. hour for 10 minutes.
2. 2 hours for 10 minutes.
3. 4 hours for 10 minutes.
4. 8 hours for 10 minutes.

(262) **14.** Psychoactive drugs should never be used for the purpose of:

1. relief of headaches.
2. insomnia.
3. discipline.
4. hallucinations.

(265) **15.** In the "roll" method of getting up from a fall, after rolling onto the right side and bending the right knee, the patient should:

1. crawl to a chair.
2. pull to a sitting position on the floor.
3. get up on all fours.
4. leverage upward to the kneeling position by pressing down on the right forearm.

(265) **16.** In the "crawl" method of getting up from a fall, after rolling to a prone position, getting up on all fours, and crawling to a sturdy couch, the patient should:

1. pull to a sitting position on the floor.
2. bring one foot forward, putting the foot flat on the floor.
3. stand up.
4. gradually move up and backward to a stair height.

(265) **17.** In the "stair shuffle" method of getting up from a fall, after pulling to a sitting position on the floor and shuffling on the buttocks to the stairs, the patient should:

1. turn around and kneel on the lowest stair.
2. get up on all fours.
3. turn around and place arms on waist-height stair to support body.
4. gradually move up and backward to a stair height suitable for standing.

(261) **18.** Keeping the bed at the lowest level and using the least restrictive restraints are interventions related to:

1. Impaired skin integrity.
2. Risk for injury.
3. Altered urinary function.
4. Risk for infection.

(263) **19.** The first step in preventing falls and injury is to determine:

1. which medications the patient is taking.
2. the hazards in the environmental setting.
3. who is at greatest risk.
4. whether the patient has alcohol or drug problems.

CHAPTER 20

Student Name ______________________________

Immobility

Answer Key: Textbook page references are provided as a guide for answering these questions. A complete answer key was provided for your instructor.

OBJECTIVES

1. Describe common problems associated with immobility.
2. Discuss the impact of exercise and positioning on preventing complications related to immobility.
3. Identify the risk factors for pressure ulcers.
4. Describe the stages of pressure ulcers.
5. Describe methods of preventing and treating pressure ulcers.
6. Discuss the effects of immobility on respiratory status, nutrition, and elimination.

LEARNING ACTIVITIES

A. Match the definition in the numbered column with the most appropriate term in the lettered column.

(267)	**1.** ________ The inability to move; imposed restriction on entire body	A.	Erythema
		B.	Pressure ulcer
		C.	Isometric exercise
		D.	Immobility
		E.	Range of motion
(269)	**2.** ________ Exercise in which each joint is moved in various directions to the farthest possible extreme	F.	Active exercise
		G.	Contracture
		H.	Shearing forces
		I.	Passive exercise
(269)	**3.** ________ Exercise of the patient that is carried out by the therapist or nurse without the assistance of the patient		

Continued next page

(269) **4.** ________ Muscle contraction without movement used to maintain muscle tone

(269) **5.** ________ Exercise carried out by the patient

(270) **6.** ________ Redness of the skin; usually a sign that capillaries have become congested because of impaired blood flow

(269) **7.** ________ Shortening of the muscles and tendons

(270) **8.** ________ Two contacting parts sliding on each other

(270) **9.** ________ An open wound caused by pressure on a bony prominence; also called a "bed sore" or "decubitus ulcer"

B. List 12 elements of a pressure sore prevention protocol.

(270) **1.** ____________________

(270) **2.** ____________________

(270) **3.** ____________________

(270) **4.** ____________________

(270) **5.** ____________________

(270) **6.** ____________________

(270) **7.** ____________________

(270) **8.** ____________________

(270) **9.** ____________________

(270) **10.** ____________________

(270) **11.** ____________________

(270) **12.** ____________________

C. Match the characteristic in the numbered column with the most appropriate stage of pressure ulcer in the lettered column. Answers may be used more than once.

(272) **1.** ________ Wound may be infected and is usually open and draining

(272) **2.** ________ Some skin loss in the epidermis and/or dermis

(272) **3.** ________ Irregular, ill-defined area of pressure reflecting the shape of the object creating the pressure

A. Stage I
B. Stage II
C. Stage III
D. Stage IV

Continued next page

Student Name____

(272) **4.** __________ Craterlike sore with a distinct outer margin

(272) **5.** __________ Ulcer is surrounded by a broad, indistinct, painful, reddened area that is hot or warmer than normal

(272) **6.** __________ Nonblanchable erythema

(272) **7.** __________ A shallow ulcer develops and appears blistered, cracked, or abraded

(272) **8.** __________ Ulcer is usually infected and may appear black with exudation, foul odor, and purulent drainage

(272) **9.** __________ Full-thickness skin loss involving damage or necrosis of the dermis and subcutaneous tissues

(272) **10.** __________ Little destruction of tissue; condition is reversible

(272) **11.** __________ Full-thickness skin loss with extensive destruction of the deeper underlying muscle and possible bone tissue

(272) **12.** __________ Pain and tenderness may be present, with swelling and hardening of the tissue and associated heat

D. In Figure 20-1, label the bony prominences (A–Z).

(271)	**A.**	______________________	*(271)*	**N.**	______________________
(271)	**B.**	______________________	*(271)*	**O.**	______________________
(271)	**C.**	______________________	*(271)*	**P.**	______________________
(271)	**D.**	______________________	*(271)*	**Q.**	______________________
(271)	**E.**	______________________	*(271)*	**R.**	______________________
(271)	**F.**	______________________	*(271)*	**S.**	______________________
(271)	**G.**	______________________	*(271)*	**T.**	______________________
(271)	**H.**	______________________	*(271)*	**U.**	______________________
(271)	**I.**	______________________	*(271)*	**V.**	______________________
(271)	**J.**	______________________	*(271)*	**W.**	______________________
(271)	**K.**	______________________	*(271)*	**X.**	______________________
(271)	**L.**	______________________	*(271)*	**Y.**	______________________
(271)	**M.**	______________________	*(271)*	**Z.**	______________________

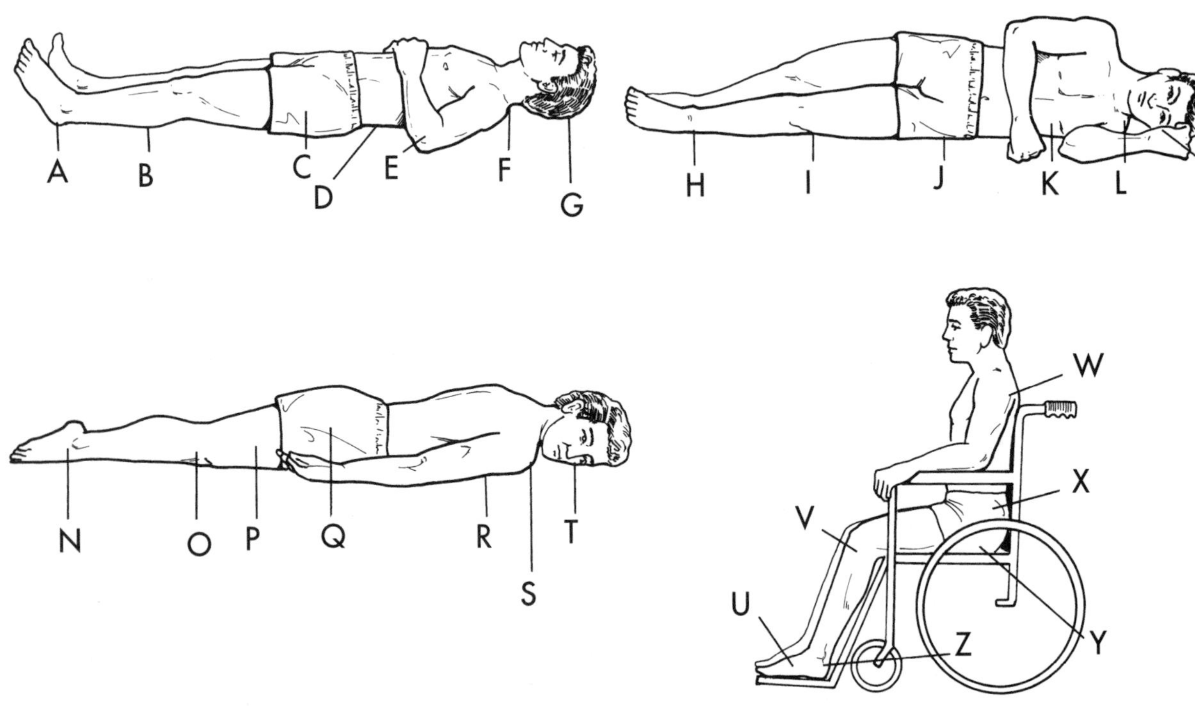

Student Name____

MULTIPLE-CHOICE QUESTIONS

E. Choose the most appropriate answer.

(269) **1.** Little or no motion of the joints results in:

1. contractures.
2. tendonitis.
3. bursitis.
4. skin breakdown.

(270) **2.** What is the most frequent site of skin breakdown?

1. ischial tuberosities
2. sacrum
3. heels
4. trochanter

(272) **3.** The best preventive measure for pressure ulcers is:

1. a high-protein diet.
2. deep breathing.
3. frequent position changes.
4. moderate exercise.

(270) **4.** The medical term used for bedsores is:

1. wound infection.
2. cellulitis.
3. pressure ulcer.
4. bony pressure.

(270) **5.** An area of redness that is the beginning of a pressure sore is called:

1. erythema.
2. inflammation.
3. a wound.
4. hemorrhage.

(270) **6.** Erythema progresses rapidly to an ulcerated stage in persons who are malnourished, obese, or aged, who have:

1. skin infection.
2. poor skin turgor.
3. lacerations.
4. circulatory disease.

(270) **7.** The action on tissues that occurs when a patient slumps down while sitting in bed is called:

1. lacerating.
2. shearing.
3. projectile.
4. slanting.

(270) **8.** Which of the following conditions is expensive to treat, results in longer hospital stays, increases the likelihood of nursing home placement, and increases mortality?

1. falls
2. use of physical restraints
3. overuse of antibiotics
4. pressure ulcers

(270, 271) **9.** A useful instrument for identifying those at risk for developing pressure ulcers is the:

1. pain scale.
2. neurologic scale.
3. Norton scale.
4. Glasgow coma scale.

(272) **10.** What is *not* recommended for pressure points?

1. sheepskin
2. massage
3. egg crate mattress
4. trapeze bars

(272) **11.** Which of the following causes concentrated areas of pressure that puts patients at higher risk for developing pressure ulcers?

1. sheepskin
2. egg crate mattress
3. trapeze bar
4. rubber ring

(274) **12.** When a person remains immobile or does not take deep breaths, which of the following is most likely to occur to the respiratory status?

1. an accumulation of carbon dioxide that collects in the alveoli
2. an accumulation of thick secretions that pool in the lower respiratory structures
3. decreased circulation to the lungs
4. decreased oxygen entering the lungs

(274) **13.** When thick secretions pool in the lower respiratory structures, they interfere with the:

1. exchange of white blood cells and red blood cells in the capillaries.
2. circulation of blood to the extremities.
3. detoxification process in the liver.
4. exchange of oxygen and carbon dioxide in the lungs.

(274) **14.** Which of the following is contraindicated in the care of patients with pressure ulcers?

1. use of moisturizers
2. heat lamp
3. egg crate mattress
4. sheepskin boots

(274) **15.** What is the most common problem associated with immobility in relation to food and fluid intake?

1. hypoproteinemia
2. hypokalemia
3. anorexia
4. nausea

(274) **16.** For patients with pressure ulcers, the diet should be high in:

1. potassium.
2. fiber.
3. protein.
4. vitamins.

(275) **17.** Inactivity, decreased fluid intake, and lack of fiber in the diet cause:

1. anorexia.
2. nausea.
3. constipation.
4. diarrhea.

(272) **18.** Which of the following is recommended for the treatment of stage I ulcers?

1. disinfectants
2. mild soap
3. alcohol
4. powder

(275) **19.** The urinary system functions best when the person is:

1. sitting.
2. upright.
3 side-lying.
4. lying prone.

(275) **20.** The most effective way to prevent urinary incontinence associated with immobility is to establish a:

1. high-protein diet.
2. coughing and deep-breathing program.
3. restriction of fluid intake.
4. schedule for toiletings.

(274) **21.** Which of the following is contraindicated in the treatment of patients with stage II ulcers?

1. mild soap
2. normal saline
3. water
4. heat lamp

CHAPTER 21

Student Name ______________________________

Confusion

Answer Key: Textbook page references are provided as a guide for answering these questions. A complete answer key was provided for your instructor.

OBJECTIVES

1. Define delirium and dementia.
2. Identify the causes of acute confusion.
3. Explain the differences between delirium and dementia.
4. Discuss nursing assessment and interventions related to delirium and dementia.

LEARNING ACTIVITIES

A. Match the definition in the numbered column with the most appropriate term in the lettered column. Answers may be used more than once.

(278)	**1.**	________	Short-term confusional state	A. Delirium B. Dementia
(278)	**2.**	________	Often irreversible confusion	
(278)	**3.**	________	Acute confusional state	
(278)	**4.**	________	Chronic confusion	
(278)	**5.**	________	Often reversible confusion	
(278)	**6.**	________	Characterized by disturbances in attention, thinking, and perception	

Continued next page

(278) **7.** ________ Characterized by impairment of intellectual function

(278, 279) **8.** ________ Caused by some underlying illness

(278) **9.** ________ Develops over a short period of time

B. List three systemic causes of delirium.

(279) **1.** ________________________________

(279) **2.** ________________________________

(279) **3.** ________________________________

C. List two concepts that should be used as a basis for providing care for patients with dementia.

(284) **1.** ________________________________

(284) **2.** ________________________________

MULTIPLE-CHOICE QUESTIONS

D. Choose the most appropriate answer.

(280) **1.** The first priority of nursing interventions for the patient with delirium is to:

1. provide safety and comfort.
2. take vital signs.
3. force fluids.
4. provide therapeutic touch.

(282) **2.** Because adequate sleep is important for the patient with delirium, which would be most appropriate to help the patient fall asleep?

1. a glass of wine, a shower, and a long walk
2. pain medication, milk and cookies, and watching a movie
3. a back rub, a glass of warm milk, and soothing conversation
4. a sedative, a large dinner, and physical activity

(280) **3.** When one is dealing with a delirious patient who is experiencing hallucinations, the best response of the nurse would be:

1. "What is it that you are seeing on the wall?"
2. "You are sick in the hospital, and what you are seeing is part of the illness."
3. "The time is 2:00 PM and the date is ______."
4. "Tell me what you are seeing."

(282) **4.** The use of physical restraints should be avoided with patients with delirium because restraints tend to:

1. increase anxiety.
2. disturb thought processes.
3. increase impaired thinking.
4. disturb sleep patterns.

Student Name____

(284) **5.** When a patient with dementia resists activities such as bathing or dressing, the nurse should:

1. orient the patient to reality.
2. avoid confrontations.
3. state clearly what needs to be done.
4. offer a variety of choices to encourage decision making.

(282, 283) **6.** Patients with dementia should be offered:

1. three full meals a day.
2. low-fiber foods.
3. a diet high in salt.
4. finger foods high in protein and carbohydrates.

(284) **7.** When you are taking care of patients with dementia, it is helpful to remember that they usually:

1. benefit from reality orientation.
2. forget things quickly.
3. do not forget things quickly.
4. are able to learn new things.

(284) **8.** If patients with dementia start to become very restless or agitated, an effective nursing intervention is to:

1. discuss the cause of their discomfort with them.
2. speak calmly and reassure them constantly.
3. orient them to time and place.
4. divert their attention and gently guide them to a new activity.

(284) **9.** Which approach may agitate people with dementia?

1. a nonconfrontational manner
2. use of calm, gentle mannerisms
3. reality orientation
4. use of simple, direct communication

(284) **10.** If a patient with dementia is afraid of bathtubs, you should:

1. reassure the patient that there is nothing to be afraid of.
2. explain the reason for taking a bath in the bathtub.
3. offer a variety of choices to the patient about taking a bath .
4. arrange another way to give personal care.

(282) **11.** In caring for a patient with delirium, you should:

1. provide frequent, routine toileting.
2. provide frequent orientation to surroundings.
3. cut the food into small portions.
4. break tasks down into individual steps to be done one at a time.

CHAPTER 22

Student Name ______________________________

Incontinence

Answer Key: Textbook page references are provided as a guide for answering these questions. A complete answer key was provided for your instructor.

OBJECTIVES

1. Identify the types of urinary and fecal incontinence.
2. Explain the pathophysiology and treatment of specific types of incontinence.
3. Identify common therapeutic measures used for the incontinent patient.
4. List nursing assessment data needed to assist in the evaluation and treatment of incontinence.
5. Assist in developing a nursing care plan for the patient with incontinence.

LEARNING ACTIVITIES

A. Match the definition in the numbered column with the most appropriate term in the lettered column.

(293) **1.** __________ Involuntary loss of urine during physical exertion

(299) **2.** __________ Uncontrolled passage of stool associated with constipation

(300) **3.** __________ Fecal incontinence caused by weak perineal muscles, loss of anal reflexes, loss of anal sphincter tone, or rectal prolapse

A. Functional incontinence
B. Transient incontinence
C. Voiding
D. Overflow incontinence (fecal)
E. Overactive bladder
F. Urinary incontinence
G. Urge incontinence
H. Credé's technique
I. Stress incontinence
J. Neurogenic bladder
K. Fecal incontinence
L. Anorectal incontinence
M. Symptomatic incontinence
N. Neurogenic incontinence
O. Overflow incontinence (urine)

Continued next page

(300) **4.** __________ Reflexive uncontrolled bowel movement, usually seen with dementia

(293) **5.** __________ Inappropriate voiding in the presence of normal bladder and urethral function

(300) **6.** __________ Incontinence associated with colorectal disease

(292) **7.** __________ Involuntary loss of urine associated with a full bladder

(286) **8.** __________ The inability to control the passage of urine

(291) **9.** __________ Temporary loss of control over voiding

(286) **10.** __________ The inability to control the passage of feces

(291) **11.** __________ Involuntary loss of urine, usually shortly after a strong urge to void

(293) **12.** __________ Condition in which the bladder does not function normally because of some disorder affecting the nerves of the bladder

(286) **13.** __________ Urination

(293) **14.** __________ Expression of urine from the bladder by applying pressure over the lower abdomen

(291) **15.** __________ Lower urinary tract disorder without pathological or metabolic causes that is characterized by urinary frequency, urgency, and urge incontinence

B. Fill in the blanks.

(286) **1.** Four factors required for normal controlled voiding include healthy bladder muscles (detrusor muscles), a patent urethra, normal transmission of nerve impulses, and

__________________ __________________________.

(291) **2.** Five methods of treatment for urge incontinence include antibiotics for infection, removal of impaction, behavioral techniques, anticholinergics, and

__________________________.

(292) **3.** Factors that contribute to overflow incontinence include obstruction to urine flow, underactive detrusor muscle, or ______________________________________.

Student Name ____________________

(293) **4.** Drugs that may cause urinary retention include antihistamines, epinephrine, theophylline, and ____________________.

(293) **5.** A common reason for urethral obstruction in males is ____________________.

(293) **6.** The two groups of patients that usually require intermittent catheterization only once or twice before normal bladder function returns are ____________________ and ____________________.

(293) **7.** Activities that may lead to stress incontinence include coughing, laughing, sneezing, and ____________________.

(293) **8.** Contributing factors to stress incontinence include pelvic floor muscle relaxation following childbirth, obesity, and ____________________.

C. List six methods of treatment for a person with stress incontinence.

(293) **1.** ____________________

(293) **2.** ____________________

(293) **3.** ____________________

(293) **4.** ____________________

(293) **5.** ____________________

(293) **6.** ____________________

D. List any seven of ten classifications of drugs that may contribute to urinary incontinence.

(293) **1.** ____________________

(293) **2.** ____________________

(293) **3.** ____________________

(293) **4.** ____________________

(293) **5.** ____________________

(293) **6.** ____________________

(293) **7.** ____________________

E. Match the definition or description in the numbered column with the most appropriate diagnostic test or procedure in the lettered column.

(287) **1.** ________ Used to evaluate the neuromuscular function of the bladder

(287) **2.** ________ May be ordered to create images of the urinary structures

(287) **3.** ________ Clean-catch urinalysis and blood urea nitrogen measurement

(287) **4.** ________ Used to determine whether the patient is emptying the bladder completely

(287) **5.** ________ Measures voiding duration and the amount and rate of urine voided

(287) **6.** ________ Uses a scope inserted through the urethra to visualize the urethra and bladder

(287) **7.** ________ Detects involuntary passage of urine when abdominal pressure increases

(287) **8.** ________ Used to assess neuromuscular function of the urinary tract

A. Postvoiding residual
B. Imaging procedures
C. Cystometry
D. Urodynamic testing
E. Cystoscopy
F. Laboratory tests
G. Provocative stress testing
H. Uroflowmetry

Student Name________________________________

F. Match the definition or description in the numbered column with the most appropriate therapeutic measure in the lettered column.

(288) **1.** ________ Intended to help the patient recognize incontinence and to ask caregivers for help with toileting

(288) **2.** ________ Voiding schedule based on the patient's usual pattern

(289) **3.** ________ Includes anticholinergics and smooth muscle relaxants

(288) **4.** ________ Uses patient education, scheduled voiding, and positive reinforcement

(289) **5.** ________ Sometimes employed by people with spinal cord injury

(288) **6.** ________ Uses electronic or mechanical sensors to give feedback about physiologic activity

(288) **7.** ________ Commonly called Kegel exercises

(288) **8.** ________ Retained in the vagina to strengthen muscles of pelvic floor

A. Pelvic muscle exercises
B. Vaginal cones
C. Bladder training
D. Habit training
E. Drug therapy
F. Biofeedback
G. Prompted voiding
H. Reflex training

G. Match the nursing diagnosis in the numbered column with the most appropriate cause in the lettered column.

(295) **1.** ________ Functional incontinence

(295) **2.** ________ Reflex incontinence

(296) **3.** ________ Risk for infection

A. Neurologic impairment
B. Chronic bladder distention or catheterization
C. Physical, cognitive, or environmental barriers

H. Match each nursing diagnosis in the numbered column with the most appropriate nursing goal in the lettered column.

(295) **1.** ________ Reflex incontinence related to neurologic impairment

(296) **2.** ________ Stress incontinence related to weak pelvic structures, and increased intra-abdominal pressure

(296) **3.** ________ Total incontinence related to neurologic dysfunction

(296) **4.** ________ Urge incontinence related to decreased bladder capacity or bladder spasms

(296) **5.** ________ Risk for impaired skin integrity related to the presence of urine on the skin

(296) **6.** ________ Risk for infection related to chronic bladder distention or catheterization

(295) **7.** ________ Deficient knowledge of causes of incontinence and corrective measures

A. Patient understanding of incontinence and its management
B. Reduce risk of skin breakdown
C. Adequate management of irreversible incontinence to prevent spillage
D. Improve control of urine flow
E. Continent voiding with appropriate support
F. Reduce risk of urinary tract infection
G. Improved self-esteem
H. Adequate management of irreversible incontinence
I. Decreased social isolation
J. Ability to hold increased volume of urine

Continued next page

Student Name____

(295) **8.** __________ Functional incontinence related to physical, cognitive, or environmental barriers

(296) **9.** __________ Social isolation related to fear of embarrassment

(296) **10.** __________ Situational low self-esteem related to loss of control over voiding

I. Match the name or classification of the drugs in the numbered column with the corresponding type of incontinence they treat in the lettered column.

(290) **1.** __________ Alpha-adrenergic blockers

(290) **2.** __________ Cholinergics

(290) **3.** __________ Beta-adrenergic blockers

(290) **4.** __________ Anticholinergics

(290) **5.** __________ Alpha-adrenergics

(290) **6.** __________ Collagen

(290) **7.** __________ Propranolol (Inderal)

(290) **8.** __________ Bethanechol chloride (Urecholine)

(290) **9.** __________ Prazosin (Minipress)

(290) **10.** __________ Ephedrine

(290) **11.** __________ Oxybutynin (Ditropan)

(290) **12.** __________ Propantheline bromide (Pro-Banthine)

A. Overflow incontinence
B. Urge incontinence
C. Stress incontinence

J. Match the cause of incontinence in the numbered column with the type of incontinence in the lettered column. Answers may be used more than one time.

(292) **1.** __________ UTI

(292) **2.** __________ Spinal cord injury above T10

(292) **3.** __________ Relaxation of pelvic floor muscles

(292) **4.** __________ Dementia

(292) **5.** __________ CVA

(292) **6.** __________ Urethral trauma

(292) **7.** __________ Post anesthesia

A. Urge
B. Overflow
C. Reflex
D. Stress
E. Functional

MULTIPLE-CHOICE QUESTIONS

K. Choose the most appropriate answer.

(293) **1.** Drugs that may cause urinary retention include:

1. chlorothiazides and loop diuretics.
2. antihypertensives and insulin.
3. anticholinergics and epinephrine.
4. antibiotics and antiviral drugs.

(287) **2.** The amount of urine remaining in the bladder after voiding is called the:

1. urodynamic series.
2. clean catch.
3. voiding duration.
4. postvoiding residual.

(292) **3.** Which treatment is contraindicated for patients with reflex incontinence?

1. cutaneous triggering
2. tapping the suprapubic area
3. stroking the inner thigh
4. Credé's method

(287) **4.** How much urine normally remains in the bladder after voiding?

1. 50 ml or less
2. 100 ml or less
3. 200 ml or less
4. 250 ml or less

(292) **5.** If the bladder becomes overdistended, the patient with reflex incontinence may have a very serious reaction called:

1. stress incontinence.
2. orthostatic hypotension.
3. autonomic dysreflexia.
4. tachycardia.

(293) **6.** Which is considered to be the last resort in the management of overflow incontinence?

1. Credé's method
2. Valsalva maneuver
3. indwelling catheter
4. anal stretch maneuver

Student Name________________________

(293) **7.** When a person voids inappropriately because of an inability to get to the toilet, this is called:

1. urge incontinence.
2. functional incontinence.
3. reflex incontinence.
4. stress incontinence.

(296) **8.** Stimuli that may encourage voiding include:

1. decreasing the fluid intake to less than 2000 ml/day.
2. drinking caffeine and cola drinks.
3. pressing down on the abdomen.
4. pouring warm water over the perineum, and drinking water while on the toilet.

(298) **9.** The patient who is incontinent of urine is at risk for:

1. urinary tract infection and urinary calculi (stones).
2. upper respiratory infection and pelvic infection.
3. bradycardia and thrombophlebitis.
4. diarrhea and skin breakdown.

(300) **10.** Which constipating drug would be effective in treating neurogenic incontinence if given once a day in the morning?

1. senna
2. milk of magnesia
3. codeine
4. Metamucil

(299) **11.** The first step in the medical management of fecal overflow incontinence is to:

1. treat the underlying medical condition.
2. teach pelvic muscle exercises and biofeedback.
3. cleanse the colon, often with enemas and suppositories.
4. schedule toileting based on the patient's usual time of defecation.

(300) **12.** What type of incontinence is present in patients with dementia who do not voluntarily delay defecation?

1. overflow
2. anorectal
3. neurogenic
4. symptomatic

(300) **13.** The treatment for fecal neurogenic incontinence is to:

1. cleanse the colon, usually with enemas and suppositories.
2. treat the underlying medical condition.
3. schedule toileting based on the patient's usual time of defecation.
4. teach pelvic muscle exercises and biofeedback.

(300) **14.** A patient has blood and mucus in his stool. This type of fecal incontinence is:

1. neurogenic.
2. symptomatic.
3. anorectal.
4. overflow.

(300) **15.** Fecal incontinence associated with nerve damage that causes the muscles of the pelvic floor to be weak is:

1. symptomatic.
2. neurogenic.
3. anorectal.
4. overflow.

(299) **16.** Causes of overflow fecal incontinence include:

1. nerve damage that causes weak pelvic muscles.
2. colon or rectal disease.
3. loss of anal reflexes in patients with dementia.
4. constipation in which the rectum is constantly distended.

(301) **17.** A patient with fecal incontinence may need laxatives to:

1. relieve constipation.
2. establish bowel control.
3. improve the loss of anal sphincter tone.
4. reverse the loss of the anal reflex.

(301) **18.** In order to prevent constipation, the patient with fecal incontinence is advised to consume increased fluids and:

1. protein.
2. fiber.
3. carbohydrates.
4. potassium.

CHAPTER 23

Student Name ______________________________

Loss, Death, and End-of-Life Care

Answer Key: Textbook page references are provided as a guide for answering these questions. A complete answer key was provided for your instructor.

OBJECTIVES

1. Describe beliefs and practices related to death and dying.
2. Describe responses of patients and their families to terminal illness and death.
3. Identify nursing diagnoses that are appropriate for the terminally ill.
4. Identify nursing goals that are appropriate for the terminally ill.
5. Identify nursing interventions to meet the needs of terminally ill and dying patients.
6. Discuss the needs of the terminally ill patient's significant others.
7. Discuss the ways nurses can intervene to meet the needs of the terminally ill patient's significant others.
8. Explore the responses of the nurse who works with the terminally ill.
9. Explore the needs of the nurse who works with terminally ill patients.
10. Identify issues related to caring for the dying patient, including advance directives, do-not-resuscitate decisions, brain death, organ donations, and pronouncement of death.

LEARNING ACTIVITIES

A. Match the definition in the numbered column with the most appropriate term in the lettered column.

(313)	**1.**	________	A wrap in which the body is placed after death for transport to the mortuary	A. Denial B. Grief C. Shroud D. Autopsy E. Advance directive F. Loss
(314)	**2.**	________	Written statement of a person's wishes regarding medical care	G. Cerebral death

Continued next page

(304) **3.** __________ A real or potential absence of someone or something that is valued

(310) **4.** __________ Absence of cerebral cortex functioning

(306) **5.** __________ A defense mechanism in which the individual thinks and behaves as if not aware of an unpleasant reality

(312) **6.** __________ Examination of a body after death to determine or confirm the cause of death

(305) **7.** __________ An emotional response to a loss

B. Match the loss in the numbered column with the most appropriate category in the lettered column.

(305) **1.** __________ Loss of dependence in young adulthood

(305) **2.** __________ Hair loss

(305) **3.** __________ Disabilities

(305) **4.** __________ Separation from family when placed in long-term care facility

(305) **5.** __________ Loss of family heirloom

(305) **6.** __________ Children leaving parents for school

(305) **7.** __________ Radical surgery

(305) **8.** __________ Loss of appointment calendar

(305) **9.** __________ Death of family member

(305) **10.** __________ Moving away from parents

(305) **11.** __________ Increased dependence in old age

A. Change in self-image
B. Loss of significant others
C. Loss of possessions
D. Developmental change

Student Name____

C. Match the definition or description in the numbered column with the most appropriate stage of grieving in the lettered column.

(306) **1.** __________ Patient or family members may become outraged with situations

(307) **2.** __________ Peaceful acknowledgment of the loss

(307) **3.** __________ Patient realizes the loss is final and the situation cannot be altered

(306) **4.** __________ Patient refuses to acknowledge the loss

(307) **5.** __________ Patient wishes for more time or wishes to avoid the loss

(307) **6.** __________ Patient expresses feelings that the loss is occurring as a punishment for past actions and may try to negotiate with a higher power for more time

(306) **7.** __________ Protects the patient and family from the reality of the loss

A. Depression
B. Anger
C. Denial
D. Acceptance
E. Bargaining

D. Match Kübler-Ross's stages in the numbered column with Martocchios's stages in the lettered column.

(307)	**1.**	________	Depression	A. Yearning and protest
				B. Anguish, disorganization, and despair
(307)	**2.**	________	Denial	C. Shock and disbelief
				D. Reorganization and restoration
(307)	**3.**	________	Acceptance	
(307)	**4.**	________	Anger/bargaining	

E. Match the belief about death in the numbered column with the most appropriate age group in the lettered column.

(307)	**1.**	________	Sees death as inevitable	A. Young adulthood
				B. Middle adulthood
				C. Older adulthood
(307)	**2.**	________	Faces death of parents and family members	
(307)	**3.**	________	Examines death as it relates to various meanings, such as freedom from discomfort	
(307)	**4.**	________	Sees death as future event	
(307)	**5.**	________	Faces death of peers	
(307)	**6.**	________	May experience death anxiety	

F. Match the definition or description in the numbered column with the most appropriate state of awareness of terminal illness in the lettered column.

(308)	**1.**	________	Patients and others involved freely discuss the impending death	A. Mutual pretense
				B. Closed awareness
				C. Open awareness
(308)	**2.**	________	Patient and family know of a terminal prognosis but do not discuss the issue openly	
(308)	**3.**	________	Patient and family recognize that patient is ill but do not understand severity of illness	

Student Name____

G. Match the action in the numbered column with the relevant fear in the lettered column.

(308)	**1.**	__________	Assure patient that medication will be given promptly, as needed	A.	Fear of loneliness
				B.	Fear of meaninglessness
				C.	Fear of pain
(309)	**2.**	__________	Express worth of dying person's life		
(309)	**3.**	__________	Simple presence of person to provide support and comfort		
(309)	**4.**	__________	Holding hands, touching, and listening		
(308)	**5.**	__________	Provide consistent pain control		
(309)	**6.**	__________	Dying person reviews his or her life		
(309)	**7.**	__________	Prayers, thoughts and feelings provide comfort		

H. Match the definition in the numbered column with the most appropriate term in the lettered column.

(311)	**1.**	__________	The body's cooling after death	A.	Rigor mortis
				B.	Livor mortis
				C.	Algor mortis
(311)	**2.**	__________	Discoloration in the skin after death		
(311)	**3.**	__________	Stiffening of the body after death		

MULTIPLE-CHOICE QUESTIONS

I. Choose the most appropriate answer.

(309) **1.** Which change occurs preceding death?

1. Blood pressure rises.
2. Breathing sounds are quiet.
3. Pulse slows.
4. Extremities turn red.

(309) **2.** Mouth breathing and the accumulation of mucus preceding death result in noisy, wet-sounding respirations called:

1. suffocation.
2. death rattle.
3. tightness in the chest.
4. pneumonia.

(311) **3.** Livor mortis is generally most obvious in the:

1. skin in extremities.
2. fingers and toes.
3. face and chest.
4. back and buttocks.

(314) **4.** Most states have replaced the idea of living wills with:

1. euthanasia acts.
2. natural death acts.
3. self-disclosure acts.
4. DNR acts.

(308) **5.** Which cultural group values stoicism at death?

1. Greeks
2. Mexicans
3. Vietnamese
4. Swedes

(309) **6.** What is the last sense to remain intact during the death process?

1. vision
2. smell
3. hearing
4. touch

(309) **7.** Where does the sense of touch decrease first in a dying person?

1. face
2. abdomen
3. arms
4. legs

(309) **8.** Why does the patient who is dying appear to stare?

1. The blink reflex is lost gradually.
2. Vision is blurred.
3. There is decreased lubrication of the eye.
4. Decreased circulation to the eye occurs progressively.

(309) **9.** Which body function ceases first in the dying person?

1. heartbeat
2. respiration
3. brain function
4. kidney function

(310) **10.** Which is *not* a criterion to determine death?

1. unresponsiveness to external stimuli that would usually be painful
2. complete absence of spontaneous breathing
3. total lack of reflexes
4. a flat EEG for 8 hours

(310) **11.** Which criterion must be present for brain death to be pronounced and life support disconnected by the physician?

1. All brain function must cease.
2. Coma or unresponsiveness must be present.
3. Absence of all brain stem reflexes must be noted.
4. Apnea must be present.

Student Name____

(311) **12.** After death, what happens to the body as it cools?

1. Respirations are noisy and labored.
2. Reflex jerking movements of the extremities occur.
3. Pupils are not reactive to light.
4. Skin loses elasticity and is easily broken.

(311) **13.** What causes a livor mortis after death?

1. Skin loses elasticity and breaks down easily.
2. There is a breakdown of red blood cells.
3. Chemical changes prevent muscle relaxation.
4. Circulation decreases and the body cools.

(313) **14.** Which religious group believes that the body should not be shrouded until sacraments have been performed?

1. Muslims
2. Orthodox Jews
3. Protestants
4. Roman Catholics

(317) **15.** The durable power of attorney for health care can be used only if the physician certifies in writing that the person is:

1. incapable of making decisions.
2. brain dead.
3. unresponsive or in a coma.
4. lacking reflexes.

(316) **16.** What decision involves the use of medications for resuscitation without the use of CPR?

1. chemical code
2. no code
3. DNR
4. advance directive

(314) **17.** The Patient Self-Determination Act requires that institutions must inform patients about:

1. rules and regulations about CPR.
2. the right to have an autopsy.
3. the right to initiate advance directives.
4. rules and regulations about the delivery of hospice care.

CHAPTER 24

Student Name ____________________

The Patient with Cancer

Answer Key: Textbook page references are provided as a guide for answering these questions. A complete answer key was provided for your instructor.

OBJECTIVES

1. Explain the differences between benign and malignant tumors.
2. List the most common sites of cancer in men and women.
3. Describe measures to reduce the risk of cancer.
4. Define terms used to name and classify cancer.
5. List nursing responsibilities in the care of patients having diagnostic tests to detect possible cancer.
6. Explain the nursing care of patients undergoing each type of cancer therapy: surgery, radiation, chemotherapy, and biotherapy.
7. Assist in developing a nursing care plan for the terminally ill patient with cancer and the patient's family.

LEARNING ACTIVITIES

A. Match the definition in the numbered column with the most appropriate term in the lettered column

(321) **1.** __________ Tending to progress in virulence; has the characteristics of becoming increasingly undifferentiated, invading surrounding tissues, and colonizing distant sites

A. Radiotherapy
B. Benign
C. Chemotherapy
D. Metastasis
E. Neoplasm
F. Alopecia
G. Oncofetal antigen
H. Malignant
I. Antineoplastic
J. Carcinogen
K. Biotherapy

Continued next page

(327) **2.** __________ A gene product that is normally suppressed in adult tissues but reappears in the presence of some types of cancer

(323) **3.** __________ Cancer-causing agent

(328) **4.** __________ The use of radiation in the treatment of cancer and other diseases

(321) **5.** __________ Process by which cancer spreads to distant sites

(331) **6.** __________ Drugs used to treat cancer, including hematopoietic growth factors, biologic response modifiers, and monoclonal antibodies

(331) **7.** __________ An agent that inhibits the maturation or reproduction of malignant cells

(320) **8.** __________ Tumor; may be benign or malignant

(330) **9.** __________ Use of chemicals to treat illness

(320) **10.** __________ Not malignant

(330) **11.** __________ Loss of hair

B. Of the following normal cells, check the six that are most sensitive to radiation. *(330)*

__________ nail beds

__________ digestive and urinary tract linings

__________ respiratory tract lining

__________ skin

__________ lymph tissue

__________ ovaries

__________ kidneys

__________ lungs

__________ testes

__________ hair follicle

__________ bone marrow

Student Name____

C. Of the following drugs, check the four types of antineoplastic drugs that are frequently used in chemotherapy. *(332)*

__________ diuretics

__________ bronchodilators

__________ hormones

__________ antihistamines

__________ narcotics

__________ alkylating agents

__________ antithyroid drugs

__________ antiemetics

__________ sedative

__________ antihypertensives

__________ antitumor antibiotics

__________ hypnotics

__________ biologic response modifiers

D. Check the three major systemic side effects of antineoplastic drugs from the following list. *(333)*

__________ dry mouth

__________ bone marrow suppression

__________ urinary retention

__________ sedation

__________ nausea and vomiting

__________ constipation

__________ dizziness

__________ alopecia

__________ electrolyte imbalance

__________ tachycardia

E. List seven warning signs of cancer.

(324) **1.** ____

(324) **2.** ____

(324) **3.** ____

(324) **4.** ____

(324) **5.** ____

(324) **6.** ____

(324) **7.** ____

F. Match the tissue affected in the numbered column with the type of tumor in the lettered column.

(323) 1. ________ Bone

(323) 2. ________ Pigment cells in the skin

(323) 3. ________ Fat tissue

(323) 4. ________ Cartilage

(323) 5. ________ Smooth muscle tissue

(323) 6. ________ Fibrous connective tissue

(323) 7. ________ Tissues in the skin, glands, and linings of the digestive, urinary, and respiratory tracts

(323) 8. ________ Blood-forming tissues

(323) 9. ________ Bone, muscle, and other connective tissue

A. Chondrosarcoma
B. Fibroma
C. Melanoma
D. Osteosarcoma
E. Leiomyoma
F. Lipoma
G. Leukemias and lymphoma
H. Sarcoma
I. Carcinoma

G. Match the definition in the numbered column with the most appropriate stage in the lettered column.

(323) 1. ________ There is limited spread of the cancer in the local area, usually to nearby lymph nodes

(323) 2. ________ The malignant cells are confined to the tissue of origin; there is no invasion of other tissues

(323) 3. ________ The cancer has metastasized to distant parts of the body

(323) 4. ________ The tumor is larger or has spread from the site of origin into nearby tissues, or both; regional lymph nodes are likely to be involved

A. Stage I
B. Stage II
C. Stage III
D. Stage IV

Student Name____

H. Match the definition or description in the numbered column with the most appropriate term in the lettered column.

(326) **1.** __________ Removal of cells from living tissue for microscopic examination

(326) **2.** __________ Used to detect cancers of digestive and urinary tracts

(326) **3.** __________ Useful for diagnosing tumors in the head or trunk

(326) **4.** __________ Insertion of lighted tubes into hollow organs or body cavities

(326) **5.** __________ Used to detect cancers of the central nervous system, spinal column, neck bones, and joints

(326) **6.** __________ Used to detect cancer cells in the cervix

(326) **7.** __________ Used to detect tissue abnormalities of cancers of the thyroid, liver, and lung

(326) **8.** __________ Used to detect solid tumors in the brain and breast

A. Magnetic resonance imaging
B. Computed tomography
C. Endoscopy
D. Papanicolaou smear
E. Biopsy
F. Positron emission tomography
G. Contrast radiographs
H. Radionuclide scans

I. Match the effect in the numbered column with the most appropriate drug in the lettered column.

(331) **1.** ________ Pulmonary inflammation and fibrosis

(331) **2.** ________ Neurotoxicity resulting in numbness and tingling of extremities

(331) **3.** ________ Toxic effects on the heart that may lead to heart failure

(331) **4.** ________ Hypersensitivity

A. Vincristine (Oncovin)
B. Doxorubicin (Adriamycin)
C. Bleomycin (Blenoxane)
D. Paclitaxel (Taxol)

J. Match the nursing diagnosis related to treatment of cancer in the numbered column with its most appropriate "related to" statement in the lettered column.

(338) **1.** ________ Impaired oral mucous membranes

(338) **2.** ________ Interrupted family processes

(338) **3.** ________ Anxiety

(338) **4.** ________ Risk for constipation

(338) **5.** ________ Imbalanced nutrition: less than body requirements

(338) **6.** ________ Dysfunctional grieving

(338) **7.** ________ Risk for infection

(338) **8.** ________ Fatigue

(338) **9.** ________ Ineffective individual coping

(338) **10.** ________ Disturbed body image

(338) **11.** ________ Risk for injury

(338) **12.** ________ Ineffective therapeutic regimen management

A. Multiple stressor or overwhelming threat to self
B. Decreased salivation or inflammation (stomatitis, mucositis)
C. Lack of knowledge, inadequate resources, denial, hopelessness
D. Effects and outcomes of treatment
E. Loss of body part or altered appearance or function
F. Decreased white blood cells or venous access devices
G. Illness and therapy
H. Alopecia, surgical scars, ostomies, and loss of function
I. Side effects of therapy
J. Anemia or effects of cancer
K. Anorexia, nausea, and vomiting
L. Decreased activity or drug side effects

Student Name____

MULTIPLE-CHOICE QUESTIONS

K. Choose the most appropriate answer.

(320) **1.** What is the second most common cause of death in the United States?

1. heart disease
2. cancer
3. accident
4. stroke

(321) **2.** The type of invasion that involves the movement of cancer cells into adjoining tissue is:

1. regional. 2. systemic.
3. localized. 4. centralized.

(322) **3.** What is the effect on cells and tissue when DNA of a normal cell is exposed to a carcinogen and irreversible changes occur in the DNA?

1. The cell appears abnormal but continues to function normally.
2. The cell is in a latent period before increased growth forms tumors.
3. A tumor develops.
4. Transformed cells relocate to remote sites.

(322) **4.** A patient whose primary tumor has grown and spread to regional lymph nodes but not to distant sites is staged:

1. T1, N2, M1.
2. T2, N1, M0.
3. T0, N3, M1.
4. T4, N0, M0.

(324) **5.** The recommended diet that may reduce the risk of some cancers is one that is:

1. high-protein.
2. high-fat.
3. high-fiber.
4. low-carbohydrate.

(323) **6.** Your patient has cancer that has been staged T1, N0, M0. You would interpret this information as:

1. minimal size and extension of tumor.
2. no sign of tumor.
3. malignancy in epithelial tissue but not in basement membrane.
4. progressively increasing size and extension.

(328) **7.** A treatment likely to be curative when tumors are confined in one area is:

1. radiotherapy.
2. chemotherapy.
3. immunotherapy.
4. surgery.

(328) **8.** The use of ionizing radiation in the treatment of disease is called:

1. biotherapy.
2. chemotherapy.
3. radiotherapy.
4. immunotherapy.

(328) **9.** Radiation has immediate and delayed effects on cells; the immediate effect is:

1. cell death.
2. alteration of DNA, which impairs cell's ability to reproduce.
3. interruption of the clotting cascade.
4. cell starvation.

(324) **10.** Androgenic steroids and certain estrogens are known to be:

1. anti-inflammatory.
2. carcinogenic.
3. biologic response modifiers.
4. appetite stimulants.

(331) **11.** A patient experiences erythema and peeling of skin while receiving radiation therapy. The appropriate nursing intervention is to:

1. increase fluid intake.
2. not use lotions.
3. watch for excessive bruising and bleeding.
4. report fever.

(331) **12.** Which side effect occurs in patients undergoing radiotherapy and also in patients taking antineoplastic drugs?

1. phlebitis at infusion site
2. erythema and peeling of skin
3. alopecia
4. cardiomyopathy

(321) **13.** The highest rate of death from prostate, colon, and breast cancer occurs among:

1. Caucasians.
2. Latinos.
3. Native Americans.
4. African-Americans.

(331) **14.** What is the most dangerous side effect of antineoplastic drugs?

1. alopecia
2. nausea and vomiting
3. electrolyte imbalance
4. bone marrow suppression

(332) **15.** A drug that boosts the body's natural defenses to combat malignant cells is:

1. vincristine.
2. interferon.
3. doxorubicin (Adriamycin).
4. paclitaxel (Taxol).

(339) **16.** The outcome criterion, a patient's completion of essential activities without dyspnea or tachycardia, is related to patients with:

1. alopecia.
2. loss of a body part.
3. anemia.
4. denial.

(339) **17.** The priority care for patients experiencing neurotoxicity from antineoplastic drugs is to:

1. monitor for edema.
2. protect the patient from infection.
3. protect extremities from injury.
4. assess skin turgor.

(339) **18.** Invasive procedures are minimized in patients with:

1. leukopenia.
2. thrombocytopenia.
3. anemia.
4. agranulocytosis.

(340) **19.** Compromised host precautions may be needed for patients with:

1. leukopenia.
2. thrombocytopenia.
3. anemia.
4. weight loss.

(342) **20.** What is appropriate teaching for the patient who is having external radiation therapy?

1. The treatment may be painful for the first 5 minutes, but the pain will subside.
2. You will be radioactive as long as the machine is turned on.
3. Skin markings made by the radiologist are used to mark areas that will not be irradiated.
4. Skin over the area being treated may become discolored and irritated.

CHAPTER 25

Student Name ______________________________

The Ostomy Patient

Answer Key: Textbook page references are provided as a guide for answering these questions. A complete answer key was provided for your instructor.

OBJECTIVES

1. List the indications for ostomy surgery to divert urine or feces.
2. Describe nursing interventions to prepare the patient for ostomy surgery.
3. Explain the types of procedures used for fecal diversion.
4. Assist in developing a nursing process to plan care for the patient with each of the following types of fecal diversion: ileostomy, continent ileostomy, ileoanal reservoir, and colostomy.
5. Explain the types of procedures done for urinary diversion.
6. Assist in developing a nursing care plan for the patient with each of the following types of urinary diversion: ureterostomy, ileal conduit, continent internal reservoir.
7. Discuss content to be included in teaching patients to learn to live with ostomies.

LEARNING ACTIVITIES

A. Match the definition in the numbered column with the most appropriate term in the lettered column.

(347) **1.** __________ Opening created to drain contents of an organ

(363) **2.** __________ Surgically created opening in the kidney to drain urine

(363) **3.** __________ Surgically created opening into the urinary bladder

A. Anastomosis
B. Colostomy
C. Continent
D. Ileostomy
E. Nephrostomy
F. Ostomy
G. Prolapse
H. Stoma
I. Ureterostomy
J. Vesicostomy

Continued next page

(347) **4.** __________ Surgical procedure that creates an opening into a body structure

(352) **5.** __________ Capable of controlling natural impulses; in relation to an ostomy, able to retain feces or urine

(358) **6.** __________ Surgically created opening in the ureter

(355) **7.** __________ Downward displacement

(358) **8.** __________ Communication or connection between two organs or parts of organs

(348) **9.** __________ Surgically created opening in the ileum

(354) **10.** __________ Surgically created opening in the colon

B. Complete the statements in the numbered column with the most appropriate term in the lettered column. Some terms may be used more that once, and some terms may not be used.

(348) **1.** When fecal matter is diverted from the colon, it may be liquid, semisolid, or formed; fecal matter in the ileum is __________.

(349) **2.** Following ileostomy surgery, the stoma is inspected for color and __________.

(348) **3.** The procedure that is required when the entire colon must be bypassed or removed is __________.

(349) **4.** Following ileostomy surgery, the base of the stoma is inspected for redness, purulent drainage, and __________.

(349) **5.** Following ileostomy surgery, a pale or bluish stoma may indicate poor __________.

(349) **6.** Following ileostomy surgery, the nurse should inform the physician if the color of the stoma is __________.

A. Ileostomy
B. Pale or blue
C. Circulation
D. Liquid
E. Red
F. Skin breakdown
G. Bleeding
H. Colostomy

Student Name____

C. Complete the statements in the numbered column with the appropriate term in the lettered column. Some terms may be used more than once, and some terms may not be used.

(359) **1.** An internal pouch created from a loop of ileum for storing fecal matter is called __________.

(355) **2.** The two main complications of colostomy are prolapse and __________.

(359) **3.** Two serious consequences of urinary tract infections following ureterostomy include kidney damage and __________.

(359) **4.** Yeast infections around the ureterostomy stoma may be treated with __________.

(356) **5.** A type of medication that can be inserted into a colostomy stoma to stimulate evacuation is __________.

(360) **6.** If odor is a problem with ureterostomy, the pouch can be soaked for 20–30 minutes in __________.

(359) **7.** Complications experienced by patients with cutaneous ureterostomies include stenosis and __________.

(355) **8.** Three contributing factors to prolapsed stoma include coughing or sneezing, a poorly attached stoma, and __________.

A. Urinary tract infections
B. Nystatin
C. Vinegar water
D. Ileostomy
E. Too small an abdominal opening
F. Continent ileostomy
G. Ureterostomy
H. Septicemia
I. Rectal suppository
J. Colostomy
K. Too large an abdominal opening
L. Stenosis
M. Lack of hand washing
N. Certain foods
O. 70% alcohol

D. Describe the signs and symptoms to observe in the postoperative ileostomy patient that would indicate electrolyte imbalances.

(350) **1.** Mental status changes

a. ______________________________

b. ______________________________

(350) **2.** Neuromuscular status changes

a. ______________________________

b. ______________________________

c. ______________________________

(350) **3.** Fluid volume changes

a. ______________________________

b. ______________________________

c. ______________________________

E. List four food groups that patients with continent ileostomies should avoid, at least initially.

(353) **1.** ______________________________

(353) **2.** ______________________________

(353) **3.** ______________________________

(353) **4.** ______________________________

Student Name______________________________

F. Using Figure 25-4 below, label each type of colostomy (A–D) and indicate which type of drainage is passed by each (E–G). Match the characteristics (H–I) to the appropriate type of colostomy. *(355)*

A. Descending colostomy
B. Ascending colostomy
C. Transverse colostomy
D. Sigmoid colostomy
E. Liquid to semisolid stool
F. Softly formed stool
G. Liquid material
H. Done for right-sided tumors
I. Often used in emergencies, such as intestinal obstruction, because it can be done quickly

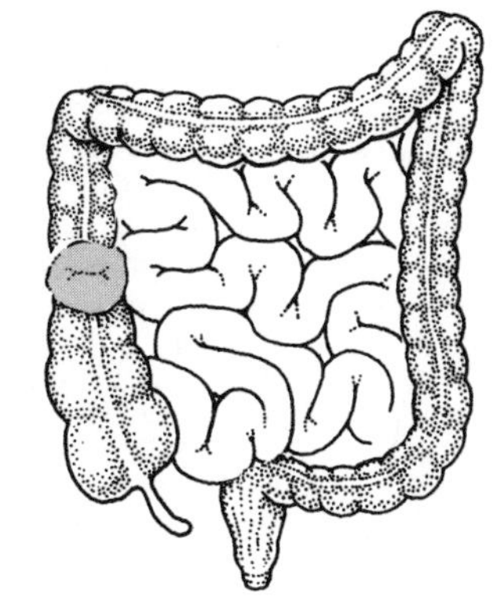

1. ______________________________
____

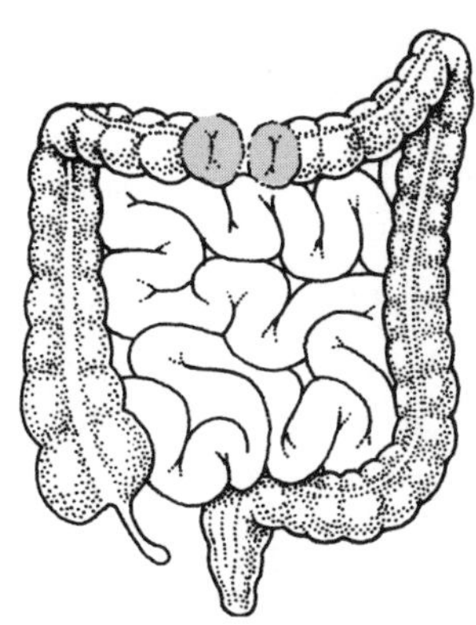

2. ______________________________
____

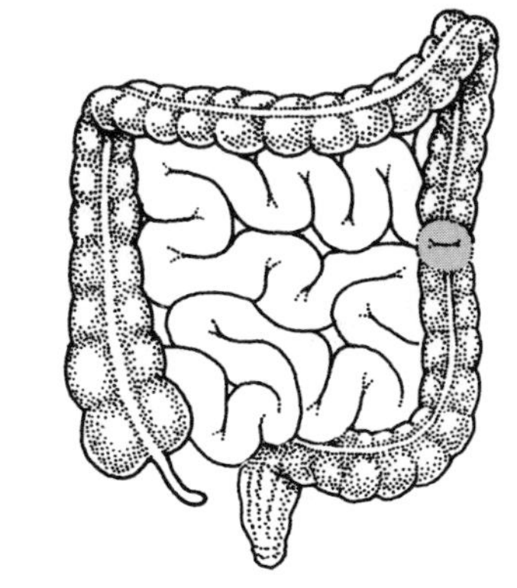

3. ______________________________
____

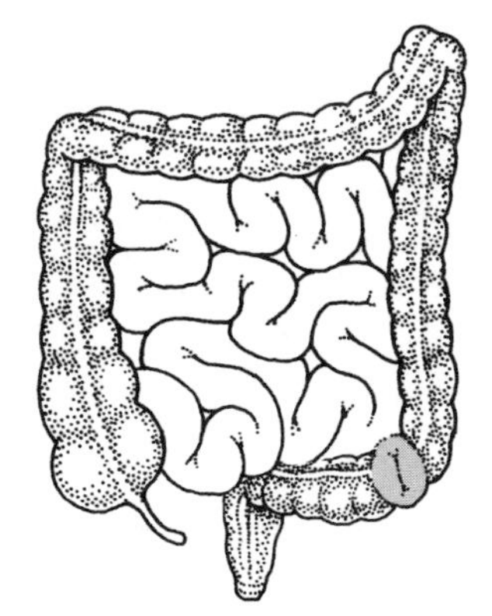

4. ______________________________
____

G. Using Figure 25-5 below, label the types of urinary diversion procedures (A–E) using the following terms. *(358)*

A. Continent internal ileal reservoir
B. Colon conduit
C. Ureterosigmoidostomy
D. Ileal conduit
E. Cutaneous ureterostomy

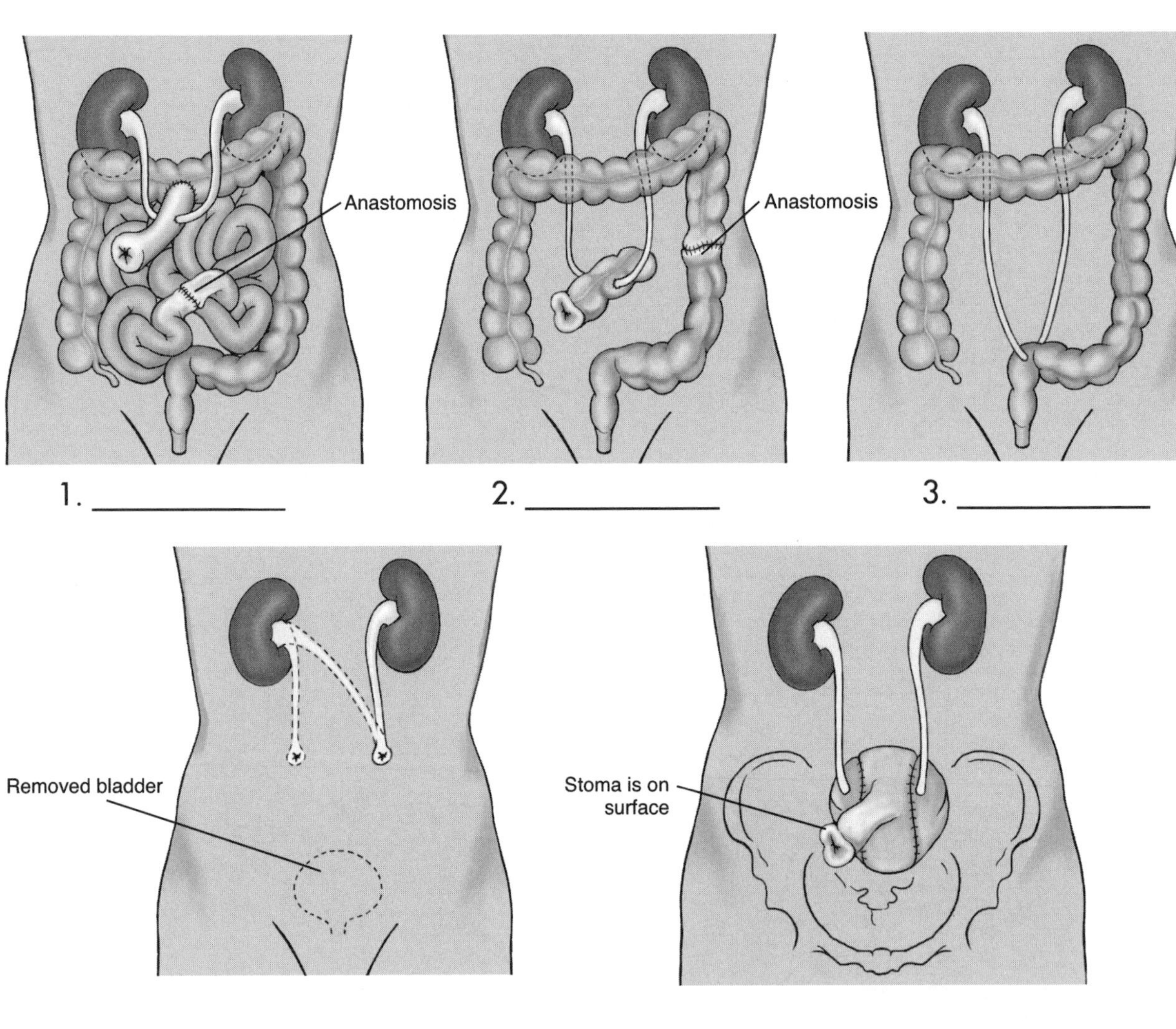

Student Name______________________________

MULTIPLE-CHOICE QUESTIONS

H. Choose the most appropriate answer.

(355) **1.** A colostomy is performed by bringing a loop of the intestine through the wall of the:

1. bladder.
2. rectum.
3. abdomen.
4. stomach.

(355) **2.** Which complication of colostomy involves the narrowing of the abdominal opening around the base of the stoma?

1. prolapse
2. stenosis
3. obstruction
4. evisceration

(356) **3.** A nursing diagnosis for the colostomy patient is Risk for injury related to:

1. hemorrhage or infection.
2. dyspnea or tachycardia.
3. hypotension or bradycardia.
4. prolapse or stenosis.

(358) **4.** If you notice that the colostomy is not draining properly:

1. place a gloved finger in the stoma to dilate it.
2. use a larger catheter to irrigate.
3. inform the physician.
4. force the catheter in 3 inches.

(350) **5.** The loss of bicarbonate in ileostomy drainage can result in:

1. hypokalemia.
2. hypercalcemia.
3. metabolic acidosis.
4. fluid volume excess.

(362) **6.** If the ileal conduit stoma turns gray or black, the physician should be notified immediately, as it may mean that:

1. ureteral obstruction has occurred.
2. circulation is impaired.
3. wound infection is present.
4. prolapse has occurred.

(362) **7.** After bowel resection for the ileal conduit procedure, you should expect:

1. necrosis of the wound.
2. temporary ileus (absence of bowel activity).
3. gray-black stoma.
4. ureteral calculi.

(362) **8.** In which procedure would the nurse expect to find mucus in the drainage?

1. ureterostomy
2. vesicostomy
3. cystostomy
4. ileal conduit

(353) **9.** A patient with a continent ileostomy develops bloody diarrhea, anorexia, and pain. You suspect this patient has:

1. peritonitis.
2. inflammation of the reservoir.
3. leaking of suture lines.
4. obstruction of pouch drainage.

(353) **10.** Abdominal distention, nausea and vomiting, and decreased bowel sounds are signs and symptoms of:

1. inflammation of the ileoanal reservoir.
2. peritonitis.
3. small bowel obstruction.
4. hemorrhage.

(353) **11.** The Kock pouch is made with a section of:

1. sigmoid colon.
2. jejunum.
3. ileum.
4. ascending colon.

(353) **12.** A patient with an ileostomy one week postoperatively has a pulse of 120, respirations 28, temperature of 101° F, and a rigid abdomen. You suspect that this patient has which complication?

1. obstruction
2. peritonitis
3. inflammation
4. evisceration of the site

(354) **13.** Which foods tend to produce thicker stools?

1. milk and cottage cheese
2. fresh fruits
3. green, leafy vegetables
4. pasta and boiled rice

(354) **14.** Why is a nasogastric tube placed in a patient with bowel obstruction?

1. dilate the digestive tract
2. decompress the bowel
3. provide method of feeding
4. improve peristalsis

(356) **15.** What is a complication of colostomy irrigation?

1. obstruction
2. diarrhea
3. infection
4. perforated bowel

(354) **16.** The reason metronidazole (Flagyl) is given to patients with an ileoanal reservoir is that it treats:

1. pain.
2. bleeding.
3. inflammation.
4. fluid volume deficit.

(356) **17.** Which condition in a patient with a colostomy requires the nurse to contact the physician immediately?

1. prolapse
2. perforated bowel
3. diarrhea
4. red stoma

(354) **18.** Which of the following is a sign of bowel obstruction?

1. bloody stools
2. fever
3. abdominal distention
4. hypotension

(355) **19.** Which of the following is a major long-term complication caused by coughing in a patient with a colostomy?

1. prolapse
2. stenosis
3. obstruction
4. inflammation

(359) **20.** Which is a complication of ureterostomy?

1. obstruction
2. perforation
3. hydronephrosis
4. prolapse

(359) **21.** Which drug is used to treat a rash around the stoma of a patient with a ureterostomy?

1. tetracycline 2. Neosporin
3. Benadryl 4. nystatin

(348) **22.** Which group has the highest rate of colon and rectal cancers?

1. Asians
2. African-Americans
3. Caucasians
4. Native Americans

CHAPTER 26

Student Name ____________________

Neurologic Disorders

Answer Key: Textbook page references are provided as a guide for answering these questions. A complete answer key was provided for your instructor.

OBJECTIVES

1. Identify common neurologic changes in the older person and the implications of these for nursing care.
2. Describe the diagnostic tests and procedures used to evaluate neurologic dysfunction and the nursing responsibilities associated with each.
3. Identify the uses, side effects, and nursing interventions associated with common drug therapies employed in patients with neurologic disorders.
4. Describe the signs and symptoms associated with increased intracranial pressure and the medical therapies used in treatment.
5. List the components of the nursing assessment of the patient with a neurologic disorder.
6. Describe the pathophysiology, signs and symptoms, complications, and medical or surgical treatment for patients with selected neurologic disorders.
7. Assist in developing a nursing care plan for the patient with a neurologic disorder.

LEARNING ACTIVITIES

A. Match the definition in the numbered column with the most appropriate term in the lettered column.

(383) **1.** ________ Abnormal extension of the upper extremities with extension of the lower extremities; accompanies increased pressure on the entire cerebrum and the motor tract structures of the brain stem

(365) **2.** ________ Biochemical messenger at nerve endings that stimulates an excitatory or inhibitory impulse

(387) **3.** ________ A peculiar sensation that precedes a set of symptoms

(382) **4.** ________ Weakness on one side of the body

(383) **5.** ________ Abnormal flexion of the upper extremities with extension of the lower extremities; accompanies increased pressure on the frontal lobes

(404) **6.** ________ Pain in a nerve or along the course of a nerve

(394) **7.** ________ An abnormal sensation

(393) **8.** ________ Inflammation of brain tissue

A. Aura
B. Dysautonomia
C. Contralateral
D. Extension (decerebrate) posturing
E. Abnormal flexion (decorticate) posturing
F. Encephalitis
G. Hemiparesis
H. Hemiplegia
I. Intracranial
J. Ipsilateral
K. Neuralgia
L. Neurotransmitter
M. Paresthesia
N. Postictal
O. Seizure

Continued next page

Student Name____

(394) **9.** __________ Effects on the autonomic nervous system

(376) **10.** __________ Affecting the same side

(382) **11.** __________ Paralysis on one side of the body

(376) **12.** __________ Affecting the opposite side

(371, 382) **13.** __________ Within the skull

(385) **14.** __________ Convulsion; series of involuntary contractions of voluntary muscles

(386) **15.** __________ After a seizure

B. List four neurotransmitters.

(367) **1.** ____________________

(367) **2.** ____________________

(367) **3.** ____________________

(367) **4.** ____________________

C. List how the four parts of the nervous system listed below change with normal aging.

(368) **1.** Nerve cells (number): ____________________

(368) **2.** Brain (weight): ____________________

(368) **3.** Ventricles (size): ____________________

(368) **4.** Nerve tissues: ____________________

D. List normal characteristics of pupils that are noted in pupillary evaluation regarding the three areas below.

(372) **1.** Size: ____________________

(372) **2.** Shape: ____________________

(372) **3.** Reactivity: ____________________

E. Indicate the measures that are taken in each of the following areas for patients with increased ICP.

(384) **1.** Positioning: ____________________

(384) **2.** Hyperventilation: ____________________

(384) **3.** Fluid restriction: ____________________

(384) **4.** Mechanical drainage: ____________________

(384) **5.** Drug therapy: ____________________

F. Complete the table below by filling in the appropriate "related to" statements and nursing goals for the patient with amyotrophic lateral sclerosis (ALS).

(401)

Nursing Diagnosis	Related To:	Nursing Goals/Outcome Criteria
Ineffective airway clearance		
Impaired physical mobility		participation in activities to maintain mobility
Imbalanced nutrition: less than body requirements	dysphagia	
Impaired verbal communication		effective communication
Impaired skin integrity		
Anticipatory grieving	progressive, fatal disease	
Situational low self-esteem		
Altered family processes		

G. In each of the physical examination areas in the numbered column, indicate the possible age-related change by matching it to a term in the lettered column. Some terms may be used more than once, and some terms may not be used.

(368) **1.** ________ Pupil of the eye

(368) **2.** ________ Pupillary response to light

(368) **3.** ________ Tracking movement of eye

(368) **4.** ________ Reflexes

(368) **5.** ________ Achilles tendon jerk

(368) **6.** ________ Reaction time

A. Slower
B. Decrease(s)
C. Remain(s) intact
D. Larger
E. Faster
F. May be absent
G. Smooth
H. Increase(s)
I. Jerky
J. Smaller

Student Name____

H. Complete the statements in the numbered column with the most appropriate term in the lettered column. Some terms may be used more than once, and some terms may not be used.

(372) **1.** Decreased responsiveness accompanied by lack of spontaneous motor activity is __________.

(372) **2.** A patient who cannot be aroused even by powerful stimuli is __________.

(371) **3.** The most accurate and reliable indicator of neurologic status is the __________.

(372) **4.** Excessive drowsiness is __________.

(372) **5.** If a patient is stuporous but can be aroused, the patient is __________.

(372) **6.** Unnatural drowsiness or sleepiness is __________.

A. Agitation
B. Level of consciousness
C. Combativeness
D. Somnolence
E. Neuromuscular response
F. Lethargy
G. Comatose
H. Pupillary evaluation
I. Semicomatose
J. Stupor

I. Complete the statements in the numbered column with the most appropriate term in the lettered column. Some terms may be used more than once, and some terms may not be used.

(384) **1.** The most common type of pain __________.

(392) **2.** Inflammation of the coverings of the brain and spinal cord caused by either viral or bacterial organisms is called __________.

(393) **3.** Inflammation of brain tissue usually caused by a virus is __________.

(393) **4.** A rapidly progressing disease that affects the motor component of the peripheral nervous system is __________.

(396) **5.** A progressive degenerative disorder that results in an eventual loss of coordination and control over involuntary motor movement is __________.

A. Meningitis
B. Parkinson's disease
C. Seizure disorder
D. Cerebral palsy
E. Guillain-Barré syndrome
F. Headache
G. Encephalitis

J. Complete the statements in the numbered column with the most appropriate term in the lettered column. Some terms may be used more than once, and some terms may not be used.

(402) **1.** The amount of acetylcholine available at the neuromuscular junction is reduced in __________.

(398) **2.** A chronic progressive degenerative disease that attacks the protective myelin sheath around axons and disrupts motor pathways of the CNS is __________.

(401) **3.** A degenerative neurologic disease, which is also known as Lou Gehrig's disease, is __________.

(398) **4.** Young adults have the highest rate of incidence, with women affected more frequently than men, in __________.

(401) **5.** A disease that affects males more than females, striking most often between 40 and 70 years of age, is __________.

(402) **6.** An inherited degenerative neurologic disorder that begins in middle adulthood with abnormal movements is __________.

(402) **7.** A chronic, progressive disease in which there is a defect at the neuromuscular junction, where electrical impulses are transmitted to muscle tissue, is __________.

A. ALS
B. Huntington's disease
C. Parkinson's disease
D. Myasthenia gravis
E. MS
F. Cerebral palsy
G. Guillain-Barré syndrome

Student Name____

K. Indicate whether the following responses are controlled by the (A) sympathetic or (B) parasympathetic nervous system.

(370)	**1.**	________	Bronchial dilation	A. Sympathetic nervous system B. Parasympathetic nervous system
(370)	**2.**	________	Pupil constriction	
(370)	**3.**	________	Increased gut peristalsis and tone in lumen	
(370)	**4.**	________	Decreased rate and force of cardiac contractions	
(370)	**5.**	________	Pupil dilation	
(370)	**6.**	________	Bronchial constriction	
(370)	**7.**	________	Decreased gut peristalsis and tone in lumen	
(370)	**8.**	________	Increased rate and force of cardiac contractions	
(368)	**9.**	________	Flight-or-fight response	
(368)	**10.**	________	Mediates rest response	

L. Match the dysfunctions in the numbered column with the corresponding part of the brain in the lettered column. Some terms may be used more than once, and some terms may not be used.

(376)	**1.**	________	Loss of steady gait	A. Cerebellum B. Hypothalamus
(376)	**2.**	________	Dysfunction occurring on the same side as the offending lesion	C. Cerebral cortex D. Spinal cord
(376)	**3.**	________	Motor dysfunction on the opposite side from the lesion	
(376)	**4.**	________	Loss of steady, balanced posture	

M. Match the intervention or description in the numbered column with the appropriate diagnostic test in the lettered column. Some diagnostic tests may be used more than once, and some tests may not be used.

(374) **1.** ________ People who are confused or claustrophobic may require mild sedation before this test

(373) **2.** ________ A shampoo is done before the test, and medications, such as anticonvulsants and stimulants, are withheld 24 to 48 hours before the test

(373, 378) **3.** ________ Tell the patient to expect to lie still on a stretcher while the dye is injected and radiographs are taken of the head

(374) **4.** ________ Keep the patient flat, and "log-roll" the patient for up to 48 hours

(378) **5.** ________ A cannula is usually inserted into the femoral artery, and a catheter is advanced to the carotid or vertebral arteries

(373) **6.** ________ Needle electrodes are placed on several points over a nerve and muscles supplied by the nerve

A. Brain scan
B. Lumbar puncture
C. Magnetic resonance imaging
D. Pneumoencephalography
E. CT scan
F. Cerebral angiography
G. Electromyography
H. Pupillary evaluation
I. Electroencephalogram

Continued next page

Student Name ______________________

(374) **7.** __________ Special infusion pumps, oxygen equipment, and ventilators are used

(373) **8.** __________ Encourage fluid intake following the procedure to minimize headache

(373, 378) **9.** __________ Inform the radiologist about any allergies to iodine, shellfish, or contrast media

(373) **10.** __________ Patient must remain on one side in a knee-to-chest position

(378) **11.** __________ Potassium chloride is given 2 hours before the isotope is given for this test to prevent excessive isotope uptake

(374) **12.** __________ Because air, blood, bone, tissue, and CSF have varying densities, they appear in various shades of gray in this test

(378) **13.** __________ A contrast dye is injected, followed by a series of radiographs

(374) **14.** __________ Tell the patient to expect to hear a noise like a muffled drumbeat while in the machine

N. Match the definition or description in the numbered column with the most appropriate term in the lettered column.

(382) **1.** __________ Surgery that requires opening the skull

(379) **2.** __________ Excision of a segment of the skull

(382) **3.** __________ Procedure done to repair a skull defect

A. Cranioplasty
B. Craniotomy
C. Craniectomy

O. Match the definition in the numbered column with the most appropriate term in the lettered column. Some terms may be used more than once, and some terms may not be used.

(387) **1.** ________ Lacerations, contusions, abrasions, and hematomas

(387) **2.** ________ Head trauma in which there is no visible injury to the skull or brain

(388) **3.** ________ Head trauma in which there is actual bruising and bleeding in the brain tissue

(388) **4.** ________ A collection of blood, usually clotted, which may be classified as subdural or epidural

(388) **5.** ________ Injuries resulting from sharp objects that penetrate the skull and brain tissue

A. Contusion(s)
B. Seizure(s)
C. Scalp injuries
D. Penetrating injuries
E. Amnesia
F. Hematoma
G. Concussion
H. Fixed pupils

P. Match the nursing diagnosis for patients with meningitis in the numbered column with the "related to" statement in the lettered column.

(393) **1.** ________ Altered cerebral tissue perfusion

(393) **2.** ________ Ineffective breathing pattern

(393) **3.** ________ Acute pain

(393) **4.** ________ Risk for injury

(393) **5.** ________ Deficient fluid volume

(393) **6.** ________ Risk for disuse syndrome

A. Confusion, seizures, restlessness
B. Irritation of the meninges
C. Bed rest
D. Increased intracranial pressure
E. Vomiting and fever
F. Depression of the respiratory center

Student Name____

Q. Match the description of symptoms of Parkinson's disease in the numbered column with the most appropriate term in the lettered column. Some terms may be used more than once, and some may not be used.

(396)	**1.**	__________	Trembling, shaking type of movement usually seen in upper extremities	A.	Bradykinesia
				B.	Tremor
				C.	Bradycardia
				D.	Rigidity
				E.	Pill-rolling
				F.	Dementia
(396)	**2.**	__________	Stiffness		
(396)	**3.**	__________	Extremely slow movements		
(396)	**4.**	__________	Movement of thumb against fingertips		

R. Match the uses of drugs in the numbered column with names of drugs used for multiple sclerosis in the lettered column.

(399)	**1.**	__________	Anti-inflammatory drug used during period of exacerbation	A.	Betaseron (interferon beta-1b)
				B.	Prednisone
				C.	Baclofen
				D.	ACTH
(399)	**2.**	__________	Anti-inflammatory drug used to encourage remission		
(399)	**3.**	__________	Drug used to decrease the frequency of recurrent neurologic episodes in relapsing-remitting MS		
(399)	**4.**	__________	Drug used to treat the spasticity experienced by MS patients		

S. Match the definition in the numbered column with the most appropriate neurologic disease in the lettered column. Some diseases may be used more than once, and some diseases may not be used.

(404) **1.** ________ A disease characterized by intense pain along nerve lines in the face

(405) **2.** ________ A disease characterized by multiple tumors of peripheral, spinal, and cranial nerves

(405) **3.** ________ Acute paralysis of the seventh cranial nerve

(406) **4.** ________ Paralysis associated with a loss in motor coordination caused by cerebral damage

(406) **5.** ________ Progressive muscle weakness, fatigue, pain, and respiratory problems years after the initial infection, illness, and recovery

A. Myasthenia gravis
B. Neurofibromatosis
C. Cerebral palsy
D. Bell's palsy
E. Parkinson's disease
F. Postpolio syndrome
G. Trigeminal neuralgia
H. Multiple sclerosis

MULTIPLE-CHOICE QUESTIONS

T. Choose the most appropriate answer.

(373) **1.** To minimize headache following a lumbar puncture, what should be increased?

1. calcium 2. fluid intake
3. potassium 4. ambulation

(382) **2.** The family should be advised that a craniotomy can take as long as:

1. 2 hours. 2. 6 hours.
3. 12 hours. 4. 24 hours.

(382) **3.** As ICP increases and perfusion is reduced, oxygen delivery to cerebral tissue is:

1. increased. 2. bypassed.
3. reduced. 4. stopped.

Student Name____

(382) **4.** Classic pupillary changes are seen in increasing ICP. Sometimes a "blown pupil" is observed, which means that the pupil:

1. is dilated.
2. is pinpoint.
3. reacts to light.
4. is unequal to the other pupil.

(382) **5.** The pupils may become dilated and fixed as ICP rises due to pressure on the:

1. oculomotor nerve.
2. cerebellum.
3. hypothalamus.
4. optic nerve.

(373, 378) **6.** The primary route for arterial blood flow to the brain is the:

1. carotid artery.
2. subclavian vein.
3. jugular vein.
4. inferior vena cava.

(385) **7.** A type of headache in which the pain is usually unilateral and has a warning is called:

1. cluster.
2. migraine.
3. tension.
4. sinus.

(385) **8.** Seizure activity involves a large number of hyperactive neurons that use excessive:

1. calcium and vitamin D
2. potassium and chloride
3. sodium and iron
4. oxygen and glucose

(392) **9.** Management of bacterial meningitis revolves around prompt recognition and treatment with:

1. corticosteroids.
2. antihistamines.
3. anticholinergics.
4. antimicrobials.

(395) **10.** One common source of anxiety for many patients with Guillain-Barré syndrome is impaired:

1. communication.
2. self-esteem.
3. circulation.
4. elimination.

(396) **11.** In order to reduce the symptoms of Parkinson's disease, L-dopa crosses the blood-brain barrier and is converted to:

1. epinephrine.
2. dopamine.
3. norepinephrine.
4. acetylcholine.

(404) **12.** Trigeminal neuralgia is characterized by:

1. hypotension.
2. tachycardia.
3. infection.
4. intense pain.

(403) **13.** In myasthenia gravis, rapid improvement of muscle strength after administration of edrophonium chloride (Tensilon) indicates an underlying:

1. hypertensive crisis.
2. adrenergic crisis.
3. myasthenic crisis.
4. cholinergic crisis.

CHAPTER 27

Student Name ______________________________

Cerebrovascular Accident

Answer Key: Textbook page references are provided as a guide for answering these questions. A complete answer key was provided for your instructor.

OBJECTIVES

1. Discuss the risk factors for cerebrovascular accident (CVA).
2. Identify the four types of CVA.
3. Describe the pathophysiology, signs and symptoms, and medical treatment for each type of CVA.
4. Describe the neurologic deficits that may result from CVA.
5. Explain the tests and procedures used to diagnose a CVA, and nursing responsibilities for patients undergoing those tests and procedures.
6. List data to be included in the nursing assessment of the CVA patient.
7. Assist in developing a nursing process for a CVA patient during the acute and rehabilitation phases.
8. Specify criteria used to evaluate the outcomes of nursing care for the CVA patient.
9. Identify resources for the CVA patient and family.

LEARNING ACTIVITIES

A. Match the definition in the numbered column with the most appropriate term in the lettered column.

(415) **1.** ________ Inability to speak clearly because of neurologic damage that impairs normal muscle control

(412) **2.** ________ Between the arachnoid and pia mater layers of the membranes covering the brain

(422) **3.** ________ Drooping of the upper eyelid

(415) **4.** ________ Difficulty speaking, reading, and writing

(410) **5.** ________ Neurologic deficits that last less than 24 hours; caused by diminished cerebral blood flow

(422) **6.** ________ Double vision

(414) **7.** ________ The inability to understand words or the inability to respond with words, or both

(416) **8.** ________ Loss of half the field of vision; loss is on the side opposite the brain lesion

(415) **9.** ________ Partial inability to initiate coordinated voluntary motor acts

(414) **10.** ________ Ability to speak clearly but without meaning

A. Intracerebral
B. Hemiplegia
C. Nonfluent aphasia
D. Dyspraxia
E. Dysarthria
F. Ptosis
G. Subarachnoid
H. Homonymous hemianopsia
I. Expressive aphasia
J. Receptive aphasia
K. Transient ischemic attack
L. Aphasia
M. Dysphagia
N. Diplopia

Continued next page

Student Name____

(412) **11.** __________ Within the cerebrum

(415) **12.** __________ Difficulty swallowing

(414) **13.** __________ Inability to comprehend words

(415) **14.** __________ Paralysis of one side of the body

B. Match the definition or description in the numbered column with the most appropriate term in the lettered column. Some terms may be used more than once, and some terms may not be used.

(408) **1.** __________ The part of the brain that controls the left side of the body

(408) **2.** __________ The part of the brain that controls the right side of the body

(408) **3.** __________ The part of the brain that controls vital basic functions, including respiration, heart rate, and consciousness

(408) **4.** __________ The part of the brain that coordinates movement, balance, and posture

(410) **5.** __________ The circulatory system in the cerebrum

(408) **6.** __________ The part of the brain that controls analytic mental processes such as language ability, mathematics, and reasoning powers

(408) **7.** __________ The part of the brain that incudes the midbrain, pons, and medulla

(408) **8.** __________ The part of the brain that controls emotional and artistic tendencies

A. Cerebellum
B. Brain stem
C. Spinal cord
D. Cerebrovascular system
E. Right hemisphere
F. Cerebrum
G. Left hemisphere

C. Match the definition or description in the numbered column with the most appropriate term in the lettered column. Some terms may be used more than once, and some terms may not be used.

(411) **1.** ________ An important warning condition for a possible later stroke

(413) **2.** ________ A buildup of fatty deposits in the blood vessels

(411) **3.** ________ The common name for cerebrovascular accident

(411) **4.** ________ A temporary neurologic deficit caused by impairment of cerebral blood flow

(411) **5.** ________ A "swooshing" noise in a clogged carotid artery that can be auscultated in diagnosing a TIA

(411) **6.** ________ Opening an obstructed blood vessel and removing the plaque

A. Bruit
B. Transient ischemic attack (TIA)
C. Angioplasty
D. Stroke
E. Endarterectomy
F. Atherosclerosis

D. Complete the statement in the numbered column with the most appropriate term in the lettered column. Some terms may be used more than once, and some terms may not be used.

(415) **1.** Three factors that create problems related to physical mobility for the stroke patient are dyspraxia, visual field disturbances, and ________.

(421) **2.** Two causes of thick secretions being retained in the respiratory tract following CVA are immobility and ________.

A. Aspiration
B. Injury
C. Homonymous hemianopsia
D. Edema
E. Oxygenation
F. Hypertension
G. Urinary tract infection
H. Dehydration
I. Hemiplegia
J. Diplopia
K. Dysphagia
L. Pneumonia

Continued next page

Student Name____

(415) **3.** Dysphagia may result in airway obstruction or pneumonia due to __________.

(416) **4.** Patients who see only half the field of vision following a stroke have __________.

(416) **5.** The most frequent cause of death following a stroke is __________.

(422) **6.** Dehydration in patients following a stroke may result in signs and symptoms of constipation, skin dryness, and __________.

(417) **7.** A priority immediately after a stroke is __________.

(422) **8.** A sensory-perceptual problem in a patient with a stroke is __________.

(422) **9.** The patient who does not feel pressure or pain due to lost sensation following a stroke is susceptible to __________.

E. Match the nursing diagnosis for the patient with a CVA in the numbered column with the most appropriate "related to" statement in the lettered column.

(420) **1.** __________ Risk for injury

(420) **2.** __________ Risk for deficient fluid volume

(420) **3.** __________ Risk for fluid volume excess

(418) **4.** __________ Imbalanced nutrition: less than body requirements

(421) **5.** __________ Interrupted family processes

(420) **6.** __________ Ineffective airway clearance

(419) **7.** __________ Impaired verbal communication

(421) **8.** __________ Impaired physical mobility

(420) **9.** __________ Ineffective breathing pattern

(421) **10.** __________ Total or functional incontinence

(421) **11.** __________ Disturbed thought processes

(421) **12.** __________ Disturbed sensory perception; ineffective thermoregulation

A. Dysphagia, inability to feed self, inability to chew
B. Impaired cough reflex, altered consciousness, impaired swallowing
C. Inadequate intake, excessive diuresis
D. Weakness, paralysis, spasticity, impaired balance
E. Seizure activity, confusion, motor impairment
F. Overhydration
G. Disruption of family roles and functions
H. Aphasia
I. Impaired cerebral circulation
J. Inability to manage a toileting process
K. Increased intracranial pressure
L. Neurologic impairment

F. Match the uses of drugs in the numbered column with the drugs used for treatment of stroke in the lettered column.

(417) **1.** ________ Used to treat cerebral edema

(417) **2.** ________ Used to treat subarachnoid hemorrhage by dilating and preventing spasms in cerebral blood vessels

(417) **3.** ________ Used to reduce intracranial pressure by reducing cerebral inflammation

(417) **4.** ________ Used to prevent strokes caused by thrombi

(417) **5.** ________ Used to dissolve clots that cause acute ischemic stroke

(417) **6.** ________ Used to treat seizures, if seizures are present with stroke

(417) **7.** ________ Used to break up clots

A. Anticonvulsants, such as phenytoin and phenobarbital
B. Platelet aggregation inhibitors, such as aspirin
C. Hyperosmotic agents, such as mannitol
D. Streptokinase
E. Calcium channel blockers, such as nimodipine
F. Tissue plasminogen activator (TPA)
G. Corticosteroids

MULTIPLE-CHOICE QUESTIONS

G. Choose the most appropriate answer.

(408) **1.** A folded layer of nerve cells that covers each hemisphere of the brain is called the:

1. cerebellum.
2. cerebrum.
3. gyrus.
4. cortex.

(419) **2.** One of the most important needs of the acute stroke patient is to be turned and repositioned at least every:

1. 2 hours.
2. 4 hours.
3. 8 hours.
4. 12 hours.

Student Name____________________

(423) **3.** Turning and repositioning the stroke patient will reduce the incidence of:

1. hypertension.
2. skin breakdown.
3. headache.
4. cerebral edema.

(411) **4.** A warning condition for a possible later stroke is:

1. TIA.
2. paralysis.
3. hemorrhage.
4. cyanosis.

(416) **5.** If increased intracranial pressure is suspected in a patient with a stroke, which diagnostic test is contraindicated?

1. CT scan
2. MRI
3. PET
4. lumbar puncture

(422) **6.** Diminished or lost sensation in body parts occurs in many stroke patients. The patient who does not feel pressure or pain is susceptible to:

1. injury.
2. infection.
3. pneumonia.
4. dyspnea.

(424) **7.** Constipation may develop in the stroke patient due to dehydration, drug therapy, and:

1. infection.
2. cerebral edema.
3. loss of sensation on one side.
4. immobility.

(426) **8.** In the acute phase following a stroke, if the patient has homonymous hemianopsia, the environment is arranged so that the important items are available on the:

1. unaffected side.
2. affected side.
3. left side.
4. right side.

(424) **9.** The main focus of the rehabilitation phase following a stroke is to:

1. cure the disease process.
2. assist the patient into remission.
3. prevent another stroke from occurring.
4. return the patient to the highest functional level possible.

(416) **10.** The most frequent cause of death in stroke patients is:

1. kidney failure.
2. pneumonia.
3. seizure.
4. heart attack.

CHAPTER 28

Student Name ______________________________

Spinal Cord Injury

Answer Key: Textbook page references are provided as a guide for answering these questions. A complete answer key was provided for your instructor.

OBJECTIVES

1. Explain the impact of spinal cord injury.
2. Describe the diagnostic tests used to evaluate spinal cord injuries and related nursing responsibilities.
3. Explain the physical effects of spinal cord injury.
4. Describe the medical and surgical treatment during the acute phase of spinal cord injury.
5. List the data to be included in the nursing assessment of the patient with a spinal cord injury.
6. Identify nursing diagnoses, goals, interventions, and outcome criteria for the patient with a spinal cord injury.
7. Describe the nursing care for the patient undergoing a laminectomy.
8. State the goals of rehabilitation for the patient with spinal cord injury.

LEARNING ACTIVITIES

A. Match the definition in the numbered column with the most appropriate term in the lettered column.

(436) **1.** ________ Loss of motor and sensory function in all four extremities due to damage to the spinal cord

(439) **2.** ________ Soft, in relation to muscle, lacking tone

(439) **3.** ________ Abnormally exaggerated response of the autonomic nervous system to a stimulus

A. Paraplegia
B. Myelinated
C. Quadriplegia; tetraplegia
D. Dermatome
E. Flaccid
F. Spastic
G. Autonomic dysreflexia

Continued next page

(436) **4.** __________ Loss of motor and sensory function due to damage to the spinal cord that spares the upper extremities but, depending on the level of the damage, affects the trunk, pelvic, and lower extremities

(439) **5.** __________ Increased muscle tone characterized by sudden, involuntary muscle spasms

(444) **6.** __________ Area of skin supplied by sensory nerve fibers from a single posterior spinal root

(433) **7.** __________ Surrounded with a sheath

B. Complete the statements in the numbered column with the most appropriate term in the lettered column. Some terms may be used more than once, and some terms may not be used.

(439) **1.** As spinal shock begins to subside and reflex activity returns, the patient is at risk for __________.

(439) **2.** Cervical injuries below the level of C4 spare the diaphragm, but they can involve the impairment of the __________.

(439) **3.** An immediate, transient response to injury in which reflex activity below the level of the injury temporarily ceases is called __________.

(439) **4.** A very serious and potentially dangerous problem for the patient with a spinal cord injury, which is described as an exaggerated response of the autonomic nervous system in the patient whose injury is at or above the T6 level, is called __________.

(440) **5.** An increase in muscle tone is called __________.

(447) **6.** When the abdomen becomes distended and bowel sounds are absent, peristalsis has ceased; a condition called __________.

A. Spinal shock
B. Respiratory arrest
C. Autonomic dysreflexia
D. Spasticity
E. Flaccidity
F. Intercostal muscles
G. Ileus
H. Coma

Student Name____

C. Match the description in the numbered column with the most appropriate stage in the lettered column. Some stages may be used more than once, and some terms may not be used.

(441)	**1.**	__________ When the patient is ready to tackle the work of rehabilitation	A.	Impact
			B.	Denial
			C.	Acknowledgment
			D.	Retreat
			E.	Reconstruction
(441)	**2.**	__________ When the patient is in emotional shock and may express a desire to die	F.	Remediation
(441)	**3.**	__________ When the patient is ready to begin to plan for the future		
(441)	**4.**	__________ When the patient begins to face the injury and deal with it realistically		
(441)	**5.**	__________ When the patient becomes aware of the devastating changes that have taken place		
(441)	**6.**	__________ The stage marked by depression and withdrawal as the patient considers the implications of the injury		

D. Complete the statements in the numbered column with the most appropriate term in the lettered column. Some terms may be used more than once, and some terms may not be used.

(443)	**1.**	Removal of all or part of the posterior arch of the vertebra is called __________.	A.	Dermatome chart
			B.	Immobilization
			C.	Spinal fusion
			D.	Proprioception
(443)	**2.**	The placement of a piece of donor bone, commonly taken from the hip, into the area between the involved vertebrae is called __________.	E.	Laminectomy
			F.	Traction

Continued next page

(444) 3. Sensory loss is best determined by the use of a __________.

(443) 4. The surgical procedure that is done to alleviate compression on the spinal cord or nerves is called __________.

E. If a patient with an upper cervical injury is fortunate enough to receive immediate attention and rapid transport to a skilled facility, what medical treatment will be instituted right away?

(441)

F. Explain why most spinal cord–injured patients can maintain bowel function.

(440)

G. List three factors that contribute to problems with the integumentary system of the spinal cord–injured patient.

(440) 1. ____

(440) 2. ____

(440) 3. ____

H. Explain why the traditional head-tilt–chin-lift method of opening the airway is inappropriate in spinal cord–injured patients.

(441)

Student Name____

I. Match the nursing diagnosis for the spinal cord–injured patient in the numbered column with the "related to" statements in the lettered column. Some statements may be used more than once.

(444)	**1.**	__________	Risk for infection
(444)	**2.**	__________	Disturbed sensory perception (kinesthetic, tactile)
(445)	**3.**	__________	Ineffective thermoregulation
(445)	**4.**	__________	Self-care deficit (feeding, dressing, grooming)
(445)	**5.**	__________	Sexual dysfunction
(444)	**6.**	__________	Dysreflexia
(444)	**7.**	__________	Risk for disuse syndrome
(444)	**8.**	__________	Bowel incontinence
(444)	**9.**	__________	Impaired urinary elimination
(445)	**10.**	__________	Ineffective individual coping
(444)	**11.**	__________	Ineffective breathing patterns
(444)	**12.**	__________	Risk for injury

A. Sensory motor impairment
B. Altered body function
C. Involuntary muscle spasms, lack of motor and sensory function, orthostatic hypotension
D. Skeletal traction pins
E. Overwhelming losses and limited potential for recovered function
F. Neurologic impairment
G. Altered sensory transmission
H. Impaired conduction of impulses
I. Bladder or bowel distention, renal calculi, pressure ulcers
J. Pathologic or prescribed immobility, or both
K. Spinal cord trauma

MULTIPLE-CHOICE QUESTIONS

J. Choose the most appropriate answer.

(441) **1.** The halo device is used to provide immobilization and alignment of the:

1. cervical vertebrae.
2. thoracic vertebrae.
3. lumbar vertebrae.
4. sacral vertebrae.

(446) **2.** For the patient maintained in cervical traction while on a conventional bed, position changes must be accomplished by:

1. assisted ambulation.
2. range-of-motion exercises.
3. "log-rolling."
4. grasping the muscles.

(446) **3.** Prompt intervention following autonomic dysreflexia (AD) must be directed toward severe:

1. hypertension.
2. hypotension.
3. infection.
4. lung compromise.

(446) **4.** Patients with skull tongs are maintained on:

1. bed rest with ambulation three times a day.
2. isolation precautions.
3. high-roughage diets.
4. strict bed rest.

(447) **5.** When the patient has spasticity, nursing management is directed toward the prevention of contractures and:

1. infection.
2. muscle atrophy.
3. dyspnea.
4. heart failure.

(440) **6.** During the time of flaccid paralysis, the nurse must be diligent in performing:

1. active range-of-motion exercises.
2. passive range-of-motion exercises.
3. coughing and deep-breathing exercises.
4. early ambulation.

(447) **7.** Following an ileus, the patient will be given oral fluids and food when:

1. the swallow reflex returns.
2. the patient is no longer anorexic.
3. bladder continence returns.
4. peristalsis returns

(444) **8.** Using the "Grading Scale for Muscle Strength," the nurse would score a finding of full active range of motion against gravity and resistance as:

1. 1. 2. 2.
3. 3. 4. 5.

(450) **9.** Which finding is reported to the physician in the postlaminectomy patient?

1. WBC of 7,000
2. blood pressure 125/80
3. clear drainage from incision site
4. respirations 18

(450) **10.** Applying pneumatic stockings, assisting patients with ROM exercises, and auscultating breath sounds are done in the postoperative laminectomy patient to promote:

1. tissue perfusion.
2. resistance to infection.
3. pain relief.
4. physical immobility.

(439) **11.** Which type of spinal cord injury will result in a loss of motor control below the waist?

1. C4 2. C7
3. T4 4. T10

(450) **12.** Which action is indicated in the management of spasticity in the spinal cord–injured patient?

1. Increase tactile stimuli.
2. Administer antihypertensive medications.
3. Perform passive ROM exercises at least four times a day.
4. Turn and reposition the patient at least every 4 hours.

Student Name____

(435) **13.** Which procedure is a visualization of the spinal cord and vertebrae through the injection of a radiopaque dye directly into the subarachnoid space of the spinal cord?

1. myelography
2. electromyography
3. lumbar puncture
4. electroencephalography

(436) **14.** Injuries at or above C5 may result in instant death because the:

1. innervation to the phrenic nerve is interrupted.
2. sympathetic innervation to the heart is blocked.
3. sensory nerves to the brain are interrupted.
4. saphenous nerve can no longer transmit impulses.

(440) **15.** The spinal cord–injured patient may have difficulty maintaining body temperature within a normal range because :

1. the hypothalamus can no longer regulate temperature.
2. regulatory mechanisms of vasoconstriction and sweating are lost.
3. the peripheral nerves to the skin are interrupted.
4. the skin is not able to lose heat through evaporation.

(441) **16.** At the scene of an accident involving a patient with spinal cord injury, emergency personnel will apply a hard cervical collar around the patient's neck to immobilize the:

1. skull.
2. spinal column.
3. brain.
4. upper part of the body.

(441, 442) **17.** Which type of traction is applied to a fiberglass jacket and is used to immobilize and align the cervical vertebrae and relieve compression of nerve roots?

1. Philadelphia collar
2. Gardner-Wells tongs
3. Crutchfield tongs
4. halo ring

(439) **18.** Which condition is an exaggerated sympathetic response to stimuli, such as bladder distention, that produces severe hypertension with the potential for seizures and stroke?

1. spinal cord injury
2. autonomic dysreflexia
3. meningitis
4. amyotrophic lateral sclerosis

CHAPTER 29

Student Name ______________________________

Acute Respiratory Disorders

Answer Key: Textbook page references are provided as a guide for answering these questions. A complete answer key was provided for your instructor.

OBJECTIVES

1. Identify data to be collected in the nursing assessment of the patient with a respiratory disorder.
2. Identify the nursing implications of age-related changes in the respiratory system.
3. Describe diagnostic tests or procedures for respiratory disorders and nursing interventions.
4. Explain nursing care of patients receiving therapeutic treatments for respiratory disorders.
5. For selected respiratory disorders, describe the pathophysiology, signs and symptoms, complications, diagnostic measures, and medical treatment.
6. Assist in developing a nursing care plan for the patient who has an acute respiratory disorder.

LEARNING ACTIVITIES

A. Match the definition in the numbered column with the most appropriate term in the lettered column.

(458) **1.** __________ Dry, rattling sound caused by partial bronchial obstruction

(456) **2.** __________ Rapid respiratory rate

(491) **3.** __________ Presence of air in the pleural cavity that causes the lung on the affected side to collapse

A. Atelectasis
B. Crackles
C. Dyspnea
D. Hemothorax
E. Hypercapnia
F. Hypoxemia
G. Hypoxia
H. Orthopnea
I. Pneumothorax
J. Rhonchus
K. Tachypnea
L. Tissue perfusion
M. Ventilation
N. Apnea

Continued next page

(457) **4.** __________ Temporary cessation of breathing

(458) **5.** __________ Low oxygen level in body tissues

(458) **6.** __________ Movement of air in and out of the lungs

(458) **7.** __________ Rales; abnormal lung sounds heard on auscultation

(457) **8.** __________ Difficulty breathing when lying down

(466) **9.** __________ Accumulation of blood in the pleural space

(458) **10.** __________ Low level of oxygen in the blood

(460) **11.** __________ Blood flow through blood vessels of tissue

(458) **12.** __________ Collapsed lung or part of a lung

(457) **13.** __________ Difficulty breathing

(482) **14.** __________ Excess carbon dioxide in the blood

B. List three characteristics of the right bronchus that explain why foreign bodies from the trachea enter the right bronchus.

(455) **1.** ______________________________

(455) **2.** ______________________________

(455) **3.** ______________________________

C. List three age-related changes that occur in the pharynx and the larynx.

(457) **1.** ______________________________

(457) **2.** ______________________________

(457) **3.** ______________________________

D. List four purposes of pulmonary function tests.

(463) **1.** ______________________________

(463) **2.** ______________________________

(463) **3.** ______________________________

(463) **4.** ______________________________

Student Name____

E. Explain why culture and sensitivity specimens should be collected before antimicrobial therapy is begun.

(464, 465)

F. Explain why smoking is not allowed when a patient is receiving oxygen therapy.

(471)

G. List one nursing goal, five nursing interventions, and three outcome criteria for the following nursing diagnosis for the patient with fractured ribs.

(487)

Nursing Diagnosis
Ineffective breathing pattern related to pain that occurs with ventilation

Nursing Goal
1.

Outcome Criteria

1.

2.

3.

Nursing Interventions

1.

2.

3.

4.

5.

H. List five signs and symptoms of pulmonary embolus (PE).

(488) **1.** ____________________ *(488)* **4.** ____________________

(488) **2.** ____________________ *(488)* **5.** ____________________

(488) **3.** ____________________

I. Match each diagnostic procedure in the numbered column with appropriate nursing implication on the right. Some nursing implications may be used more than once.

(462) **1.** __________ CT scan

(461) **2.** __________ Fiberoptic bronchoscopy

(461) **3.** __________ Thoracentesis

(463) **4.** __________ MRI

(461) **5.** __________ Pulmonary function tests

A. Tell patient not to move or cough during procedure to prevent damage to pleural tissue.
B. Advise patient not to smoke or eat for 4 to 6 hours before test.
C. Determine whether patient is allergic to iodine.
D. Tell patient not to wear metal-containing clothes or jewelry.
E. Advise patient of NPO status until the gag reflex returns.

J. Match the definition or description in the numbered column with the most appropriate term in the lettered column.

(472) **1.** __________ Tube used with a surgically created opening through the neck into the trachea

(472) **2.** __________ Curved tube used to maintain an airway temporarily

(472) **3.** __________ Soft rubber tube inserted through the nose and extended to the base of the tongue

(472) **4.** __________ Long tube inserted through the mouth or nose into the trachea

A. Endotracheal tube
B. Nasal airway
C. Tracheostomy tube
D. Oral airway

Student Name____

K. Match the definition or description in the numbered column with the most appropriate term in the lettered column.

(476)	**1.** __________	Suppress the cough reflex	
(476)	**2.** __________	Dry up nasal secretions	
(476)	**3.** __________	Relax smooth muscle in the bronchial airways and blood vessels	
(476)	**4.** __________	Side effect of antihistamines	
(477)	**5.** __________	Prevent acute asthma attacks (not used to stop them after they've started)	
(477)	**6.** __________	Inhibit allergic response; prevent asthmatic attacks	
(476)	**7.** __________	Cause constriction of nasal blood vessels and reduce swelling of mucous membranes	
(477)	**8.** __________	Treat asthma (anti-inflammatory drugs)	
(476)	**9.** __________	Thin respiratory secretions so that they are more readily mobilized	
(476)	**10.** __________	Possible side effect of antimicrobials	
(476)	**11.** __________	Possible side effect of decongestants	
(468)	**12.** __________	Side effect of bronchodilators	

A. Decongestants
B. Hypertension
C. Allergic response
D. Antitussives
E. Expectorants
F. Antihistamines
G. Drowsiness
H. Mast cell stabilizers
I. Bacterial infection
J. Bronchodilators
K. Restlessness
L. Corticosteroids
M. Leukotriene inhibitors

L. Match the definition or description in the numbered column with the most appropriate term in the lettered column.

(474)	**1.** ________ Surgical incision of the chest wall	A.	Tidal volume
(474)	**2.** ________ Removal of an entire lung	B.	Thoracotomy
(474)	**3.** ________ Stripping of the membrane that covers the visceral pleura	C.	Pneumonectomy
(475)	**4.** ________ Performed by inserting an endoscope through a small thoracic incision	D.	Thoracoplasty
(474)	**5.** ________ Removal of ribs	E.	Atelectasis
(472)	**6.** ________ Preset amount of oxygenated air delivered during each ventilator breath	F.	Decortication of lung
(471)	**7.** ________ Collapsed alveoli	G.	Thoracoscopy

Student Name____

M. Label the structures in Figure 29-2 (A–E).

(455)

A. _________________________ **D.** _________________________

B. _________________________ **E.** _________________________

C. _________________________

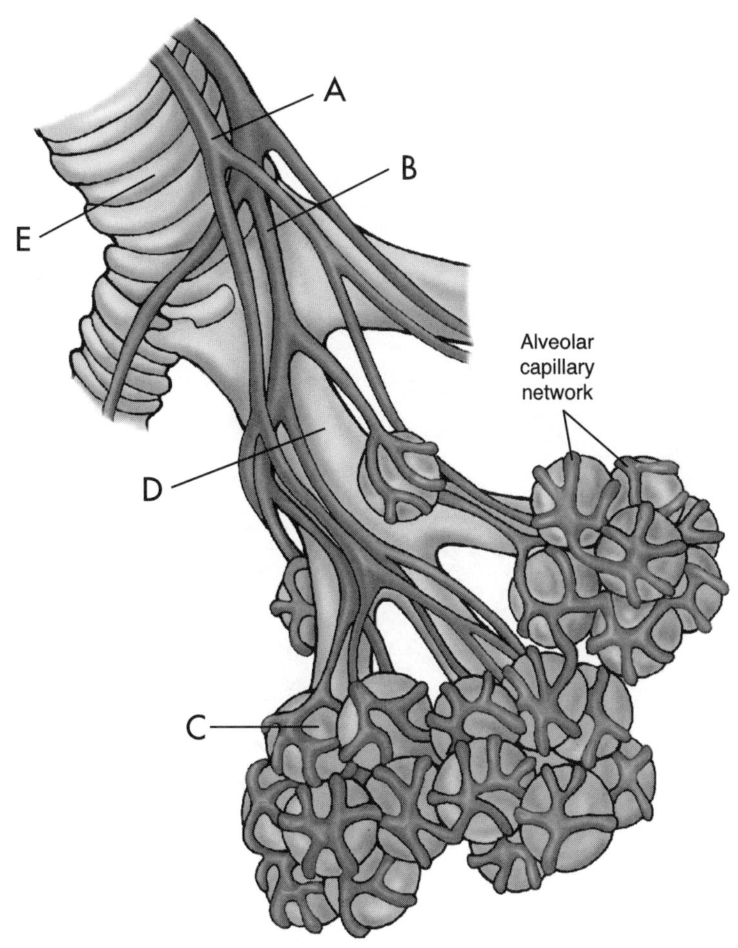

N. Using Figure 29-1B, label the structures (A–I).

(454)

A. ______________________

B. ______________________

C. ______________________

D. ______________________

E. ______________________

F. ______________________

G. ______________________

H. ______________________

I. ______________________

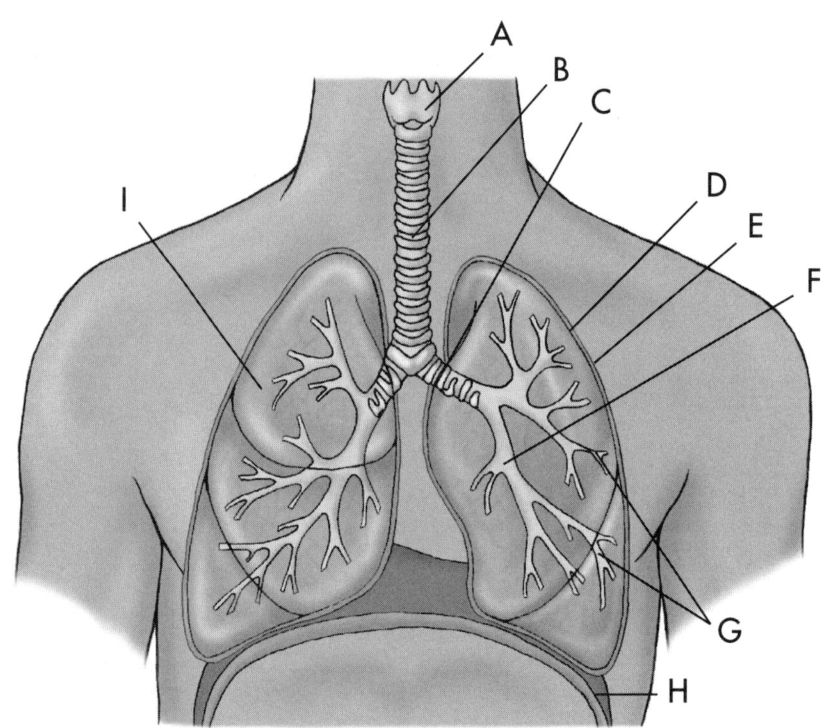

MULTIPLE-CHOICE QUESTIONS

O. Choose the most appropriate answer.

(480) **1.** Who is at risk for having aspiration pneumonia?

1. chronically ill patients
2. patients with tube feedings
3. immunosuppressed patients
4. smokers

(460) **2.** One of the most frequently used methods of respiratory screening and diagnosis is:

1. the lung scan.
2. fluoroscopy.
3. the chest radiograph.
4. MRI.

Student Name ______________________________

(460) **3.** An examination that gives information about the speed and degree of lung expansion and structural defects in the bronchial tree is:

1. the lung scan.
2. fluoroscopy.
3. the chest radiograph.
4. MRI.

(460) **4.** A test to assess lung ventilation and lung perfusion is:

1. the lung scan.
2. fluoroscopy.
3. the chest radiograph.
4. MRI.

(480) **5.** The mucous membrane lining of the lower respiratory tract responds to acute inflammation by increasing the production of:

1. blood cells. 2. secretions.
3. hormones. 4. neurons.

(465) **6.** A test done to determine the presence of the bacteria that cause tuberculosis is:

1. MRI.
2. the lung scan.
3. spirometry.
4. the acid-fast test.

(462) **7.** A test done to determine the presence of malignant cells is:

1. the acid-fast test.
2. the lung scan.
3. sputum cytology.
4. spirometry.

(467) **8.** Chest physiotherapy should be performed:

1. eight times each day.
2. after meals.
3. before meals.
4. at bedtime.

(468) **9.** The technique of positioning the patient to facilitate gravitational movement of respiratory secretions toward the bronchi and trachea for expectoration is:

1. postural drainage.
2. chest percussion.
3. chest vibration.
4. clapping.

(468) **10.** If excessive secretions that the patient cannot expectorate accumulate in the oral or nasal airway, what may be required?

1. spirometry
2. the lung scan
3. MRI
4. suctioning

(468) **11.** Humidity is necessary in the respiratory tract to prevent secretions from becoming:

1. inspissated. 2. moist.
3. wet. 4. warm.

(471) **12.** With simple oxygen masks for patients, flow rates from the flowmeter should be adjusted to:

1. 1–6 liters/min.
2. 6–10 liters/min.
3. 10–12 liters/min.
4. 15–20 liters/min.

(472) **13.** Ventilators are most commonly required for patients with:

1. oxygen toxicity.
2. tachycardia.
3. hypoxemia.
4. hyperventilation.

(472) **14.** The preset amount of oxygenated air delivered during each ventilator breath is called the:

1. vital capacity.
2. nebulizing dose.
3. tidal volume.
4. respiratory rate.

(472) **15.** The total number of breaths delivered per minute is called the:

1. oxygen level setting.
2. tidal volume setting.
3. pressure setting.
4. respiratory rate setting.

(472) **16.** What is prescribed to keep the pressure in the lungs above the atmospheric pressure at the end of expiration?

1. the oxygen level setting
2. the tidal volume setting
3. positive end-expiratory pressure (PEEP)
4. negative inspiratory pressure

(478) **17.** A drug used to prevent acute asthma attacks but that is not useful in stopping an attack once it has begin is called:

1. a mast cell stabilizer.
2. an antitussive.
3. an expectorant.
4. an antihistamine.

(458) **18.** Which group of people abstain from using tobacco?

1. Greek Orthodox
2. Protestants
3. Mormons
4. Orthodox Jews

(465) **19.** Which procedure is performed by inserting a flexible scope into the bronchial tree?

1. video thoracoscopy
2. fiberoptic bronchoscopy
3. incentive spirometry
4. pneumonectomy

(480) **20.** Which herb is taken to decrease the duration and severity of a cold?

1. ginkgo 2. ginseng
3. kava kava 4. echinacea

CHAPTER 30

Student Name ______________________________

Chronic Respiratory Disorders

Answer Key: Textbook page references are provided as a guide for answering these questions. A complete answer key was provided for your instructor.

OBJECTIVES

1. Identify examples of chronic inflammatory, obstructive, and restrictive pulmonary diseases.
2. Explain the relationship between cigarette smoking and chronic respiratory disorders.
3. For selected chronic respiratory disorders, describe the pathophysiology, signs and symptoms, complications, diagnostic measures, and medical treatment.
4. Assist in developing a nursing care plan for the patient who has a chronic respiratory disorder.

LEARNING ACTIVITIES

A. Match the definition in the numbered column with the most appropriate term in the lettered column.

(507) **1.** __________ One of many occupational diseases caused by inhalation of particles of industrial substances

(503) **2.** __________ Permanent dilation of a portion of the bronchi or bronchioles

A. Granuloma
B. Asthma
C. Brachytherapy
D. Pneumoconiosis
E. Asbestosis
F. Bronchiectasis
G. Pneumonitis
H. Bronchitis
I. Emphysema

Continued next page

(507) **3.** __________ A collection of inflammatory cells commonly surrounded by fibrotic tissue that represents a chronic inflammatory response to infectious or noninfectious agents

(493) **4.** __________ A condition characterized by episodes of bronchospasm that causes wheezing and dyspnea; reactive airway disease

(496) **5.** __________ Abnormal accumulation of air in body tissues; in the lung, a disorder characterized by loss of lung elasticity with trapping of air, retained carbon dioxide, and dyspnea

(507) **6.** __________ Inflammation of the lung

(509) **7.** __________ Placement of a radiation source in the body to treat a malignancy

(496) **8.** __________ Bronchial inflammation

(507) **9.** __________ Interstitial fibrosis caused by inhalation of asbestos fibers

B. Complete the statement in the numbered column with the most appropriate term in the lettered column. Some terms may be used more than once, and some terms may not be used.

(493) **1.** Chronic obstructive pulmonary disease (COPD) is characterized as varying combinations of asthma, chronic bronchitis, and __________.

(493) **2.** Constriction of the airways is called __________.

(494) **3.** Severe, persistent bronchospasm is called __________.

A. Cor pulmonale
B. Acute bronchitis
C. Emphysema
D. Congestive heart failure
E. Bronchospasm
F. Status asthmaticus
G. Chronic bronchitis
H. Status epilepticus

Continued next page

Student Name ____________________

(496) **4.** Bronchial inflammation characterized by increased production of mucus and chronic cough that persist for at least 3 months of the year for 2 consecutive years is called __________.

(493) **5.** A degenerative, nonreversible disease characterized by the breakdown of the alveolar walls distal to the terminal bronchioles is __________.

(496) **6.** The term used to describe right-sided heart failure secondary to pulmonary disease is __________.

C. Match the definition or description in the numbered column with the most appropriate term in the lettered column. Some terms may be used more than once, and some terms may not be used.

(503) **1.** __________ An abnormal dilation and distortion of the bronchi and bronchioles that is usually confined to one lung lobe or segment

(504) **2.** __________ A hereditary disorder that is characterized by dysfunction of the exocrine glands and the production of thick, tenacious mucus

(504) **3.** __________ An infection spread by droplets emitted by infected people during coughing, laughing, sneezing, and singing

A. Chronic bronchitis
B. Cystic fibrosis
C. Sarcoidosis
D. Tuberculosis
E. Bronchiectasis

D. Complete the statements in the numbered column with the most appropriate term in the lettered column. Some terms may be used more than once, and some terms may not be used.

(508) **1.** The leading cause of lung cancer is __________.

(509) **2.** Four types of lung surgery procedures include a wedge resection, segmental resection, pneumonectomy, and __________.

(508) **3.** The four warning signs of lung cancer are recurring pneumonia, chest pain, persistent cough, and __________.

(508) **4.** The four major types of lung cancer are small-cell (oat cell) carcinoma, adenocarcinoma, large-cell carcinoma, and __________.

A. Hemoptysis
B. Squamous cell carcinoma
C. Fever
D. Lobectomy
E. Bronchitis
F. Cigarette smoking

E. List 10 signs and symptoms of impending respiratory failure to watch for with patients experiencing impaired gas exchange.

(495) **1.** ______________________

(495) **2.** ______________________

(495) **3.** ______________________

(496) **4.** ______________________

(496) **5.** ______________________

(496) **6.** ______________________

(496) **7.** ______________________

(496) **8.** ______________________

(496) **9.** ______________________

(496) **10.** ______________________

F. Explain why the red blood cell count is typically elevated in patients with chronic hypoxemia. *(497)*

Student Name____

G. In the treatment of COPD, the initial flow of oxygen is usually 1–3 liters/min. Why are high levels of oxygen not administered to COPD patients?

(499)

H. Tuberculosis was a leading cause of death in the United States until effective drugs became available in the 1940s and 1950s. The incidence declined until 1986, when the numbers of reported cases began to rise. List three reasons for this rise.

(504) **1.** ____

(504) **2.** ____

(504) **3.** ____

I. List four diagnostic tests that are done to confirm the diagnosis of tuberculosis.

(505) **1.** ____________________ *(505)* **3.** ____________________

(505) **2.** ____________________ *(505)* **4.** ____________________

J. List seven examples of offending substances that may lead to occupational lung diseases.

(507) **1.** ____________________ *(507)* **5.** ____________________

(507) **2.** ____________________ *(507)* **6.** ____________________

(507) **3.** ____________________ *(507)* **7.** ____________________

(507) **4.** ____________________

K. Match the definition in the numbered column with the most appropriate term in the lettered column. Some terms may be used more than once, and some terms may not be used.

(493) **1.** __________ The patient's ability to inhale or to exhale by force

(493) **2.** __________ Vital capacity, inspiratory capacity, expiratory reserve volume, residual volume, and total lung capacity

(493) **3.** __________ Measurement of the ability of gases to diffuse across the alveolar capillary membrane

A. Air flow limitation
B. Lung volumes
C. Airway dynamics
D. Diffusing capacity
E. Osmosis

L. Match the nursing diagnosis for the patient with bronchial asthma in the numbered column with the "related to" statement in the lettered column.

(495) **1.** __________ Ineffective breathing pattern

(496) **2.** __________ Impaired gas exchange

(496) **3.** __________ Anxiety

A. Bronchospasm, air trapping, increased secretions
B. Air trapping
C. Perceived threat of suffocation, hypoxemia

M. Match the signs and symptoms in the numbered column with their respective conditions in the lettered column. Some conditions may be used more than once, and some may not be used.

(497) **1.** __________ Productive cough, exertional dyspnea, and wheezing

(505) **2.** __________ Cough, night sweats, chest pain and tightness, fatigue, and anorexia

(497) **3.** __________ Dyspnea on exertion; may display use of accessory muscles of respiration; barrel chest

A. Emphysema
B. Chronic bronchitis
C. Tuberculosis

Student Name____

N. Match the nursing diagnosis for the patient with COPD in the numbered column with the "related to" statement in the lettered column.

(499) **1.** __________ Impaired gas exchange

(500) **2.** __________ Ineffective airway clearance

(500) **3.** __________ Anxiety

(501) **4.** __________ Altered nutrition: less than body requirements

(500) **5.** __________ High risk for infection

(501) **6.** __________ Activity intolerance

(501) **7.** __________ Decreased cardiac output

A. Decreased ciliary action, increased secretions, weak cough
B. Alveolar destruction, bronchospasm, air trapping
C. Anorexia, dyspnea
D. Right-sided heart failure
E. Increased secretions, weak cough
F. Inability to meet oxygen needs
G. Hypoxemia

MULTIPLE-CHOICE QUESTIONS

O. Choose the most appropriate answer.

(493) **1.** The basic pathology with asthma is the narrowing of the bronchi or bronchioles as a result of:

1. dilated smooth muscle around the airways.
2. contracted smooth muscle around the airways.
3. rapid, shallow respirations.
4. slow, deep respirations.

(493) **2.** The opening of the airways decreases in size in patients with asthma due to contracted smooth muscle and:

1. redness.
2. increased temperature.
3. infection.
4. inflammation.

(493) **3.** A serious complication of bronchoconstriction is:

1. hypoxemia. 2. hypotension.
3. drowsiness. 4. headache.

(494) **4.** Signs and symptoms of an asthma attack include dyspnea, productive cough, and:

1. tachycardia.
2. bradycardia.
3. slow respirations.
4. apnea.

(501) **5.** The best position for patients with bronchial asthma is:

1. supine. 2. prone.
3. side-lying. 4. Fowler's.

(496) **6.** Findings that should be reported to the physician if they occur in patients with impaired gas exchange include:

1. PaO_2 decreases, pH increases.
2. PaO_2 increases, pH increases.
3. PaO_2 decreases, $PaCO_2$ increases.
4. PaO_2 increases, $PaCO_2$ increases.

(496) **7.** A nasal cannula is preferred over a face mask because the mask may increase the patient's feeling of:

1. insecurity.
2. safety.
3. suffocation.
4. self-esteem.

(497) **8.** In patients with emphysema, the lungs often become hyperinflated, causing the diaphragm to flatten and increasing the reliance on:

1. coughing and deep-breathing exercises.
2. accessory muscles for breathing.
3. extra fluids to thin secretions.
4. increased heart rate.

(497) **9.** The most serious complications of chronic obstructive pulmonary disease are respiratory failure and:

1. kidney failure.
2. heart failure.
3. brain hemorrhage.
4. paralytic ileus.

(497) **10.** The term *blue bloater* is used to describe patients with:

1. advanced emphysema.
2. pneumonia.
3. adult respiratory distress syndrome.
4. advanced chronic bronchitis.

(498) **11.** The term *pink puffer* is used to describe patients with emphysema because skin color is apt to be normal because of:

1. normal arterial blood gases.
2. unlabored respirations.
3. barrel chest formation.
4. normal body temperature.

(498) **12.** The most reliable diagnostic test for COPD is:

1. the chest radiograph.
2. MRI.
3. the pulmonary function test.
4. the CBC (complete blood count).

(498) **13.** Drugs that are ordered to decrease airway resistance and the work of breathing for patients with COPD are called:

1. vasoconstrictors.
2. diuretics.
3. calcium channel blockers.
4. bronchodilators.

(498) **14.** The preferred route of administration of drugs for patients with COPD is by:

1. mouth.
2. inhalation.
3. intramuscular injection.
4. intravenous injection.

(499) **15.** During the physical examination of patients with COPD, the nurse observes the neck for:

1. edema.
2. distended veins.
3. enlarged lymph nodes.
4. cyanosis.

Student Name________________________________

(496) **16.** Because good hydration helps to thin secretions in patients with impaired gas exchange, what is the recommended daily fluid intake?

1. 600–800 ml
2. 1000–1500 ml
3. 2500–3000 ml
4. 4000–5000 ml

(496) **17.** The feeling of not being able to breathe is frightening; in addition, feelings of restlessness and anxiety are increased in the asthma patient due to decreased:

1. arterial oxygen.
2. arterial carbon dioxide.
3. heart rate.
4. respiratory rate.

(498) **18.** During the physical examination of patients with COPD, the thorax is inspected for the classic:

1. pink color.
2. blue tinge.
3. pulmonary edema.
4. barrel chest shape.

(502) **19.** The patient with COPD is monitored for signs and symptoms of airway obstruction, which include tachycardia, abnormal breath sounds, and:

1. headache.
2. oliguria.
3. constipation.
4. dyspnea.

(502) **20.** Patients with COPD are encouraged to drink extra fluids each day in order to:

1. improve urinary output.
2. increase circulation.
3. liquefy secretions.
4. prevent kidney stones.

(502) **21.** The work of breathing is increased with COPD, which in turn increases the patient's:

1. caloric requirements.
2. requirements for calcium.
3. requirements for sodium.
4. dietary roughage requirements.

(502) **22.** The recommended diet for the patient who is dyspneic is a soft diet with:

1. three large meals.
2. a low-protein emphasis.
3. a low-calorie emphasis.
4. frequent, small meals.

(503) **23.** If the COPD patient becomes excessively dyspneic or develops tachycardia during activity, the patient should:

1. increase the activity slowly.
2. stop the activity.
3. sit down briefly and then resume activity.
4. drink a full glass of water.

(503) **24.** Patients with chronic bronchitis and emphysema are at risk for heart failure and decreased cardiac output; the nurse monitors for signs of heart failure, which include increasing dyspnea, dependent edema, and:

1. bradycardia.
2. tachycardia.
3. increased urine output.
4. dehydration.

(505) **25.** A persistent, productive cough with bloody sputum (hemoptysis) is a common symptom of:

1. emphysema.
2. cystic fibrosis.
3. sinusitis.
4. tuberculosis.

(505) **26.** The most common preventive drug therapy for tuberculosis is:

1. prednisone.
2. isoniazid.
3. gamma globulin.
4. aminophylline.

(506) **27.** The patient who is thought to have active tuberculosis is isolated at first. Which of the following is *not* necessary related to the care of the patient?

1. good hand washing
2. wearing masks
3. wearing gowns
4. universal precautions

CHAPTER 31

Student Name ______________________________

Hematologic Disorders

Answer Key: Textbook page references are provided as a guide for answering these questions. A complete answer key was provided for your instructor.

OBJECTIVES

1. List the components of the hematologic system and describe their role in oxygenation and hemostasis.
2. Identify data to be collected when assessing a patient with a disorder of the hematologic system.
3. Describe tests and procedures used to diagnose disorders of the hematologic system, and nursing considerations for each.
4. Describe nursing care for patients undergoing common therapeutic measures for disorders of the hematologic system.
5. For selected disorders of the hematologic system, describe the pathophysiology, signs and symptoms, medical diagnosis and medical treatment.
6. Assist in planning nursing care for a patient with a disorder of the hematologic system.

LEARNING ACTIVITIES

A. Match the definition in the numbered column with the most appropriate term in the lettered column.

(520) **1.** __________ Person with type AB-positive blood who can receive transfusions with any type of blood because all the common antigens (A, B and Rh) are present in the blood

A. Anemia
B. Oxygenation
C. Ecchymosis
D. Orthostatic vital sign changes
E. Petechia
F. Purpura
G. Universal donor
H. Universal recipient
I. Hemostasis

Continued next page

(516) **2.** ________ A purplish skin lesion resulting from blood leaking outside the blood vessels

(522) **3.** ________ A reduction in the number of red blood cells or in the quantity of hemoglobin

(516) **4.** ________ A small (1–3 mm) red or reddish-purple spot on the skin resulting from blood capillaries breaking and leaking small amounts of blood into the tissues

(512) **5.** ________ A primary function of the hematologic system

(520) **6.** ________ Person with type O-negative blood who can donate blood to anyone because none of the common antigens is present in the blood

(515) **7.** ________ Changes in blood pressure and pulse as person moves from lying to sitting to standing positions

(516) **8.** ________ Red or reddish-purple skin lesions 3 mm or more in size that result from blood leaking outside of the blood vessels

(512) **9.** ________ Control of bleeding

B. Match the definition in the numbered column with the appropriate red blood cell disorder in the lettered column. Answers may be used more than once.

(522) **1.** ________ Results from complete failure of bone marrow

(522) **2.** ________ Condition in which too many red blood cells are produced

(522) **3.** ________ Occurs when a person does not absorb vitamin B_{12} from the stomach

(522) **4.** ________ A genetic disease carried on a recessive gene

A. Autoimmune hemolytic anemia
B. Aplastic anemia
C. Polycythemia vera
D. Pernicious anemia
E. Sickle cell anemia
F. Iron deficiency anemia

Continued next page

Student Name ____

(522) **5.** __________ Person often has a ruddy (reddish) complexion

(522) **6.** __________ Symptoms include headache, dizziness, ringing in the ears, and blurred vision

(522) **7.** __________ Person has high bilirubin levels in the blood

(522) **8.** __________ Symptoms include fatigue, severe pain, and cardiomegaly

(522) **9.** __________ Blood becomes more viscous and does not circulate freely through the body

(522) **10.** __________ May be caused by drugs (such as streptomycin and chloramphenicol) and exposure to toxic chemicals and radiation

(522) **11.** __________ Symptoms include weakness, sore tongue, and numbness of hands or feet

(522) **12.** __________ Misshapen red blood cells become fragile and rupture easily

(522) **13.** __________ Symptoms include fatigue, shortness of breath, hypotension, and jaundice

(522) **14.** __________ Bone marrow makes adequate amounts of blood cells, but they are destroyed once they are released into the circulation

(522) **15.** __________ Symptoms include pallor, extreme fatigue, tachycardia, shortness of breath, bleeding, and frequent infections

(522) **16.** __________ Results from diet low in iron or inability of the body to absorb enough iron from GI tract

C. List three ways the body compensates when a person is anemic.

(522) **1.** ____

(522) **2.** ____

(522) **3.** ____

D. List five symptoms of thrombocytopenia.

(526) **1.** ____________________

(526) **2.** ____________________

(526) **3.** ____________________

(526) **4.** ____________________

(526) **5.** ____________________

E. Match the descriptions in the numbered column with the appropriate type of coagulation disorder in the lettered column. Answers may be used more than once.

(526) **1.** __________ Diagnosis is made with blood tests and bone marrow biopsy

(526) **2.** __________ Treatment may include platelet transfusions

(526) **3.** __________ Causes include cancer chemotherapy and radiation

(526) **4.** __________ Diagnosis is made with prothrombin time (PT) and PTT

(526) **5.** __________ Secondary disorder to another pathologic process, such as sepsis, shock, burns, or obstetric complications

(526) **6.** __________ Treated with transfusion of fresh frozen plasma or cryoprecipitate

(526) **7.** __________ Hypercoagulable state with thrombosis and hemorrhage

(526) **8.** __________ Genetic disease in which a person lacks blood-clotting factors normally found in the plasma

(526) **9.** __________ Diagnosis is made with factors VIII and IX

A. Thrombocytopenia
B. Disseminated intravascular coagulation (DIC)
C. Hemophilia

Continued next page

Student Name____

F. Match the blood component in the numbered column with the indications for its use (A–D) and the usual amount prescribed (E–H) on the right.

(519) **1.** __________ Platelets

(519) **2.** __________ Cryoprecipitate

(519) **3.** __________ Packed red blood cells (PRBC)

(519) **4.** __________ Fresh frozen plasma (FFP)

A. Clotting deficiencies, hemophilia, for rapid reversal of warfarin (Coumadin), with massive red blood cell transfusions
B. Symptoms from low hematocrit or hemoglobin such as shortness of breath, tachycardia, decreased blood pressure, chest pain, lightheadedness, and fatigue
C. Hemophilia A, DIC
D. Bleeding from thrombocytopenia
E. 10–15 ml/bag; usually 10 bags are pooled together
F. 60–80 ml/pack; usually four to six packs are pooled together
G. 180–270 ml/unit
H. 250–300 ml/unit

G. Match the drug in the numbered column with its action (A–D) and the appropriate nursing intervention (E–I) on the right. Some interventions may not be used.

(522) **1.** __________ Vitamin B_{12}

(522) **2.** __________ Ferrous sulfate

(522) **3.** __________ Epoetin alfa

(522) **4.** __________ Iron dextran

A. Replaces iron
B. Replaces vitamin
C. Stimulates the bone marrow to produce red blood cells
D. Suppresses immune system
E. Intramuscular injection; must be given every month the rest of the person's life
F. Have the patient take the drug with food but not with milk, eggs, or caffeinated drinks because the milk and caffeine inhibit drug absorption; if the patient is taking a liquid form, dilute the drug and administer through a straw to prevent the drug from staining the teeth
G. May be given by intravenous or subcutaneous injection; patient is usually treated three times per week until the hematocrit is 30–33
H. Give these drugs with meals; an H_2-receptor antagonist such as ranitidine (Zantac) may be prescribed to decrease gastric acid production; if the patient takes these drugs for an extended period of time, the drug should not be stopped abruptly; instead, the drug dose should be gradually decreased over time under a physician's direction
I. Test dose before starting treatment; give intramuscular injections only in the upper outer quadrant of the buttock using the Z-track technique.

MULTIPLE-CHOICE QUESTIONS

H. Choose the most appropriate answer.

(522) **1.** A condition in which there are too many blood cells is called:

1. pernicious anemia.
2. aplastic anemia.
3. hemolytic anemia.
4. polycythemia vera.

(523) **2.** The treatment for acquired hemolytic anemia is:

1. vitamin B_{12} injections.
2. a ferrous sulfate and high-iron diet.
3. an iron dextran and high-carbohydrate diet.
4. corticosteroids and transfusions.

(523) **3.** The treatment for aplastic anemia is:

1. vitamin B_{12} injections.
2. a ferrous sulfate and high-iron diet.
3. an iron dextran and high-carbohydrate diet.
4. transfusions, antibiotics, and corticosteroids.

(524) **4.** Treatment for sickle cell crisis includes:

1. a ferrous sulfate and high-iron diet.
2. an iron dextran and high-carbohydrate diet.
3. aggressive intravenous hydration and IV morphine.
4. corticosteroids and transfusions.

(518) **5.** For each unit of packed RBCs transfused, the patient's hemoglobin should increase approximately:

1. 10 g/dl.
2. 5 g/dl.
3. 3 g/dl.
4. 1 g/dl.

(516) **6.** Red or reddish-purple spots that are the result of blood vessels breaking, which are 3 mm or larger are:

1. petechiae.
2. purpura.
3. ecchymoses.
4. nodes.

(522) **7.** Patients with low red blood cell counts may have:

1. bradycardia.
2. hypotension.
3. bleeding problems.
4. tachycardia.

(516) **8.** If a patient is orthostatic and tilt-positive, which should be increased?

1. carbohydrates
2. fluids
3. fiber
4. vitamins

(520) **9.** Once blood is picked up from the blood bank, the transfusion should be started within:

1. 5 minutes.
2. 30 minutes.
3. 1 hour.
4. 6 hours.

Student Name____

(520) **10.** Platelets are generally administered when a patient's platelet count drops below:

1. 10,000/mm^3
2. 20,000/mm^3
3. 150,000/mm^3
4. 300,000/mm^3

(520) **11.** If platelets are ordered before a procedure such as a lumbar puncture or endoscopy to prevent postprocedure bleeding, the platelets should be administered:

1. 1 week before the procedure.
2. 1 day before the procedure.
3. 6 hours before the procedure.
4. immediately before the procedure.

(527) **12.** The treatment for hemophilia is:

1. plasma and cryoprecipitate transfusions.
2. red blood cell transfusions and antibiotics.
3. white blood cell transfusions and potassium.
4. platelet and anticoagulant transfusions.

(526) **13.** Symptoms of thrombocytopenia include:

1. fatigue and pallor.
2. petechiae and purpuras.
3. nausea and vomiting.
4. tachycardia and palpitations.

(526) **14.** Treatment for thrombocytopenia includes:

1. red blood cell transfusions and iron.
2. white blood cell transfusions and antibiotics.
3. corticosteroids and platelet transfusions.
4. cryoprecipitate transfusions and anticonvulsants.

(526) **15.** The condition in which a person has too few platelets circulating in the blood is called:

1. leukemia.
2. anemia.
3. lymphoma.
4. thrombocytopenia.

(521) **16.** Four types of blood transfusion reactions include hemolytic, circulatory overload, febrile, and:

1. thrombocytopenic.
2. anaphylactic.
3. anemic.
4. leukopenic.

(515) **17.** Feverfew, garlic, and ginkgo are herbs that affect:

1. wound healing.
2. blood clotting.
3. resistance to infection.
4. kidney function.

CHAPTER 32

Student Name ______________________________

Immunologic Disorders

Answer Key: Textbook page references are provided as a guide for answering these questions. A complete answer key was provided for your instructor.

OBJECTIVES

1. List the components of the immune system and describe their role in innate immunity, acquired immunity, and tolerance.
2. List the data to be collected when assessing a patient with a disorder of the immune system.
3. Describe the tests and procedures used to diagnose disorders of the immune system and nursing considerations for each.
4. Describe the nursing care for patients undergoing common therapeutic measures for disorders of the immune system.
5. For selected disorders of the immune system, describe the pathophysiology, signs and symptoms, medical diagnosis, and medical treatment.
6. Assist in developing a nursing care plan for a patient with a disorder of the immune system.

LEARNING ACTIVITIES

A. Match the definition or description in the numbered column with the most appropriate term in the lettered column.

(533) **1.** __________ Resistance to or protection from a disease

(533) **2.** __________ Certain white blood cells (neutrophils, monocytes, and macrophages) that engulf and destroy invading pathogens, dead cells, and cellular debris

A. Acquired immunity
B. Antibody
C. Antibody-mediated acquired immunity
D. Antigen
E. Cell-mediated acquired immunity
F. Compromised host precautions
G. Eicosanoid
H. Immunity
I. Immunoglobulin
J. Innate immunity
K. Leukemia
L. Pathogen
M. Phagocytes

Continued next page

(533) **3.** ________ Class of fatty acids that regulates blood vessel vasodilation, temperature elevation, white blood cell activation, and other physiologic processes

(533) **4.** ________ Freely circulating Y-shaped antigen-binding protein produced by B lymphocytes and plasma cells

(530) **5.** ________ Disease-causing microorganism

(533) **6.** ________ A substance, usually a protein, that is capable of stimulating a response from the immune system

(533) **7.** ________ Defensive system that is operational at all times, consisting of anatomic and physiologic barriers, the inflammatory response, and the ability of certain cells to phagocytose invaders

(534) **8.** ________ Defensive response by T_C cells aimed at intracellular defects such as viruses and cancer

(533) **9.** ________ Antibody-mediated or cell-mediated response that is specific to a particular pathogen and is activated when needed

(533) **10.** ________ Defensive response by B cells assisted by TH cells, aimed at invading microorganisms such as bacteria

(532–533) **11.** ________ Membrane-bound, Y-shaped binding protein produced by B lymphocytes; called antibody when released from the cell membrane

(544) **12.** ________ Actions taken to help protect patients with low white blood cell counts from infection

(535) **13.** ________ Cancer of the white blood cells in which the bone marrow produces too many immature white blood cells

Student Name____

B. Match the organ in the numbered column with its function in the lettered column.

(530)	**1.**	__________	Lymph nodes	A.	Participate(s) in the maturation of T lymphocytes
(532)	**2.**	__________	Bone marrow	B.	Act(s) as filter to remove microorganisms from the lymph fluid before it returns to the blood
(531)	**3.**	__________	Spleen	C.	Filter(s) and destroy(s) microorganisms in the blood
(532)	**4.**	__________	Thymus	D.	Produce(s) white blood cells

C. Match the type of white blood cell in the numbered column with its function in the lettered column.

(532)	**1.**	__________	Basophils	A.	Called macrophages when they enter tissue; powerful phagocytes
(533)	**2.**	__________	B lymphocytes	B.	Initiate inflammatory response; circulate in blood and release histamine
(532)	**3.**	__________	Neutrophils	C.	Fight bacterial infections; most numerous type of the white blood cells
(532)	**4.**	__________	Monocytes	D.	Combat parasitic infections; associated with allergies
(532)	**5.**	__________	Eosinophils	E.	Manufacture immunoglobulins and stimulate the production of antibodies
(532)	**6.**	__________	Mast cells	F.	Store histamine; located in body tissues
(533)	**7.**	__________	T lymphocytes	G.	Secrete cytokines, facilitating body's immune system

D. Match the definition or description in the numbered column with the appropriate type of immunoglobulin in the lettered column.

(533)	**1.**	__________	Present in secretions such as mucus and mother's milk	A.	IgG
(533)	**2.**	__________	First immunoglobulin to be secreted during the primary immune response to an antigen	B.	IgM
(533)	**3.**	__________	Secreted during secondary immune response and is specific to a particular antigen	C.	IgA
(533)	**4.**	__________	Attaches to cell membranes of basophils and mast cells, where it triggers the cell to release histamine	D.	IgE

E. Match the definition or description in the numbered column with the most appropriate term in the lettered column.

(533) **1.** ________ Process of ingesting and digesting invading pathogens, dead cells, and cellular debris

(534) **2.** ________ Process of self-recognition that occurs as part of normal neonatal growth and development

(533) **3.** ________ Response initiated when IgM immunoglobulins on the surface of B lymphocytes detect a foreign antigen

(533) **4.** ________ System activated only when needed in response to a specific antigen; can be antibody-mediated or cell-mediated

(534) **5.** ________ Response aimed at intracellular defects caused by viruses and cancer; responsible for delayed hypersensitivity reactions and transplant organ tissue rejection

(533) **6.** ________ System that consists of anatomic and physiologic barriers, inflammatory response, and action of phagocytic cells

A. Acquired immunity
B. Innate immunity
C. Tolerance
D. Phagocytosis
E. Antibody-mediated immunity
F. Cell-mediated immunity

Student Name____

F. Explain how the following anatomic and physiologic barriers function as the body's first line of defense.

(533) **1.** Skin: ____

(533) **2.** Sweat glands: ____________________________________

(533) **3.** GI and GU mucosae: ________________________________

(533) **4.** Respiratory and gastrointestinal secretions: __________________________

G. Match the definition or description in the numbered column with the appropriate immunity type in the lettered column. Some answers may be used more than once.

(533) **1.** __________ Defense systems present at birth

(533) **2.** __________ Initiated when the IgM immunoglobulins on the surface of B lymphocytes detect a foreign antigen

(533) **3.** __________ Defense systems specific to a particular pathogen

(533) **4.** __________ Anatomic and physiologic barriers, inflammatory response, and phagocytic ability of certain cells

(533) **5.** __________ Occurs when an antibody produced by a person is transferred to another person

(533) **6.** __________ Occurs when a person produces his or her own antibodies in response to a pathogen

A. Innate immunity
B. Acquired immunity
C. Antibody-mediated immunity
D. Cell-mediated immunity
E. Active acquired antibody immunity
F. Passive acquired antibody immunity

Continued next page

(533) **7.** __________ Occurs when a person receives a vaccination

(533) **8.** __________ Permanent type of immunity

(534) **9.** __________ Primary component is T_c cells, which recognize foreign antigen in cells

(534) **10.** __________ Immunity responsible for delayed hypersensitivity reactions

(533) **11.** __________ Immunity aimed at invading microorganisms such as bacteria

(533) **12.** __________ Immunity lasts only 1–2 months after antibodies have been received

(534) **13.** __________ Immunity responsible for rejection of transplanted tissue

(533) **14.** __________ Occurs when a person has an infection and produces his or her own antibodies

(533) **15.** __________ Immunity obtained by babies through breast milk

(534) **16.** __________ Immunity aimed at intracellular defects caused by viruses and cancer

(533) **17.** __________ Immunity obtained from gamma globulin injections given to persons exposed to hepatitis

H. List the age-related changes of the immune system that occur in the following.

(534) **1.** Bone marrow: ______________________________

(534) **2.** Immunologic function: ______________________________

(534) **3.** Lymphatic tissue: ______________________________

I. List two conditions that may cause a "shift to the right" on a CBC.

(536) **1.** ______________________________

(536) **2.** ______________________________

Student Name____

J. Match the diagnostic test in the numbered column with the disease or disorder it is used to diagnose in the lettered column. Answers may be used more than once.

(536) **1.** __________ Serum protein electrophoresis

(536) **2.** __________ Antinuclear antibody test

(536) **3.** __________ Western blot test

(536) **4.** __________ Urine protein electrophoresis

(536) **5.** __________ Bone marrow biopsy

(539) **6.** __________ Lymphangiography

(539) **7.** __________ Liver-spleen scan

(539) **8.** __________ Skin tests

A. HIV infection
B. Hodgkin's disease
C. Hypersensitivities
D. Leukemia
E. Multiple myeloma
F. SLE

K. List four indications for bone marrow transplant.

(541) **1.** ____

(541) **2.** ____

(541) **3.** ____

(541) **4.** ____

L. Match the definition or description of bone marrow transplants in the numbered column with the appropriate type of transplant in the lettered column. Answers may be used more than once.

(541) **1.** __________ Requires a matched donor

(541) **2.** __________ Procedure in which a patient's own bone marrow is returned to the patient

A. Allogeneic bone marrow transplant
B. Autologous bone marrow transplant
C. Peripheral blood stem cell transplant

Continued next page

(541) **3.** ________ Procedure in which colony-stimulating factors are administered to the patient to stimulate the bone marrow to produce white blood cells

(541) **4.** ________ Procedure that reduces the duration of neutropenia

(541) **5.** ________ Best option for patients with a solid tumor that has not metastasized to the bone marrow, such as patients with breast cancer or lymphoma

(541) **6.** ________ Following harvesting of stem cells through apheresis, the patient is treated with chemotherapy and radiation therapy

(541) **7.** ________ Type of transplant that has been done the longest

(541) **8.** ________ Used to restore bone marrow function in patients with leukemia

(541) **9.** ________ Newest type of transplant, which is becoming the most common type

(541) **10.** ________ High doses of chemotherapy and radiation therapy are given to destroy bone marrow, followed by bone marrow transfusion from a human leukocyte antigen (HLA) donor to restore bone marrow function

(541) **11.** ________ Procedure in which a patient's own bone marrow is harvested before chemotherapy and radiation therapy

M. List five major complications of bone marrow and peripheral blood stem cell transplants.

(541) **1.** ____________________

(541) **2.** ____________________

(541) **3.** ____________________

(541) **4.** ____________________

(541) **5.** ____________________

Student Name____

N. List 5 causes of neutropenia.

(544) **1.** ____

(544) **2.** ____

(544) **3.** ____

(544) **4.** ____

(544) **5.** ____

O. Explain why a patient with leukemia may have signs of anemia, such as fatigue, paleness, tachycardia, and tachypnea. *(544)*

P. List six common nursing diagnoses for patients with acute leukemia.

(545) **1.** ____

(545) **2.** ____

(545) **3.** ____

(545) **4.** ____

(545) **5.** ____

(545) **6.** ____

Q. Match the definition or description in the numbered column with the appropriate immune system disorder in the lettered column.

(544) **1.** ________ Cancer of the white blood cells

(552) **2.** ________ Cancer of the lymph system staged as low, intermediate, or high grade

(552) **3.** ________ Cancer of the lymph system characterized by the presence of Reed-Sternberg cells in the lymph nodes

(552) **4.** ________ Cancer of the plasma cells in the bone marrow

(547) **5.** ________ Autoimmune disease that affects multiple organs

(549) **6.** ________ Retrovirus

A. HIV infection
B. Hodgkin's disease
C. Leukemia
D. Non-Hodgkin's lymphoma
E. Multiple myeloma
F. SLE

R. Match the example of an antigen in the numbered column with the appropriate classification of hypersensitivity reaction in the lettered column. Answers may be used more than once.

(547) **1.** ________ Autoimmune reactions

(547) **2.** ________ Contact dermatitis

(547) **3.** ________ Tuberculin skin testing

(547) **4.** ________ Systemic lupus erythematosus (SLE)

(547) **5.** ________ Insect stings

(547) **6.** ________ Pollen

(547) **7.** ________ Organ transplant cells; transplanted graft rejection

(547) **8.** ________ Blood transfusion cells; mismatched blood transfusion

(547) **9.** ________ Dust

A. Type I immediate hypersensitivity reaction mediated by IgE
B. Type II immediate hypersensitivity reaction mediated by antibodies
C. Type III immediate hypersensitivity reaction resulting in tissue damage
D. Type IV delayed hypersensitivity reaction

Student Name_______________

S. Explain why patients with HIV infection are at increased risk for cancer. *(549)*

T. List four major complications of HIV infection.

(549)	**1.**	______________	*(549)*	**3.**	______________
(549)	**2.**	______________	*(549)*	**4.**	______________

U. List four types of diagnostic blood work that may aid in the diagnosis of HIV infection.

(549)	**1.**	______________	*(549)*	**3.**	______________
(549)	**2.**	______________	*(549)*	**4.**	______________

V. Match the intervention in the numbered column with the appropriate goal in the lettered column. Answers may be used more than once.

(541) **1.** __________ Bone marrow transplant

(543) **2.** __________ Zidovudine (AZT)

(542) **3.** __________ Filgrastim (Neupogen)

(545) **4.** __________ Chemotherapy

(543) **5.** __________ Protease inhibitors

A. Boosts immune system
B. Destroys diseased bone marrow
C. Slows replication and progression of HIV
D. Stimulates bone marrow to produce white blood cells

W. List seven common nursing diagnoses for patients with HIV infection.

(550)	**1.**	______________	*(550)*	**5.**	______________
(550)	**2.**	______________	*(550)*	**6.**	______________
(550)	**3.**	______________	*(550)*	**7.**	______________
(550)	**4.**	______________			

X. List 16 nursing actions for the patient at risk for injury from infection related to compromised host precautions in the following areas.

(540) **1.** Hand washing: ____________________

(540) **2.** Hematopoietic growth factors: ____________________

(540) **3.** Vital signs: ____________________

(540) **4.** Invasive procedures: ____________________

(540) **5.** Aseptic technique: ____________________

(540) **6.** Stethoscope and thermometer use: ____________________

(540) **7.** Staff use of masks: ____________________

(540) **8.** Cleaning tabletops, equipment, and floor: ____________________

(540) **9.** Personal hygiene of patient: ____________________

(540) **10.** Cough and deep-breathe: ____________________

(540) **11.** Dietary concerns: ____________________

(540) **12.** Scheduling of patient appointments: ____________________

(540) **13.** Patient's use of masks: ____________________

(540) **14.** Flowers and plants: ____________________

(540) **15.** Use of humidifiers: ____________________

(540) **16.** Patient teaching: ____________________

Student Name ______________________________

Y. Using Figure 32-1, label the parts of the lymphatic system.

(531)	**A.**	____________	*(531)*	**D.**	____________
(531)	**B.**	____________	*(531)*	**E.**	____________
(531)	**C.**	____________			

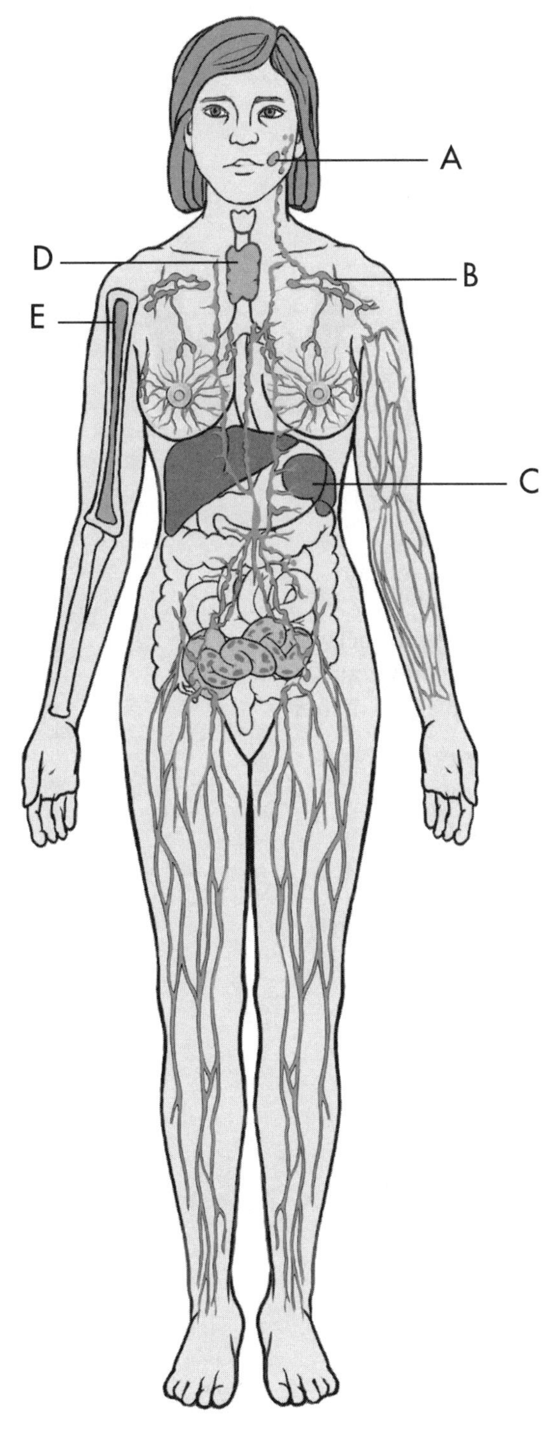

MULTIPLE-CHOICE QUESTIONS

Z. Choose the most appropriate answer.

(530) **1.** The body's defense network against infection is the:

1. cardiovascular system.
2. respiratory system.
3. immune system.
4. circulatory system.

(530) **2.** Which filters microorganisms from the lymph fluid before it is returned to the bloodstream?

1. thymus
2. bone marrow
3. spleen
4. lymph node

(533) **3.** The body's first line of defense is:

1. skin and inflammation.
2. phagocytosis and kidney.
3. blood vessels and kidney.
4. skin and mucous membranes.

(534) **4.** Which is responsible for delayed hypersensitivity reactions and rejection of transplanted tissue?

1. humoral immunity
2. interferon immunity
3. cell-mediated immunity
4. antibody-mediated immunity

(543) **5.** Antiviral medications are given to patients with HIV infection to:

1. prevent viral replication and destroy infected cells.
2. destroy viral cells that are infected.
3. slow viral replication and progression.
4. destroy bacteria and prevent infection.

(532) **6.** The most numerous white blood cells are the:

1. neutrophils.
2. basophils.
3. lymphocytes.
4. eosinophils.

(533) **7.** Interferon, interleukin, and erythropoietin are examples of:

1. lymphocytes.
2. immunoglobulins.
3. cytokines.
4. eicosanoids.

(533) **8.** A class of fatty acids that regulates blood vessel vasodilation, temperature elevation, white blood cell activation, and other immune processes includes:

1. cytokines.
2. eicosanoids.
3. lymphocytes.
4. neutrophils.

(533) **9.** Substances that make the antigen more recognizable to neutrophils, monocytes, and macrophages are:

1. eicosanoids.
2. eosinophils.
3. antibodies.
4. cytokines.

(534) **10.** When there is a breakdown of tolerance, what type of diseases occur?

1. autoimmune
2. viral
3. bacterial
4. cancers

Student Name____

(534) **11.** Rheumatoid arthritis, SLE, Graves' disease, ITP, and type 1 diabetes mellitus are examples of what type of disease?

1. lymphoma
2. pyrogenic
3. allergic
4. autoimmune

(534) **12.** The body's ability to determine self from nonself is called:

1. tolerance.
2. phagocytosis.
3. immunity.
4. inflammation.

(536) **13.** A "shift to the left" on a CBC indicates that more than 60% of white blood cells are:

1. lymphocytes.
2. basophils.
3. eosinophils.
4. neutrophils.

(536) **14.** A blood test that measures the amount of immunoglobulin proteins present in the blood is serum:

1. creatinine.
2. potassium.
3. protein electrophoresis.
4. plasmapheresis.

(540) **15.** Drugs that have revolutionized the treatment of patients with cancer receiving chemotherapy by shortening the duration of neutropenia and reducing the patient's risk of infection are:

1. prednisone and dexamethasone (Decadron).
2. doxorubicin (Adriamycin) and 5-fluoracil (5-FU).
3. vitamin B_{12} and ferrous sulfate (Feosol).
4. Sargramostim (Leukine) and filgrastim (Neupogen).

(540) **16.** The function of colony-stimulating factors (CSFs) is to stimulate the:

1. bone marrow to produce more blood cells.
2. heart to increase the force of contraction.
3. kidney to promote the reabsorption of water.
4. bronchi of the lung to dilate.

(541) **17.** A complication of allogeneic bone marrow transplants in which T lymphocytes in the transplanted bone marrow identify the patient's tissue as foreign and try to destroy the patient's tissues is:

1. hepatic veno-occlusive disease.
2. graft-versus-host disease.
3. renal insufficiency.
4. thrombocytopenia.

(544) **18.** A condition that puts a patient at increased risk of infection is:

1. anemia.
2. thrombocytopenia.
3. eosinophilia.
4. neutropenia.

(544) **19.** A cancer of the white blood cells in which the bone marrow produces too many immature WBCs is:

1. Hodgkin's disease.
2. non-Hodgkin's lymphoma.
3. leukemia.
4. multiple myeloma.

(544) **20.** Which disease is related to myelogenous and lymphocytic types?

1. leukemia
2. SLE
3. HIV infection
4. Hodgkin's disease

(545) **21.** The leading cause of death in persons with leukemia is:

1. cardiac arrest.
2. infection.
3. hemorrhage.
4. shock.

(545) **22.** Which change in vital signs may indicate sepsis, a common complication of leukemia?

1. tachycardia
2. dyspnea
3. hypertension
4. decreased temperature

(545) **23.** The reason pus may not be seen even though infection is present in a patient with leukemia is that patients with leukemia do not have normal:

1. platelets.
2. red blood cells.
3. white blood cells.
4. cytokines.

(546) **24.** When a patient's absolute neutrophil count falls below $1000/mm^3$, what precautions are instituted?

1. enteric precautions
2. droplet precautions
3. compromised host precautions
4. transmission-based precautions

(546) **25.** A common finding in patients with leukemia is a hematocrit below 30 and hemoglobin below 10 gm/dl, indicating the condition of:

1. anemia.
2. thrombocytopenia.
3. leukopenia.
4. sepsis.

(553) **26.** What minimizes the chance of the recipient's immune system attacking the transplanted organ?

1. administration of steroids
2. tissue matching of donor to recipient
3. administration of antibiotics
4. administration of platelets

(547) **27.** Exaggerated immune responses that are uncomfortable and potentially harmful are:

1. hypersensitivity reactions.
2. bacterial lung infections.
3. tachycardiac reactions.
4. peripheral neuropathy reactions.

CHAPTER 33

Student Name ______________________________

Cardiac Disorders

Answer Key: Textbook page references are provided as a guide for answering these questions. A complete answer key was provided for your instructor.

OBJECTIVES

1. Label the major parts of the heart.
2. Describe the flow of blood through the heart and coronary vessels.
3. Name the elements of the heart's conduction system.
4. State the order in which normal impulses are conducted through the heart.
5. Explain the nursing considerations for patients having procedures to detect or evaluate cardiac disorders.
6. Identify nursing implications for common therapeutic measures, including drug, diet, or oxygen therapy; pacemakers and cardioverters; cardiac surgery; and cardiopulmonary resuscitation.
7. For selected cardiac disorders, explain the pathophysiology, risk factors, signs and symptoms, complications, and treatment.
8. List the data to be obtained in assessing the patient with a cardiac disorder.
9. Assist in developing nursing care plans for patients with cardiac disorders.

LEARNING ACTIVITIES

A. Match the definition or description in the numbered column with the most appropriate term in the lettered column.

(560) **1.** ________ Slow heart rate, usually defined as fewer than 60 beats per minute (bpm)

(560) **2.** ________ Rapid heart rate, usually defined as greater than 100 bpm

(579) **3.** ________ Abnormal thickening and hardening of the arterial walls caused by fat and fibrin deposits

(581) **4.** ________ Obstruction of a blood vessel with a blood clot transported through the bloodstream

(561) **5.** ________ A sound heard on auscultation of the heart that usually indicates turbulent blood flow across heart valves

(579) **6.** ________ Abnormal thickening, hardening, and loss of elasticity of the arterial walls

(559) **7.** ________ The amount of blood in a ventricle at the end of diastole; the pressure generated at the end of diastole

(581) **8.** ________ Disturbance of rhythm; arrhythmia

A. Murmur
B. Thromboembolism
C. Hemodynamics
D. Regurgitation
E. Syncope
F. Atherosclerosis
G. Bradycardia
H. Perfusion
I. Preload
J. Infarct
K. Palpitation
L. Tachycardia
M. Afterload
N. Arteriosclerosis
O. Dysrhythmia

Continued next page

Student Name____

(599) **9.** __________ Study of the movement of blood and the forces that affect it

(560) **10.** __________ A heartbeat that is strong, rapid, or irregular enough that the person is aware of it

(576) **11.** __________ Fainting

(559) **12.** __________ The amount of resistance the ventricles must overcome to eject the blood volume

(594) **13.** __________ Backward flow

(580) **14.** __________ An area of ischemic necrosis caused by disruption of circulation

(576) **15.** __________ Passage of blood through the vessels of an organ

B. Match the definition or description in the numbered column with the most appropriate term in the lettered column.

(577) **1.** __________ The delivery of a synchronized electric shock to the myocardium to restore normal sinus rhythm

(591) **2.** __________ The percentage of ventricular end-diastolic volume ejected with each contraction of the left ventricle

(557) **3.** __________ The ability of a cell to respond to an electrochemical stimulus

(559) **4.** __________ The amount of blood (measured in liters) ejected by each ventricle per minute

(585) **5.** __________ Adaptations made by the heart and circulation to maintain normal cardiac output

A. Cardiac output
B. Systole
C. Conductivity
D. Ejection fraction
E. Compensation
F. Defibrillation
G. Contractility
H. Cardioversion
I. Diastole
J. Hypertrophy
K. Excitability
L. Thrombosis
M. Septum
N. Automaticity

Continued next page

(568) **6.** __________ The ability of a cell to generate an impulse without external stimulation

(591) **7.** __________ The ability of cardiac muscle to shorten and contract

(585) **8.** __________ Enlargement of existing cells, resulting in increased size of an organ or tissue

(555) **9.** __________ A wall that divides a body cavity

(594) **10.** __________ Termination of fibrillation, usually by electric shock

(559) **11.** __________ Contraction phase of the cardiac cycle

(562, 568) **12.** __________ The ability of the cell to transmit electrical impulses rapidly and efficiently to distant regions of the heart

(581) **13.** __________ Formation of a blood clot

(559) **14.** __________ Relaxation phase of the cardiac cycle

C. Indicate whether each of the following functions of the heart are (A) increased or (B) decreased by the sympathetic and parasympathetic nervous systems.

(559) **1.** Heart rate

__________ Sympathetic

__________ Parasympathetic

(559) **2.** Speed of conduction through the AV node

__________ Sympathetic

__________ Parasympathetic

(559) **3.** Force or contractions

__________ Sympathetic

__________ Parasympathetic

D. List two factors that increase preload and three factors that decrease preload.

(559) **1.** Increase preload: __________

(559) **2.** Decrease preload: __________

E. Indicate the age-related changes in:

(559) **1.** Density of heart muscle connective tissue: __________

(559) **2.** Elasticity of myocardium: __________

Student Name ______________________________

(559) **3.** Cardiac contractility: ______________________________

(559) **4.** Valves: ______________________________

(559) **5.** Emptying of chambers: ______________________________

(559) **6.** Number of pacemaker cells in the SA node: ______________________________

(559) **7.** Number of nerve fibers in ventricles: ______________________________

(559) **8.** Cardiac response to stress: ______________________________

F. Indicate age-related changes to blood vessels for the areas listed below.

(560) **1.** Elastic fibers: ______________________________

(560) **2.** Systolic blood pressure: ______________________________

(560) **3.** Pulse pressure: ______________________________

(560) **4.** Veins: ______________________________

G. Match the characteristic of laboratory tests in the numbered column with the appropriate test in the lettered column. Some terms may be used more than once, and some may not be used.

(567) **1.** ________ Indicates the body's ability to defend itself against infection and inflammation; elevated with acute myocardial infarction

(567) **2.** ________ Determines ability of the blood to carry oxygen from the lungs to the tissues and carbon dioxide from the tissues to the lung

(567) **3.** ________ Percentage of packed RBCs in the total sample of whole blood

A. Lipid profile
B. Erythrocyte sedimentation rate
C. Hematocrit
D. WBC
E. Arterial blood gas
F. RBC
G. Hemoglobin
H. Platelet
I. Creatine phosphokinase (CPK)
J. Lactate dehydrogenase (LDH)

Continued next page

(567) **4.** __________ Measurement of main component of the RBCs whose function is to transport oxygen to the cells

(567) **5.** __________ Measurement of formed elements in the blood needed for coagulation

(566) **6.** __________ Indicates damage to myocardial cells

(567) **7.** __________ Intracellular enzyme elevated in acute myocardial infarction

(565) **8.** __________ Determination of body's ability to maintain acid-base balance

H. The pain of heart problems may radiate or may be referred to other areas. List three areas to which pain may radiate.

(581) **1.** ____________________

(581) **2.** ____________________

(581) **3.** ____________________

I. Match the drug classification in the numbered column with its use and action in the lettered column.

(568) **1.** __________ Diuretics

(568) **2.** __________ Antianginals

(568) **3.** __________ Antiplatelets

(568) **4.** __________ Cardiac glycosides

(568) **5.** __________ Thrombolytics

A. Increase cardiac output
B. Dissolve clots
C. Prevent strokes
D. Decrease fluid retention
E. Relieve pain

J. List four words that patients with angina use to describe anginal pain.

(580) **1.** ____________________

(580) **2.** ____________________

(580) **3.** ____________________

(580) **4.** ____________________

Student Name____

K. List three reasons, related to the characteristics below, why percutaneous transluminal coronary angioplasty (PTCA) may be a preferred treatment over bypass surgery.

(582) **1.** Type of anesthesia: ______________________________

(582) **2.** Invasiveness: ______________________________

(582) **3.** Recovery time: ______________________________

L. Indicate the findings the nurse would expect to observe in patients with mitral stenosis regarding the areas listed below.

(596) **1.** Heart rate: ______________________________

(596) **2.** Respirations: ______________________________

(596) **3.** Pulse pressure: ______________________________

(596) **4.** Jugular vein: ______________________________

(596) **5.** Auscultated lung sounds: ______________________________

(596) **6.** Sounds of murmur: ______________________________

M. Match the characteristic in the numbered column with the appropriate heart chamber in the lettered column. Some chambers may be used more than once, and some chambers may not be used.

(555) **1.** __________ Contains the highest pressure in the heart

(555) **2.** __________ Receives blood through the tricuspid valve

(555) **3.** __________ Cone-shaped, has the thickest muscle mass of the four chambers

(555) **4.** __________ Receives blood saturated with oxygen from the four pulmonary veins

(555) **5.** __________ Receives blood from the inferior and superior vena cava

A. Right atrium (RA)
B. Right ventricle (RV)
C. Left atrium (LA)
D. Left ventricle (LV)

N. Indicate whether each of the following factor(s) (A) increases or (B) decreases preload, contractility, or afterload.

A. Increase(s)
B. Decrease(s)

(559) **1.** Dehydration, hemorrhage, and venous vasodilation __________ preload.

(559) **2.** Increased venous return to the heart and overhydration __________ preload.

(574) **3.** Catecholamines __________ contractility.

(570) **4.** Beta blockers __________ contractility.

(559) **5.** Vasodilation __________ afterload.

(559) **6.** Hypertension, vasoconstriction, and aortic stenosis __________ afterload.

O. Match the definition or description in the numbered column with the appropriate diagnostic test or procedure in the lettered column. Some answers may be used more than once, and some answers may not be used.

(562) **1.** __________ An ambulatory ECG that provides continuous monitoring

(562, 563) **2.** __________ A transducer is used that picks up sound waves and converts them to electrical impulses

(564) **3.** __________ A high-resolution, three-dimensional image of the heart; cardiac tissue is imaged without lung or bone interference

A. Stress test
B. Cardiac catheterization
C. EEG
D. Echocardiogram
E. Electrophysiology study (EPS)
F. MRI
G. Holter monitor
H. TEE
I. MUGA
J. Thallium imaging
K. Pulse oximetry

Continued next page

Student Name____

(565) **4.** __________ An exercise tolerance test that is a recording of an individual's cardiovascular response during a measured exercise challenge

(556) **5.** __________ Study of electrical activity of the heart

(565) **6.** __________ A procedure in which a catheter is advanced into the heart chambers or coronary arteries under fluoroscopy

(563) **7.** __________ Images of the heart obtained with a probe in the esophagus

(565) **8.** __________ Test that may determine pressures in the RA, RV, and pulmonary artery

(565) **9.** __________ Electrodes placed on the surface of the skin pick up the electrical impulses of the heart

(565) **10.** __________ The patient ambulates on a treadmill or a stationary bicycle while connected to a monitor

(562) **11.** __________ Heart sonogram that is a visualization and recording of the size, shape, position, and behavior of the heart's internal structures

(565) **12.** __________ Injection of technetium 99m that concentrates in necrotic myocardial tissue to measure ventricular failure

(566) **13.** __________ Noninvasive measurement of oxygen saturation

(565) **14.** __________ Evaluates patency of coronary artery bypass grafts

(565) **15.** __________ Use of catheters with multiple electrodes inserted through the femoral vein to record the heart's electrical activity

P. Match the description of complications of coronary artery disease in the numbered column with the most appropriate term in the lettered column. Some terms may be used more than once, and some terms may not be used.

(581) **1.** __________ Disturbances in heart rhythm

(581) **2.** __________ When the injured left ventricle is unable to meet the body's circulatory demands

(581) **3.** __________ The most frequent cause of death after an AMI; marked by hypotension and decreasing alertness

(581) **4.** __________ When clots form in the injured heart chambers, they may break loose and travel to the lung

(581) **5.** __________ A fatal complication in which weakened areas of the ventricular wall bulge and burst

A. Ventricular rupture
B. Mitral stenosis
C. Dysrhythmias
D. Hemorrhage
E. Cardiogenic shock
F. Thromboembolism
G. Cardiac failure

Q. Complete the statement in the numbered column with the most appropriate term in the lettered column. Some terms may be used more than once, and some terms may not be used.

(594) **1.** The narrowing of the opening in the valve that impedes blood flow from the left atrium into the left ventricle is called __________.

(594) **2.** The leading cause of mitral stenosis is __________.

(594) **3.** In patients with mitral stenosis, the chamber of the heart that dilates to accommodate the amount of blood not ejected is the __________.

A. Tricuspid stenosis
B. Commissurotomy
C. Angioplasty
D. Mitral stenosis
E. Heart murmur
F. Rheumatic heart disease
G. Left ventricle
H. Left atrium
I. Right ventricle

Continued next page

Student Name____

(594) **4.** Excision of parts of the leaflets of the mitral valve to enlarge the opening is called __________.

(594) **5.** When collecting data for the assessment of the patient with mitral stenosis, the nurse takes the vital signs and auscultates for __________.

R. Match the drug used for cardiac disorders in the numbered column with its classification in the lettered column. Some classifications may be used more than once, and some may not be used.

(570) **1.** __________ Nitroglycerin

(575) **2.** __________ Aspirin, dipyridamole (Persantine), and clopidogrel (Plavix)

(575) **3.** __________ Heparin and warfarin (Coumadin)

(581) **4.** __________ Morphine and meperidine hydrochloride (Demerol)

(568) **5.** __________ Furosemide (Lasix) and hydrochlorothiazide (Esidrix, HCTZ, and Oretic)

(575) **6.** __________ Streptokinase, sotalol hydrochloride (Betapace), and tissue plasminogen activator

(568) **7.** __________ Digoxin (Lanoxin) and digitoxin

A. Anticholinergics
B. Vasodilators
C. Narcotic analgesics
D. Antiplatelet agents
E. Antidysrhythmics
F. Diuretics
G. Antithrombolytic agents
H. Anticoagulants
I. Cardiac glycosides

S. Match the nursing diagnosis for the postoperative cardiac surgery patient in the numbered column with the most appropriate "related to" statement in the lettered column.

(578) 1. ________ Ineffective thermoregulation

(578) 2. ________ Decreased cardiac output

(578) 3. ________ Risk for infection

A. Altered skin integrity
B. Cooling during surgery
C. Fluid loss or decreased fluid intake

T. Match the ECG change in the numbered column with the feature of acute myocardial infarction in the lettered column.

(582) 1. ________ The T wave is inverted

(582) 2. ________ There is ST segment elevation

(582) 3. ________ A significant Q wave is present; the Q wave is greater than one-third the height of the R wave

A. Ischemia
B. Infarction
C. Injury

U. Match the use(s) of AMI drug therapy in the numbered column with the specific drug in the lettered column. Some drugs may be used more than once, and some may not be used.

(581) 1. ________ Used for chest pain

(582) 2. ________ Administered through an IV or into the coronary arteries to dissolve thrombi

(582) 3. ________ Following the administration of antithrombolytics, this drug is administered to prevent further clot formation

(582) 4. ________ Administered for ventricular tachycardia

(582) 5. ________ Increases myocardial contractility and decreases the heart rate

A. Furosemide (Lasix)
B. Streptokinase
C. Digitalis
D. Morphine sulfate
E. Atropine sulfate
F. Lidocaine
G. Heparin

Student Name____

V. Match the nursing diagnosis for a patient with acute myocardial infarction in the numbered column with the "related to" statement in the lettered column.

(583) **1.** __________ Anxiety

(583) **2.** __________ Pain

(583) **3.** __________ Decreased cardiac output

A. Dysrhythmia
B. Feeling of impending doom
C. Lack of oxygen to the myocardium

W. For the following signs and symptoms of congestive heart failure, indicate whether they are indicative of (A) right-sided or (B) left-sided failure.

(587) **1.** __________ Dependent edema

(585) **2.** __________ Decreasing BP readings

(587) **3.** __________ Increased central venous pressure

(585) **4.** __________ Anxious, pale, and tachycardiac

(587) **5.** __________ Jugular vein distention

(587) **6.** __________ Abdominal engorgement

(587) **7.** __________ Crackles, wheezes, dyspnea, and cough

(587) **8.** __________ Pulmonary edema

(587) **9.** __________ Decreased urinary output

A. Right-sided
B. Left-sided

X. Match the actions of drugs used to treat CHF in the numbered column with the drug or drug classification in the lettered column. Some answers may be used more than once, and some answers may not be used.

(587) **1.** ________ Improve(s) pump function by increasing contractility and decreasing heart rate

(587) **2.** ________ Decrease(s) circulating fluid volume and decrease(s) preload

(587) **3.** ________ Decrease(s) anxiety, dilate(s) the vasculature, and reduce(s) myocardial consumption in the acute stage

A. Heparin
B. Morphine
C. Diuretics
D. Streptokinase
E. Cardiac glycosides or inotropic agents, such as digoxin

Y. Match the nursing diagnosis for the patient with CHF in the numbered column with the "related to" statement in the lettered column.

(588) **1.** ________ Fluid volume excess

(588) **2.** ________ Impaired gas exchange

(588) **3.** ________ Anxiety

(588) **4.** ________ Decreased cardiac output

(588) **5.** ________ Activity intolerance

A. Inability to perform activities
B. Decreased pulmonary perfusion
C. Mechanical failure
D. Ineffective cardiac pumping
E. Edema and inability to breathe

Student Name____

Z. In Figure 33-2 below, label the parts (A–M) of the heart.

(557, and see A&P text)

A.	__________________	**H.**	__________________
B.	__________________	**I.**	__________________
C.	__________________	**J.**	__________________
D.	__________________	**K.**	__________________
E.	__________________	**L.**	__________________
F.	__________________	**M.**	__________________
G.	__________________		

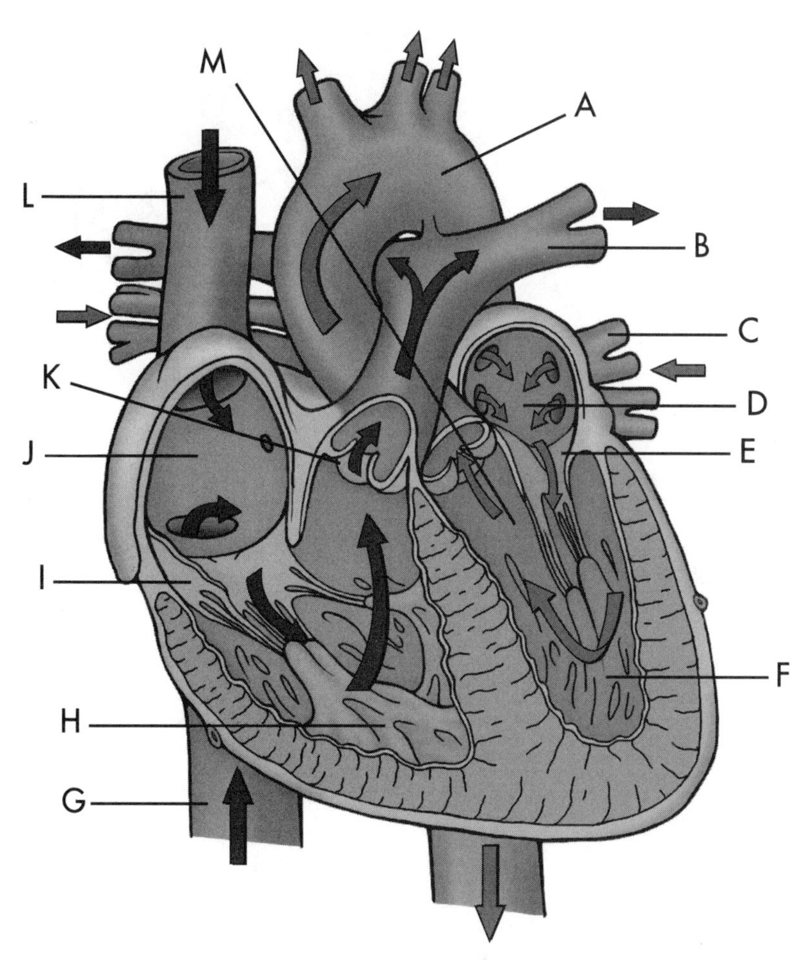

AA. In Figure 33-4 below, label the parts (A–E) of the conduction system of the heart.

(558)

A. ____________________

B. ____________________

C. ____________________

D. ____________________

E. ____________________

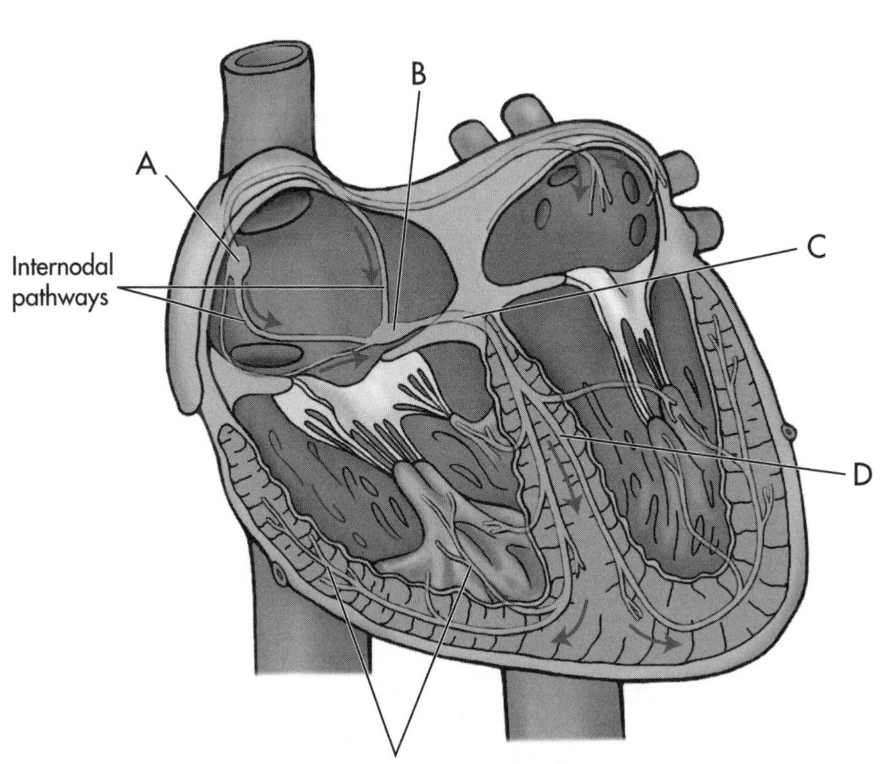

MULTIPLE-CHOICE QUESTIONS

BB. Choose the most appropriate answer.

(556) **1.** The pressure is highest in which heart chamber?

1. right atrium
2. left atrium
3. right ventricle
4. left ventricle

(559) **2.** Afterload is decreased by :

1. vasodilation.
2. overhydration.
3. vasoconstriction.
4. increased venous return to heart.

(556) **3.** The first branches of the systemic circulation are the:

1. subclavian arteries.
2. coronary arteries.
3. carotid arteries.
4. brachial arteries.

(557) **4.** The ventricles contract when the electrical impulse reaches the:

1. SA node.
2. AV node.
3. Purkinje fibers.
4. bundle of His.

Student Name____

(559) **5.** Stroke volume, the amount of blood ejected with each ventricular contraction, depends on myocardial:

1. contractility.
2. excitability.
3. conductivity.
4. automaticity.

(561) **6.** If the valves of the heart do not close properly, the patient is said to have:

1. infarction. 2. murmur.
3. necrosis. 4. tachycardia.

(559) **7.** Ways to increase oxygen supply to the myocardium are to administer supplemental oxygen and to increase coronary blood flow by:

1. coronary artery vasoconstriction.
2. increased myocardial contraction.
3. coronary artery vasodilation.
4. decreased myocardial contraction.

(560) **8.** Thrombophlebitis and varicosities are more common in:

1. adolescents.
2. young adults.
3. middle-aged people.
4. older people.

(560) **9.** Which of the following is more likely to occur in older persons as the cardiovascular system adapts more slowly to changes in position?

1. tachycardia
2. bradycardia
3. postural hypotension
4. headache

(560) **10.** In asking cardiac patients about their diets, the nurse should especially record information about which two areas of intake?

1. calcium and vitamin D
2. salt and fat
3. protein and iron
4. vitamin C and vitamin E

(560) **11.** A noninvasive measure of cardiac output is:

1. cardiac catheterization.
2. pulse pressure.
3. angioplasty.
4. blood gas measurement.

(561) **12.** The sound produced by turbulent blood flow across the valves is called a(n):

1. heart murmur.
2. ventricular gallop.
3. atrial gallop.
4. orthopnea.

(562) **13.** A common diagnostic test that measures the electrical activity of the heart is the:

1. CT scan.
2. echocardiogram.
3. ECG.
4. stress test.

(562) **14.** A normal ECG finding is documented as a normal:

1. tachycardia
2. sinus rhythm
3. bradycardia
4. ventricular gallop

(565) **15.** The stress test must be stopped immediately if which of the following symptoms occur?

1. angina and falling blood pressure
2. increased heart rate and increasing respirations
3. diaphoresis and thirst
4. slower respirations and hunger

(559) **16.** The normal cardiac output is:

1. 1–3 liters/min.
2. 4–8 liters/min.
3. 10–13 liters/min.
4. 15–20 liters/hour.

(574) **17.** Patients with acute myocardial infarction often exhibit:

1. respiratory acidosis.
2. respiratory alkalosis.
3. metabolic acidosis.
4. metabolic alkalosis.

(566) **18.** A noninvasive measurement of arterial oxygen saturation is:

1. blood pressure.
2. blood gases.
3. pulse pressure.
4. pulse oximetry.

(575) **19.** What type of diet is generally recommended for cardiac patients?

1. low-fat, high-calcium
2. low-fat, high-fiber
3. low-sodium, low-protein
4. high-sodium, low-potassium

(575) **20.** If fluid retention accompanies the cardiac problem, the physician may order restriction of:

1. potassium. 2. sodium.
3. fat. 4. calcium.

(575) **21.** Diuretics, such as furosemide, may cause a deficiency of:

1. sodium. 2. calcium.
3. fiber. 4. potassium.

(576) **22.** The purpose of temporary and permanent pacemakers is to improve cardiac output and tissue perfusion by restoring regular:

1. blood volume.
2. blood pressure.
3. impulse conduction.
4. myocardial contractility.

(577) **23.** The delivery of a synchronized shock to terminate atrial or ventricular tachyarrhythmias is called:

1. a pacemaker.
2. cardiac catheterization.
3. angioplasty.
4. cardioversion.

(577) **24.** During open-heart surgery, the patient's core temperature is reduced to decrease the body's need for:

1. oxygen. 2. sodium.
3. potassium. 4. ATP.

(579) **25.** Smoking, high blood pressure, and obesity are risk factors for:

1. mitral valve stenosis.
2. atherosclerosis.
3. pericarditis.
4. endocarditis.

(580) **26.** The most frequent symptom of coronary artery disease, which represents lack of oxygen to tissues, is:

1. fever. 2. cyanosis.
3. indigestion. 4. pain.

(580) **27.** The substernal pain resulting from lack of oxygen to the myocardium is called:

1. heartburn.
2 dyspnea.
3. pleurisy.
4. angina pectoris.

(580) **28.** Modifiable risk factors for acute myocardial infarction include hypertension, obesity, and:

1. diabetes mellitus.
2. male gender.
3. smoking.
4. family history.

Student Name____

(580) **29.** What drugs are used to prevent angina in patients with CAD?

1. diuretics
2. analgesics
3. calcium channel blockers
4. antiplatelet agents

(591) **30.** Nurses should be alert to complaints of decreased exercise tolerance and dyspnea in African-American males because they are at risk for:

1. hypertension
2. cardiomyopathy
3. endocarditis
4. mitral valve stenosis

(581) **31.** Cardiogenic shock is marked by hypotension, cool moist skin, oliguria, and:

1. decreasing alertness.
2. restlessness.
3. headache.
4. cyanosis.

(581) **32.** Which drug is administered to dilate coronary arteries and increase blood flow to the damaged area?

1. nitroglycerin
2. furosemide
3. dipyridamole (Persantine)
4. streptokinase

(583) **33.** Veins generally used in coronary artery bypass surgery as grafts to the coronary arteries include the internal mammary and _______ veins.

1. subclavian
2. femoral
3. jugular
4. saphenous

(588) **34.** In order to decrease cardiac workload and increase oxygenation to the myocardium, the recommended position for patients with CHF is:

1. prone.
2. supine.
3. side-lying.
4. semi-Fowler's or high-Fowler's.

(588) **35.** The most common adverse effects of diuretic therapy for patients with CHF are:

1. hypertension and tachycardia.
2. fluid and electrolyte imbalances.
3. headache and oliguria.
4. confusion and weakness.

(587) **36.** A common finding in patients with right-sided heart failure is:

1. increased urinary output.
2. dependent edema.
3. weight loss.
4. cough.

(587) **37.** Drugs that may be given to patients with CHF include diuretics, vasodilators, and:

1. inotropics.
2. anticonvulsants.
3. antihistamines.
4. cholinergics.

(589) **38.** The most common site for organisms to accumulate in patients with infective endocarditis is the:

1. mitral valve.
2. tricuspid valve.
3. aortic valve.
4. pulmonary valve.

(589) **39.** Symptoms of endocarditis include weight loss, malaise, and:

1. oliguria.
2. hypertension.
3. fever.
4. convulsions.

(590) **40.** An important diagnostic test for patients with endocarditis is the:

1. RBC count.
2. WBC count.
3. hematocrit.
4. hemoglobin.

(590) **41.** The main drugs used for endocarditis are:

1. cardiac glycosides.
2. diuretics.
3. calcium channel blockers.
4. antimicrobials.

(590) **42.** The hallmark symptom of pericarditis is:

1. chest pain.
2. headache.
3. hypertension.
4. indigestion.

(590) **43.** The patient with pericarditis is treated with analgesics, anti-inflammatory agents, antibiotics, and:

1. diuretics.
2. anticonvulsants.
3. antipyretics.
4. anticholinergics.

(582) **44.** A procedure in which a peripherally inserted catheter is passed into an occluded artery and a balloon inflated to dilate the artery is:

1. percutaneous transluminal angioplasty.
2. coronary atherectomy.
3. intracoronary stent placement.
4. laser angioplasty.

(591) **45.** Disease of the heart muscle that generally has an unknown cause and leads to heart failure is called:

1. myocardial infarction.
2. congestive heart failure.
3. cardiomyopathy.
4. pericarditis.

(591) **46.** Which type of cardiomyopathy is associated with a high incidence of sudden death?

1. hypertrophic
2. dilated
3. restrictive
4. congestive heart failure

(593) **47.** Lifelong medications that must be given to patients with heart transplants include:

1. antihistamines.
2. analgesics.
3. antimicrobials.
4. immunosuppressives.

(594) **48.** The two major valve problems of the heart are stenosis and:

1. inflammation.
2. regurgitation.
3. emboli.
4. hemorrhage.

(575) **49.** Heparin dosage for the patient with a cardiac disorder is adjusted according to the patient's:

1. hemoglobin.
2. prothrombin time.
3. partial thromboplastin time.
4. hematocrit.

Student Name________________________________

(568) **50.** Diuretics such as furosemide and hydrochlorothiazide are used with cardiac conditions to treat:

1. hypokalemia.
2. fluid retention.
3. dehydration.
4. dysrhythmias.

(568) **51.** Before each dose of digitalis, the apical pulse is counted for 1 full minute; the drug is withheld and the physician notified if the pulse is below:

1. 60 bpm. 2. 70 bpm.
3. 72 bpm. 4. 80 bpm.

(569) **52.** Elderly people are more susceptible to adverse drug effects because they:

1. metabolize drugs more quickly.
2. have decreased elasticity of vessels.
3. excrete drugs more slowly.
4. are hypersensitive to more drugs.

(593) **53.** Patients taking immunosuppressive drugs to prevent rejection of transplanted tissue have reduced:

1. circulation.
2. resistance to infection.
3. metabolism of drugs.
4. red blood cell counts.

(568) **54.** Antidysrhythmic drugs work by slowing impulse conduction, increasing resistance to premature contraction, or:

1. increasing contractility.
2. enhancing inotropism.
3. depressing automaticity.
4. stimulating the SA node.

(580) **55.** A major part of treatment for persons with heart disease is the reduction of dietary fat and:

1. sugar. 2. protein.
3. cholesterol. 4. vitamin E.

(594) **56.** An automatic implantable cardioverter-defibrillator is used to:

1. improve contractility in people with cardiomyopathy.
2. decrease the risk of sudden cardiac death in people with recurrent life-threatening dysrhythmias.
3. convert patients in cardiac arrest to normal sinus rhythm.
4. support cardiac function in patients awaiting heart transplants.

(594) **57.** The internal cardiac defibrillator (ICD) is used to treat patients with life-threatening, recurrent:

1. hypertension.
2. aortic stenosis.
3. ventricular fibrillation.
4. endocarditis.

(607) **58.** A Swan-Ganz catheter is inserted into the pulmonary artery to measure:

1. tricuspid valve function.
2. right-sided heart pressure.
3. mitral valve stenosis.
4. aortic stenosis.

(599) **59.** Measurements below normal from a central venous catheter threaded into the right atrium indicates:

1. hypovolemia.
2. hypervolemia.
3. hypotension.
4. low cardiac output.

(560) **60.** How should you document a pulse that is easily obliterated by slight finger pressure, which returns as the pressure is released?

1. absent
2. nonpalpable
3. weak or thready
4. bounding

(561) **61.** Which heart sound is normal in children and young adults but is pathologic if it is heard after the age of 30?

1. S_1
2. S_2
3. S_3, ventricular gallop
4. S_4, atrial gallop

(575) **62.** What type of drug therapy is used after an AMI to prevent strokes?

1. cardiac glycosides
2. antidysrhythmics
3. antiplatelets
4. nitrates

(580) **63.** Calcium channel blockers, vasodilators, and beta-adrenergic blockers are used to treat:

1. CHF.
2. angina.
3. AMI.
4. heart murmurs.

(568) **64.** Drugs that slow down the rate of impulse conduction in the heart are:

1. antidysrhythmics.
2. nitrates.
3. calcium channel blockers.
4. antiplatelets.

(575) **65.** The dosage of heparin is based on measurements of the patient's:

1. aPTT. 2. INR.
3. PT. 4. CBC.

(561) **66.** When the pericardium is inflamed, a sound heart along the left sternal border is the:

1. heart murmur.
2. friction rub.
3. atrial gallop.
4. ventricular gallop.

(587) **67.** The most widely used drugs in the treatment of CHF are:

1. cardiac glycosides.
2. antianginals.
3. antidysrhythmics.
4. adrenergic beta-blockers.

(580) **68.** The first medication given to patients with chest pain is:

1. morphine.
2. aspirin.
3. Demerol.
4. nitroglycerin.

(576) **69.** Which herb taken to lower plasma lipids may increase the effects of anticoagulants and insulin?

1. kava kava 2. ephedra
3. garlic 4. aloe

(576) **70.** Chambers paced, chambers sensed, and mode of response are three settings for a:

1. defibrillator.
2. pacemaker.
3. holter monitor.
4. cardioverter.

Student Name____

(577) **71.** Patient teaching for a person with a permanent pacemaker includes:

1. teaching patients how to count their pulse for 1 full minute daily.
2. showing patients how to take and document weekly weights.
3. encouraging patients to avoid foods high in vitamin K.
4. limiting exercise to walking twice a week.

(594) **72.** The leading cause of mitral stenosis is:

1. hypertension.
2. acute myocardial infarction.
3. infective endocarditis.
4. rheumatic heart disease.

(594) **73.** As left atrial pressure increases in mitral stenosis, this change leads to:

1. right ventricular hypertrophy.
2. decreased pulmonary pressures.
3. decreased workload on the right side of the heart.
4. increased peripheral edema.

(573) **74.** If dietary control does not reduce cholesterol sufficiently, treatment may include:

1. antihypertensives.
2. antidysrhythmics.
3. antianginals.
4. antilipemics.

(573) **75.** Questran, Lopid, and niacin are drugs classified as:

1. cardiac glycosides.
2. nitrates.
3. antilipemics.
4. antiplatelets.

CHAPTER 34

Student Name ______________________________

Vascular Disorders

Answer Key: Textbook page references are provided as a guide for answering these questions. A complete answer key was provided for your instructor.

OBJECTIVES

1. Identify specific anatomic and physiologic factors that affect the vascular system and tissue oxygenation.
2. Indicate appropriate parameters for assessing a patient with peripheral vascular disease, aneurysm, and aortic dissection.
3. Discuss tests and procedures used to diagnose selected vascular disorders and the nursing considerations for each.
4. State the pathophysiology, signs and symptoms, complications, and medical or surgical treatments for selected vascular disorders.
5. Assist in developing a plan of care for patients with selected vascular disorders.

LEARNING ACTIVITIES

A. Match the definition in the numbered column with the most appropriate term in the lettered column.

(624) **1.** __________ Sudden obstruction of an artery by a floating clot or foreign material

(614) **2.** __________ An abnormal sensation

(613) **3.** __________ Concentration of the blood

(632) **4.** __________ Development of a clot in the presence of venous inflammation

A. Thrombophlebitis
B. Thrombosis
C. Phlebothrombosis
D. Embolism
E. Vasoconstriction
F. Paresthesia
G. Bruit
H. Ischemia
I. Aneurysm
J. Hemoconcentration
K. Poikilothermia
L. Vasodilation
M. Viscosity

Continued next page

(624) **5.** ________ Deficient blood flow due to obstruction or constriction of blood vessels

(613) **6.** ________ Increase in blood vessel diameter

(632) **7.** ________ Development of venous thrombi without venous inflammation

(612) **8.** ________ Decrease in blood vessel diameter

(614) **9.** ________ Coolness in an area of the body due to decreased blood flow

(615) **10.** ________ Thickness of the blood

(632) **11.** ________ Development or presence of a thrombus

(629) **12.** ________ Dilated segment of an artery caused by weakness and stretching of the vessel wall

(615) **13.** ________ Murmur detected by auscultation

B. Match the definition or description in the numbered column with the most appropriate term in the lettered column. Some terms may be used more than once, and some may not be used.

(612) **1.** ________ Vessels that return blood to the heart

(612) **2.** ________ The two main trunks of these vessels are the thoracic duct and the right lymphatic duct

(610) **3.** ________ Thick-walled, elastic structures

(612) **4.** ________ Equipped with valves that aid in the transportation of blood against gravity

(611) **5.** ________ Formed by a single layer of endothelial cells

(610) **6.** ________ Vessels that carry blood away from the heart

A. Veins
B. Valves
C. Leaflets
D. Capillaries
E. Lymph vessels
F. Arteries
G. Lymph nodes

Student Name____

(611) **7.** __________ Transfer of oxygen and nutrients between the blood and the tissue cells occurs here

(612) **8.** __________ Thin-walled vessels that collect and drain fluid from the peripheral tissues and transport the fluid to the venous system

C. Indicate for each factor in the numbered column whether it (A) increases or (B) decreases peripheral resistance.

(612) **1.** __________ Sympathetic nervous system stimulation

(612) **2.** __________ Epinephrine

(612, 613) **3.** __________ Angiotensin

(613) **4.** __________ Kinins, histamine, and prostaglandins

(613) **5.** __________ Viscous blood

(620) **6.** __________ Heat

(618) **7.** __________ Cold

(618) **8.** __________ Emotional stress

A. Increases
B. Decreases

D. List the 6 Ps—characteristics of peripheral vascular disease.

(613) **1.** ____

(613) **2.** ____

(613) **3.** ____

(613) **4.** ____

(613) **5.** ____

(613) **6.** ____

E. Complete the statement in the numbered column with the most appropriate term in the lettered column. Some terms may be used more than once, and some may not be used.

(615) **1.** A test to evaluate the pain response in the calf area to determine venous thrombosis is called __________.

(615) **2.** A test used to determine the patency of the ulnar and radial artery is called __________.

(615) **3.** When blood flowing through the arteries sounds like turbulent, fast-moving fluid, these sounds are called __________.

(614) **4.** Brown pigmentation sites with flaky skin over the edematous areas of the ankles are described as __________.

A. Bruits
B. Babinski's reflex
C. Allen's test
D. Moro's reflex
E. Homans' sign
F. Stasis dermatitis

F. Complete the statements in the numbered column with the most appropriate term in the lettered column. Some terms may be used more than once, and some terms may not be used.

(617) **1.** A noninvasive, inexpensive diagnostic tool in which sound waves are directed toward the artery or vein being tested is __________.

(617) **2.** A noninvasive examination that measures the blood volume and graphs changes in the flow of blood is __________.

(617) **3.** The segmental limb pressure test and pulse volume measurement test are examples of __________.

(617) **4.** An invasive procedure that requires the injection of dye into the vascular system is called __________.

(631) **5.** A noninvasive test that demonstrates backward flow of venous blood is __________.

A. MRI
B. Pressure measurement
C. Brodie-Trendelenburg test
D. Angiography
E. Doppler ultrasound
F. Plethysmography
G. ECG

Student Name____

G. Match the description or definition in the numbered column with the most appropriate term in the lettered column. Some terms may be used more than once, and some terms may not be used.

(620, 621) **1.** __________ The injection of a chemical that irritates the venous endothelium for patients with varicose veins

(620) **2.** __________ A procedure that is done to relieve arterial stenosis in people who are poor surgical risks

(620) **3.** __________ A procedure used to remove varicose veins

(620) **4.** __________ An incision into the obstructed vessel to strip away emboli and atherosclerotic plaque followed by surgical closure of the vessel

(620) **5.** __________ The excision of the sympathetic ganglia; used for patients with intermittent claudication

(620) **6.** __________ The removal of a blood clot located in a large vessel

A. Sympathectomy
B. Percutaneous transluminal angioplasty
C. Thermotherapy
D. Embolectomy
E. Sclerotherapy
F. Intermittent pneumatic compression
G. Vein ligation and stripping
H. Endarterectomy

H. Complete the statements relating to signs and symptoms of deep vein thrombosis in the numbered column with the most appropriate term in the lettered column. Some terms may be used more than once, and some terms may not be used.

(632) **1.** The affected extremity appears __________.

(632) **2.** Superficial veins are __________.

(632) **3.** The affected area of compromise may be __________.

(632) **4.** Homans' sign is __________.

A. Warm and tender
B. Negative
C. Cool
D. Prominent
E. Positive
F. Edematous
G. Lack of sensation

I. Match the nursing diagnosis in the numbered column for a patient with venous thrombosis with the appropriate "related to" statement in the lettered column.

(632) 1. ________ Impaired skin integrity

(632) 2. ________ Acute pain

(632) 3. ________ Activity intolerance

(632) 4. ________ Ineffective tissue perfusion

A. Impaired circulation and tissue ischemia
B. Venous stasis
C. Ineffective peripheral circulation
D. Leg pain or swelling

J. Explain why care must be taken when using heat on patients with peripheral vascular disease.

(620)

K. List four classifications of drugs that are used in the general management of peripheral vascular disease to improve peripheral circulation.

(621) 1. ____________________

(621) 2. ____________________

(621) 3. ____________________

(621) 4. ____________________

L. List two primary anticoagulants and their antidotes.

(621) 1. Oral drug and antidote: ____________________

(621) 2. Parenteral drug and antidote: ____________________

M. List four complications of aneurysms.

(629) 1. ____________________

(629) 2. ____________________

(629) 3. ____________________

(629) 4. ____________________

Student Name____

N. Using figure 34-2, label the structures of the artery, vein, and capillary using the following numbers.

1. Tunica adventitia
2. Endothelial cells
3. Tunica media
4. External elastic membrane
5. Tunica intima
6. Internal elastic membrane
7. Valve

(611)

A. _____________________

B. _____________________

C. _____________________

D. _____________________

E. _____________________

F. _____________________

G. _____________________

H. _____________________

I. _____________________

J. _____________________

Artery

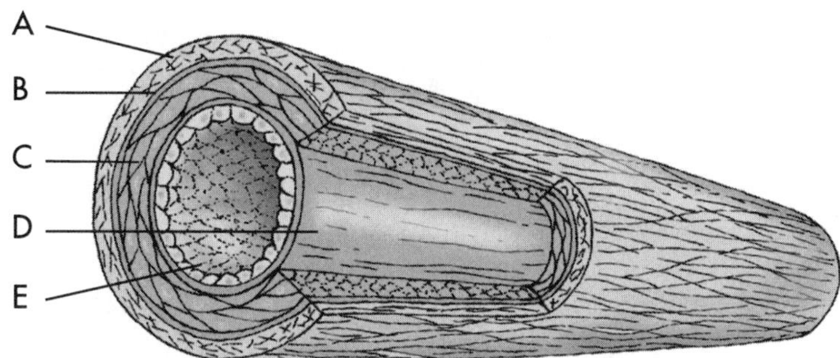

Vein

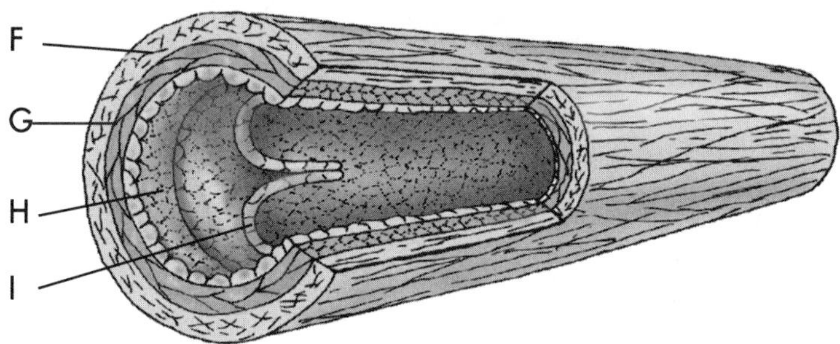

Capillary

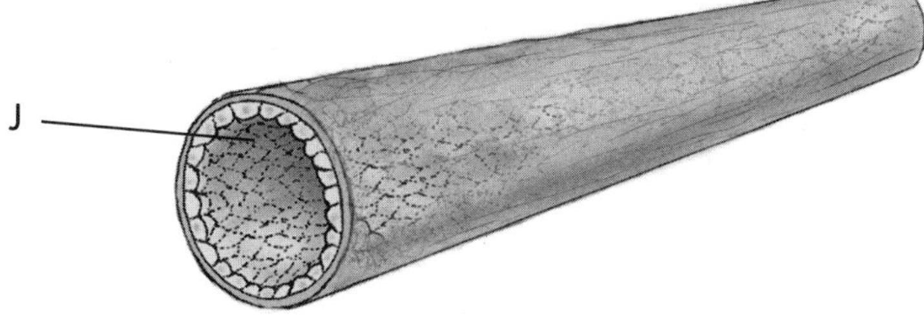

O. Using Figure 34-8, label the veins involved in varicosities using the following numbers.

1. Small saphenous veins
2. Great saphenous veins
3. External iliac veins
4. Femoral veins

(631)

A. ____________________ **C.** ____________________

B. ____________________ **D.** ____________________

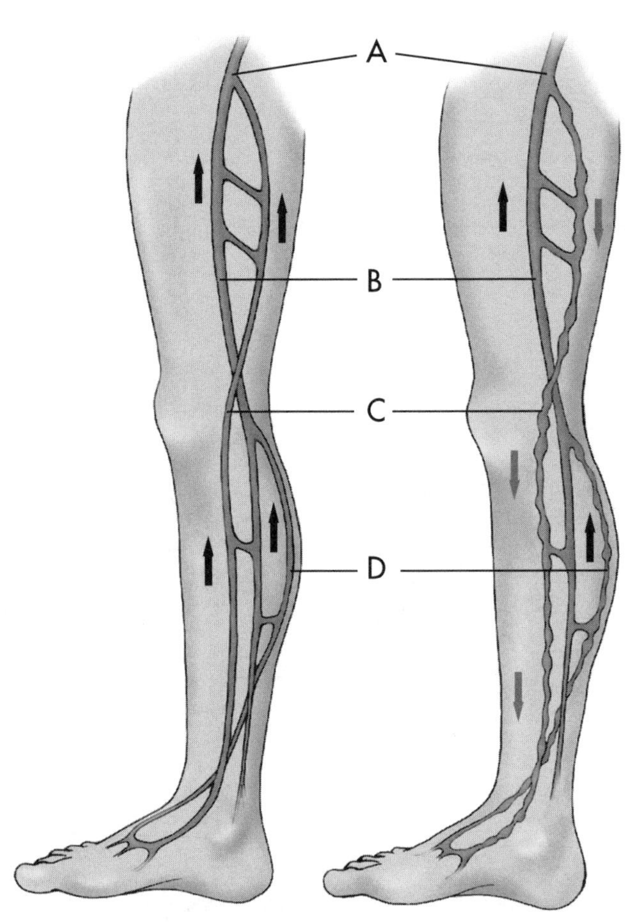

MULTIPLE-CHOICE QUESTIONS

P. Choose the most appropriate answer.

(610) **1.** Any interruption of the blood flow to the distal regions of the body, as occurs in peripheral vascular disease (PVD), results in:

1. kidney failure.
2. cardiac shock.
3. dyspnea.
4. hypoxia.

(610) **2.** The nervous system that acts on the smooth muscles of vessels, resulting in dilation and constriction of the artery walls, is the:

1. autonomic.
2. somatic.
3. central.
4. cranial.

Student Name____

(613) **3.** The primary result of aging on the peripheral vessels is:

1. vasoconstriction of arteries.
2. vasodilation of veins.
3. increased elasticity of vessel walls.
4. stiffening of vessel walls.

(613) **4.** Aging in the vascular system causes a slowing of the heart rate and a decrease in the stroke volume, resulting in decreased:

1. cardiac output.
2. tachycardia.
3. peripheral resistance.
4. hypertension.

(613) **5.** The transportation of oxygen is compromised in the aging patient by the decreased:

1. hematocrit.
2. WBC count.
3. hemoglobin.
4. cardiac enzymes.

(610) **6.** PVD is a common complication of:

1. pneumonia.
2. myocardial infarction.
3. diabetes.
4. influenza.

(614) **7.** If PVD causes limb-threatening ischemia, amputation of a limb may be necessary because of the development of:

1. cyanosis.
2. tissue necrosis.
3. fractures.
4. hypersensitivity.

(614) **8.** Skin temperature is palpated in patients with PVD to determine the existence of:

1. infection. 2. bleeding.
3. cyanosis. 4. ischemia.

(614) **9.** In the evaluation of edema, when the thumb is depressed in the area for 5 seconds and the depression of the thumb remains in the edematous area, the edema is said to be:

1. 1+. 2. 2+.
3. 3+. 4. pitting.

(618) **10.** If pain or severe skin color changes occur during exercises with PVD patients, the nurse should:

1. encourage the exercises to be done gradually.
2. stop the exercises immediately.
3. ambulate the patient to promote venous return.
4. administer muscle relaxants as ordered.

(618) **11.** It is important for patients with PVD to stop smoking because smoking causes:

1. intermittent claudication.
2. skin ulceration.
3. vasoconstriction.
4. vasodilation.

(619) **12.** The primary function of intermittent pneumatic compression devices is to prevent:

1. infection.
2. hemorrhage.
3. deep vein thrombosis.
4. cyanosis.

(620) **13.** Which position should be avoided by patients with PVD?

1. extended standing
2. elevation of lower extremities
3. lowering extremities below the level of the heart
4. elevation of extremities to a nondependent position

(620) **14.** Which works as a vasodilator that promotes arterial flow to the peripheral tissues?

1. TED hose
2. intermittent pneumatic compression
3. heat
4. cold

(621) **15.** Elevation of the extremity following surgery for patients with PVD aids in the prevention of:

1. hemorrhage.
2. edema.
3. hypotension.
4. ulceration.

(621) **16.** Disappearance of a peripheral pulse during the postoperative care of patients with PVD alerts the nurse to the development of a:

1. thrombotic occlusion.
2. massive hemorrhage.
3. severe infection.
4. varicose vein.

(621) **17.** The main adverse action of anticoagulants is:

1. bleeding.
2. infection.
3. hypertension.
4. oliguria.

(621) **18.** Thrombolytic therapy is employed to:

1. shorten the clotting time.
2. increase clot formation.
3. prevent the formation of new clots.
4. dissolve an existing clot.

(624) **19.** The use of vasodilators results in increased blood flow by relaxing the vascular smooth muscle and causing:

1. increased clotting time.
2. decreased elasticity in vessels.
3. decreased resistance in vessels.
4. increased narrowing in vessels.

(632) **20.** A grave risk with a diagnosis of deep vein thrombosis is the development of:

1. hemorrhage.
2. pneumonia.
3. pulmonary embolus.
4. infection.

(632) **21.** Three precipitating factors (called Virchow's triad) for a thrombus to form include hypercoagulability, damage to the vessel walls, and:

1. hemorrhage.
2. stasis of the blood.
3. decreased hematocrit.
4. damaged blood cells.

(632) **22.** The primary diagnostic examinations used in the detection of thrombus formation are plethysmography, Doppler ultrasound, and:

1. venography.
2. an ECG.
3. myelography.
4. angioplasty.

(633) **23.** Patients with thrombosis should not be massaged or rubbed because of the possible development of:

1. severe infection.
2. hemorrhage.
3. skin breakdown.
4. pulmonary emboli.

Student Name ____________________

(633) **24.** The placement of antiembolism hose on patients with thrombosis is done to improve circulation and to prevent:

1. infection.
2. stasis.
3. hemorrhage.
4. ulceration.

(624) **25.** A life-threatening event that requires immediate attention is:

1. arterial embolism.
2. thrombophlebitis.
3. varicose vein disease.
4. thrombosis.

(626) **26.** The absence of a peripheral pulse below the occlusive area is a clinical manifestation of:

1. Raynaud's disease.
2. aneurysms.
3. peripheral arterial occlusive disease.
4. thrombophlebitis.

(630) **27.** During repair of an abdominal aneurysm, the aorta is clamped for a period of time. This poses a risk of:

1. dyspnea.
2. renal failure.
3. pneumonia.
4. incontinence.

(630) **28.** Varicose veins develop as a result of faulty:

1. elasticity.
2. smooth muscle.
3. thickness.
4. valves.

(637) **29.** Chronic venous insufficiency may develop from:

1. varicose veins.
2. plaque formations.
3. thrombophlebitis.
4. aortic dissection.

(633) **30.** Signs of chronic venous insufficiency include edema of lower legs and:

1. redness.
2. infection.
3. stasis dermatitis.
4. cyanosis.

(636) **31.** The medical management of lymphangitis necessitates the administration of:

1. antimicrobial agents.
2. thrombolytic agents.
3. anticoagulants.
4. analgesics.

(636) **32.** Elastic support hose are utilized for several months following an acute attack of lymphangitis to prevent the formation of:

1. infection.
2. hemorrhage.
3. lymphedema.
4. dermatitis.

(613) **33.** The primary age-related change in peripheral vessels is:

1. thrombosis.
2. arteriosclerosis.
3. varicose vein disease.
4. chronic venous insufficiency.

(613) **34.** Aging in the vascular system causes:

1. increased hemoglobin.
2. increased stroke volume.
3. increased heart rate.
4. decreased cardiac output.

(626) **35.** A patient complains of severe aching pain in his left foot after lying quietly in bed. This type of pain is a symptom of:

1. severe arterial occlusion.
2. PVD.
3. deep vein thrombosis.
4. Raynaud's disease.

(617, 618) **36.** A priority in caring for patients with PVD is:

1. pain management.
2. stress management.
3. regular exercise.
4. a low-sodium diet.

(618) **37.** When intermittent claudication occurs, the patient should:

1. stop smoking.
2. avoid constrictive clothing.
3. use antiembolism hose.
4. stop exercise.

(619) **38.** Intermittent pneumatic compression is used for patients:

1. with paresthesia.
2. with intermittent claudication.
3. on bed rest following surgery.
4. on moderate exercise programs.

(621) **39.** Which medications intensify anticoagulant effects?

1. antacids
2. barbiturates
3. oral contraceptives
4. NSAIDs

(621) **40.** Which herbal remedy decreases the effectiveness of warfarin?

1. garlic
2. ginger root
3. St. John's wort
4. ginkgo

(623) **41.** Patients taking vasodilators for PVD must be monitored for:

1. hypotension.
2. hemorrhage.
3. increased vascular resistance.
4. hypocalcemia.

(626) **42.** Intermittent claudication is the classic sign of:

1. hypertension.
2. arterial embolism.
3. deep vein thrombosis.
4. PVD.

(628) **43.** Buerger's disease (thromboangiitis obliterans) is uncommon in persons living in:

1. India.
2. Korea.
3. Japan.
4. the United States.

(628) **44.** Chronically cold hands and numbness are symptoms of :

1. Buerger's disease.
2. Raynaud's disease.
3. atherosclerosis.
4. deep vein thrombosis.

(628) **45.** An alternative therapy for vasospastic episodes of Raynaud's disease is:

1. guided imagery.
2. meditation.
3. biofeedback.
4. yoga.

(630) **46.** Occupations requiring prolonged standing and the aging process increase the risk for:

1. PVD.
2. varicosities.
3. aneurysms.
4. aortic dissection.

(636) **47.** Which food should be avoided in patients with PVD?

1. grapefruit
2. ham
3. milk
4. pasta

CHAPTER 35

Student Name ____________________

Hypertension

Answer Key: Textbook page references are provided as a guide for answering these questions. A complete answer key was provided for your instructor.

OBJECTIVES

1. Define hypertension.
2. Explain the physiology of blood pressure regulation.
3. Discuss the risk factors, signs and symptoms, diagnosis, treatment, and complications of hypertension.
4. Identify the nursing considerations when administering selected antihypertensive drugs.
5. List the data to be obtained in the nursing assessment of a person with known or suspected hypertension.
6. Identify the nursing diagnoses, goals, and outcome criteria for the patient with hypertension.
7. Describe the nursing interventions for the patient with hypertension.

LEARNING ACTIVITIES

A. Match the definition in the numbered column with the most appropriate term in the lettered column.

(648) **1.** __________ Sudden drop in systolic blood pressure when changing from a lying or sitting position to a standing position

(641) **2.** __________ Stationary blood clot

(641) **3.** __________ Nosebleed

A. Hypertension
B. Syncope
C. Thrombus
D. Hyperlipidemia
E. Orthostatic hypotension
F. Epistaxis
G. Hypertrophy

Continued next page

(639) **4.** __________ Persistent elevation of arterial blood pressure of 140/90 mm Hg or greater

(648) **5.** __________ Fainting

(641) **6.** __________ Enlargement

(641) **7.** __________ Excess insoluble fats in the blood

B. Complete the statements in the numbered column with the most appropriate term in the lettered column. Some terms may be used more than once, and some terms may not be used.

(641) **1.** Epinephrine constricts blood vessels, increases blood pressure, and __________ the heart rate.

(646) **2.** When body position is altered from supine to standing, the diastolic blood pressure normally __________ .

(640) **3.** In response to decreased ability of the aorta to distend, pulse pressure __________.

(640) **4.** In response to increased peripheral vascular resistance, the systolic pressure __________.

(640) **5.** Epinephrine constricts blood vessels and increases the force of cardiac contraction, causing blood pressure to __________.

(640) **6.** When there is a narrowing of the arteries and arterioles, peripheral vascular resistance __________.

A. Increase(s)/rise(s)
B. Decrease(s)/fall(s)
C. Widen(s)
D. Narrow(s)

Student Name____

C. Complete the statements in the numbered column with the most appropriate term in the lettered column. Some terms may be used more than once, and some terms may not be used.

(645) **1.** An important side effect of alpha-adrenergic receptor blockers is __________.

(646) **2.** When body position is altered from supine to standing, the systolic blood pressure normally __________.

(640) **3.** Epinephrine __________ cardiac output.

(645) **4.** Flushing, dizziness, and headaches are common side effects of __________.

(645) **5.** The __________ are more susceptible to orthostatic hypotension because their blood vessels respond more slowly to position changes.

(645) **6.** Elderly patients are at risk for adverse effects of medications because of reduced liver and __________ function.

(640) **7.** Norepinephrine stimulates the blood vessels to __________.

(640) **8.** Increased cardiac output, increased peripheral resistance, and increased blood volume will result in __________ blood pressure.

(648) **9.** Symptoms of orthostatic hypotension include lightheadedness, dizziness, and __________.

(640) **10.** Aldosterone stimulates the kidney to reabsorb water and __________.

(648) **11.** A sudden drop in systolic blood pressure, usually 20 mm Hg, when going from a lying or sitting to a standing position is called __________.

A. Constrict(s)
B. Elderly
C. Diuretics
D. Orthostatic hypotension
E. Increased
F. Kidney
G. Sodium
H. Increase(s)
I. Calcium channel blockers
J. Decrease(s) about 10 mm Hg
K. Syncope

D. Complete the statements in the numbered column with the most appropriate term in the lettered column. Some terms may be used more than once, and some terms may not be used.

(640) **1.** The center for blood pressure regulation in the brain is the __________.

(648) **2.** If antihypertensive drugs are stopped suddenly, __________ may occur.

(648) **3.** Symptoms of hypertensive crisis include blurred vision, nausea, restlessness, and __________.

(649) **4.** Without appropriate treatment for hypertensive crisis, the patient may develop damage to the cardiac and __________ systems.

(643) **5.** Signs of hypokalemia include confusion, irritability, and __________.

(643) **6.** The group of antihypertensive drugs that must be used cautiously in patients with asthma, diabetes, and chronic obstructive pulmonary disease is __________.

(648) **7.** In order to prevent orthostatic hypotension, patients are encouraged to __________.

(640) **8.** With aging, atherosclerotic changes reduce elasticity of arteries, decrease cardiac output, and __________ peripheral vascular resistance.

(641) **9.** Three stimulants that may contribute to hypertension include amphetamines, nicotine, and __________.

A. Muscle weakness
B. Rise slowly from a lying or sitting position
C. Beta blockers
D. Norepinephrine
E. Caffeine
F. Rebound hypertension
G. Medulla oblongata
H. Increase
I. Severe headache
J. Renal

Student Name____

E. Complete the statements in the numbered column with the most appropriate term in the lettered column. Some terms may be used more than once, and some terms may not be used.

(641) **1.** Nicotine in cigarettes acts as a __________.

(641) **2.** Hyperlipidemia is excess __________ in the blood.

(641) **3.** Hyperlipidemia is a contributing factor for __________.

(640) **4.** Norepinephrine and epinephrine are __________.

(641) **5.** A serious complication of hypertension in which nocturia and azotemia occur is __________.

(641) **6.** The long-term effects of hypertension on the eyes include narrow arterioles, retinal hemorrhage, and __________.

(641) **7.** The long-term effects of hypertension on the heart include coronary artery disease, angina, and __________.

(640) **8.** Factors that contribute to hypertension include cardiac stimulation, retention of fluid, and __________.

(641) **9.** The long-term effects of hypertension on the brain include transient ischemic attacks and __________.

A. Vasoconstriction
B. Myocardial infarction
C. Vasoconstrictor(s)
D. Cerebrovascular accidents/strokes
E. Insoluble fats
F. Renal failure
G. Atherosclerosis
H. Papilledema

F. Complete the statements in the numbered column with the most appropriate term in the lettered column. Some terms may be used more than once, and some terms may not be used.

(643) 1. Patients on diuretics must be monitored for __________ imbalances.

(641) 2. People with hypertension are at risk for myocardial infarction and __________.

(643) 3. A plan for selecting drugs to treat hypertension, beginning with the administration of a single, relatively safe drug and progressing to combinations of drugs, is called a __________ approach.

(642) 4. Optimal blood pressure is generally defined as a diastolic blood pressure of __________ or less.

(642) 5. A nonpharmacologic approach to the treatment of hypertension includes weight reduction, smoking cessation, and __________.

(643) 6. The first step of a stepped-care approach to the treatment of hypertension recommends starting the patient on a low dose of beta blockers, ACE inhibitors, or __________.

A. Exercise
B. Diuretic(s)
C. Fluid and electrolyte(s)
D. Stepped-care
E. Stroke(s)
F. 120 mm Hg
G. 80 mm Hg
H. Progressive

G. Match the description in the numbered column with the correct lifestyle modification in the lettered column. Some modifications may be used more than once, and some may not be used.

(642) 1. __________ Reduces water in the body, decreasing the circulating blood volume

(642) 2. __________ Decreases blood glucose and cholesterol levels, increasing sense of well-being

A. Weight reduction
B. Smoking cessation
C. Sodium reduction
D. Exercise
E. Relaxation therapy or biofeedback

Continued next page

Student Name____

(642) **3.** __________ Eliminates vasoconstriction caused by nicotine

(643) **4.** __________ Reduces stress and lowers blood pressure

(642) **5.** __________ Improves cardiac efficiency by increasing cardiac output and decreasing peripheral vascular resistance

(642) **6.** __________ Reduces blood pressure by reducing the workload of the heart

H. Match the actions of the drugs in the numbered column with the correct classification of drugs in the lettered column. Some classifications may be used more than once, and some may not be used.

(645) **1.** __________ Block alpha receptor effects, lowering blood pressure by reducing peripheral resistance

(645) **2.** __________ Decrease fluid retention by decreasing the production of aldosterone

(643) **3.** __________ Reduce blood pressure by blocking the beta effects of catecholamines

(645) **4.** __________ Inhibit impulses from the vasomotor center in the brain, reducing peripheral resistance and lowering blood pressure

(645) **5.** __________ Block receptors for angiotensin II and reduce aldosterone secretion

A. Central-adrenergic blockers
B. Calcium channel blockers
C. Alpha-adrenergic receptor blockers
D. ACE inhibitors
E. Direct vasodilators
F. Beta-adrenergic receptor blockers
G. Diuretics
H. Angiotensin II receptor antagonists

Continued next page

(643) **6.** _________ Reduce blood volume through promotion of renal excretion of sodium and water

(645) **7.** _________ Block the movement of calcium into cardiac and vascular smooth muscle cells, reducing heart rate, decreasing force of cardiac contraction, and dilating peripheral blood vessels

(643) **8.** _________ Relax arteriolar smooth muscle

(645) **9.** _________ Prevent the conversion of angiotensin I to angiotensin II, a potent vasoconstrictor, decreasing peripheral resistance

I. Match the side effect or caution in the numbered column with the correct classification of drugs in the lettered column. Some classifications may be used more than once.

(645) **1.** _________ Palpitations, dizziness, headache, drowsiness

(643) **2.** _________ Hypoglycemia

(643) **3.** _________ Hypovolemia and hypokalemia

(645) **4.** _________ Flushing, dizziness, headache

(645) **5.** _________ Skin rash, renal failure

(643) **6.** _________ Use cautiously in patients with asthma, diabetes, and COPD

(643) **7.** _________ Fluid and electrolyte imbalances

(644) **8.** _________ Dizziness

A. Angiotensin II receptor antagonists
B. Beta blockers
C. Calcium channel blockers
D. Alpha-adrenergic receptor blockers
E. Diuretics
F. ACE inhibitors

Student Name____

J. Match the names of the drugs in the numbered column with the correct classification of drugs in the lettered column.

(644) **1.** __________ Prazosin (Minipress)

(644) **2.** __________ Hydrochlorothiazide (HCTZ) and spironolactone (Aldactone)

(644) **3.** __________ losartan potassium (Cozaar)

(644) **4.** __________ Clonidine (Catapres) and methyldopa (Aldomet)

(644) **5.** __________ Propranolol (Inderal)

(644) **6.** __________ Hydralazine (Apresoline) diazoxide (Hyperstat), and sodium nitroprusside (Nitropress)

(644) **7.** __________ Captopril (Capoten) and enalapril (Vasotec)

(644) **8.** __________ Verapamil (Calan)

A. Calcium channel blockers
B. Beta blockers
C. Direct vasodilators
D. Angiotensin II receptor antagonists
E. Diuretics
F. Alpha-adrenergic receptor blockers
G. Centrally acting drugs (alpha 2 agonists)
H. ACE inhibitors

K. Using this figure, list four body structures (A–D) damaged by long-term blood pressure elevation:

(641) **A.** ____________________

(641) **B.** ____________________

(641) **C.** ____________________

(641) **D.** ____________________

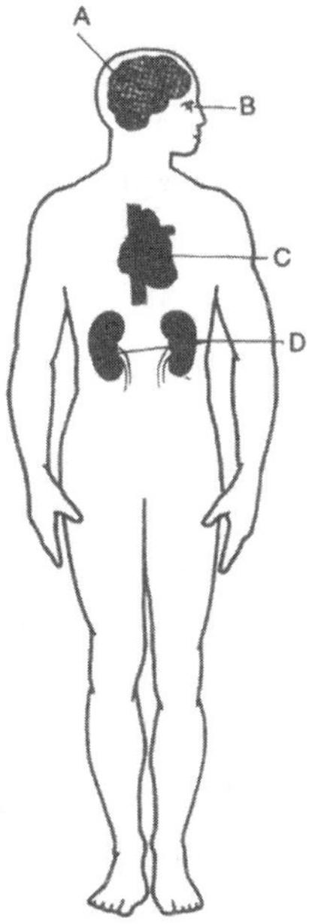

MULTIPLE-CHOICE QUESTIONS

L. Choose the most appropriate answer.

(639) **1.** The most common cardiovascular problem in the United States today is:

1. arteriosclerosis.
2. coronary artery disease.
3. myocardial infarction.
4. hypertension.

(639) **2.** The cause of primary (essential) hypertension is:

1. kidney disease.
2. drugs.
3. pregnancy.
4. unknown.

(639) **3.** Hypertension is usually detected in which age group?

1. 20–29 2. 30–50
3. 51–60 4. over 60

(639) **4.** A blood pressure of 135/87 is considered to be:

1. low normal.
2. normal.
3. high normal.
4. high.

(639) **5.** In which risk group is a hypertensive patient who smokes half a pack of cigarettes a day and who has no heart disease or heart damage, classified?

1. risk A. 2. risk B.
3. risk C. 4. risk D.

(639) **6.** Isolated systolic blood pressure elevations of 160 mm Hg in the elderly are most often due to:

1. decreased cardiac output.
2. atherosclerosis.
3. increased peripheral vascular resistance.
4. increased pulse pressure.

(640) **7.** The diameter of blood vessels is regulated primarily by:

1. the heart muscle.
2. adrenal gland hormones.
3. the vasomotor center.
4. thyroid gland hormones.

(643) **8.** Which drugs decrease the sensitivity of blood vessels to catecholamines, reducing vascular resistance?

1. diuretics
2. adrenergics
3. antihistamines
4. analgesics

(643) **9.** An older patient taking furosemide (Lasix) for hypertension complains of muscle weakness, confusion, and irritability. Which patient teaching is correct for this patient?

1. Decrease sodium in the diet.
2. Increase potassium in the diet.
3. Increase fluid intake.
4. Decrease vitamin K intake.

(643) **10.** Beta blockers are contraindicated in patients with:

1. hypertension.
2. edema.
3. osteoporosis.
4. asthma.

(643) **11.** When people with diabetes are taking beta blockers for hypertension, the only sign of hypoglycemia may be:

1. diaphoresis.
2. fatigue.
3. hunger.
4. excessive thirst.

Student Name____________________

(643) **12.** Elderly patients taking beta blockers are at greater risk than younger people for:

1. bradycardia.
2. hypoglycemia.
3. bronchoconstriction.
4. GI upset.

(643) **13.** Which group of patients responds better to diuretics as treatment for hypertension?

1. Caucasians
2. African-Americans
3. Asians
4. Hispanics

(645) **14.** Older patients taking antihypertensives are more susceptible to orthostatic hypotension, increasing their risk for:

1. confusion.
2. myocardial infarction.
3. falls.
4. congestive heart failure.

(646) **15.** When body position is changed from supine to standing, the systolic pressure normally:

1. rises about 5 mm Hg.
2. rises about 10 mm Hg.
3. falls about 5 mm Hg.
4. falls about 10 mm Hg.

(646) **16.** If a patient's diastolic pressure is 120 mm Hg, the nurse should:

1. reassess it in 10 minutes.
2. reassess it in 30 minutes.
3. notify the physician.
4. encourage the patient to stay on bed rest.

(648) **17.** What is the danger of suddenly stopping antihypertensive drugs?

1. orthostatic hypotension
2. bradycardia
3. hypokalemia
4. rebound hypertension

(648) **18.** People with increased blood pressure should not take over-the-counter:

1. analgesics.
2. cold remedies.
3. antacids.
4. laxatives.

(648) **19.** A common side effect of many antihypertensives is:

1. GI distress.
2. sexual dysfunction.
3. respiratory depression.
4. rebound hypertension.

(649) **20.** Without appropriate treatment, the patient in hypertensive crisis may develop:

1. cerebrovascular accident.
2. hyperglycemia.
3. respiratory acidosis.
4. adrenal insufficiency.

Student Name ______________________________

Digestive Tract Disorders

Answer Key: Textbook page references are provided as a guide for answering these questions. A complete answer key was provided for your instructor.

OBJECTIVES

1. Identify the nursing responsibilities in the care of patients undergoing diagnostic tests and procedures for disorders of the digestive tract.
2. List the data to be included in the nursing assessment of the patient with a digestive disorder.
3. Describe the nursing care of patients with gastrointestinal intubation and decompression, tube feedings, total parenteral nutrition, digestive tract surgery, and drug therapy for digestive disorders.
4. Describe the pathophysiology, signs and symptoms, complications, and medical treatment of selected digestive disorders.
5. Assist in developing nursing care plans for patients receiving treatment for digestive disorders.

LEARNING ACTIVITIES

A. Match the definition in the numbered column with the most appropriate term in the lettered column.

(676) **1.** __________ Difficulty swallowing

(654) **2.** __________ Indigestion

(671) **3.** __________ Inflammation of the oral mucosa

(670) **4.** __________ Cracking of the lips and corners of the mouth

A. Stomatitis
B. Dysphagia
C. Cheilosis
D. Dyspepsia

B. Complete the statements in the numbered column with the most appropriate term in the lettered column. Some terms may be used more than once, and some terms may not be used.

(660) **1.** The head of the bed is elevated during tube feedings in order to prevent ___________.

(683) **2.** An inflammation of the lining of the stomach is called ___________.

(656) **3.** The most serious complication of gastric endoscopy is ___________.

(683) **4.** The best means of diagnosing gastritis is ___________.

(705) **5.** Opiates (such as morphine) are not given to patients with diverticulosis to avoid the common side effect of ___________.

(662) **6.** A complication that occurs when tube feedings of concentrated formula are given rapidly is ___________.

(685) **7.** The most serious complication of gastric ulcers is ___________.

A. Gastroscopy
B. Hemorrhage
C. Headache
D. Constipation
E. Perforation of the digestive tract
F. Dumping syndrome
G. Diarrhea
H. Aspiration
I. Drowsiness
J. Gastritis

C. Complete the statements in the numbered column with the most appropriate term in the lettered column. Some terms may be used more than once, and some terms may not be used.

(680) **1.** Acidic gastric fluids can cause inflammation of the esophagus, called ___________.

(654) **2.** The procedure used to assess bowel sounds is ___________.

(680) **3.** Hiatal hernia is thought to be caused by weakness in the ___________.

(680) **4.** The opening in the diaphragm through which the esophagus passes is the esophageal ___________.

(657) **5.** Direct examination of the esophagus with an endoscope is called ___________.

(655) **6.** The procedure used to detect the presence of air, fluid, or masses in tissues is known as ___________.

A. Hiatus
B. Pyloric sphincter
C. Hiatal hernia
D. Esophagoscopy
E. Gastrectomy
F. Esophagitis
G. Heartburn
H. Palpation
I. Stomatitis
J. Auscultation
K. Fundoplication
L. Percussion
M. Lower esophageal sphincter

Continued next page

Student Name ____________________

(680) **7.** The protrusion of the lower esophagus and stomach upward through the diaphragm, into the chest, is __________.

(681) **8.** A surgical procedure that strengthens the LES by suturing the fundus of the stomach around the esophagus and anchoring it below the diaphragm is __________.

(680) **9.** Many patients with hiatal hernia report a feeling of burning and tightness rising from the lower sternum to the throat, which is called __________.

D. Complete the statements in the numbered column with the most appropriate term in the lettered column. Some terms may be used more than once, and some terms may not be used.

(705) **1.** Two tests that allow the physician to confirm the presence of diverticula are colonoscopy and __________.

(702) **2.** Ulcerative colitis and Crohn's disease are types of __________.

(684) **3.** A loss of tissue from the lining of the digestive tract is __________.

(702) **4.** Regional enteritis is also known as __________.

(685) **5.** A break in the wall of the stomach or the duodenum that permits digestive fluids to leak into the peritoneal cavity is __________.

(685) **6.** A common complication of peptic ulcers is __________.

(684) **7.** Normally, the barrier that protects the digestive tract lining from digestive juices is __________.

(702) **8.** The most common symptoms of inflammatory bowel disease are bloody diarrhea and __________.

(704) **9.** A condition characterized by small sac-like pouches in the intestinal wall is called __________.

(705) **10.** A complication of diverticulitis in which an abnormal opening develops between the colon and the bladder is called __________.

(704) **11.** Most diverticula are found in the __________.

A. Crohn's disease
B. Hemorrhage
C. Hiatal hernia
D. Sigmoid colon
E. Diverticulosis
F. Barium enema
G. Mucus
H. Perforation
I. Duodenum
J. Fistula
K. MRI
L. Inflammatory bowel disease
M. Abdominal pain
N. Peptic ulcer

E. Complete the statements in the numbered column with the most appropriate term in the lettered column. Some terms may be used more than once, and some terms may not be used.

(692) **1.** Creating a small upper pouch and connecting the pouch to the jejunum so stomach capacity and food absorption are decreased is called __________.

(692) **2.** When a person weighs twice as much as his or her ideal weight, this is called __________.

(693) **3.** The removal of adipose tissue from selected sites through a suction cannula used mainly for cosmetic surgery is __________.

(692) **4.** The primary treatment of obesity is a weight reduction program accompanied by __________.

(692) **5.** Excessive body fat resulting in increased body weight that is more than 20% higher than the ideal is called __________.

A. Gastrectomy
B. Obesity
C. Roux-en-Y gastric bypass
D. Exercise
E. Bulimia
F. Morbid obesity
G. Psychotherapy
H. Liposuction

F. Complete the statement in the numbered column with the most appropriate term in the lettered column. Some terms may be used more than once, and some terms may not be used.

(694) **1.** A common symptom of malabsorption is the presence of excessive fat in the stool, which is called __________.

(697) **2.** A condition in which the large intestine loses the ability to contract effectively enough to propel the fecal mass toward the rectum is __________.

(694) **3.** The passage of loose, liquid stools with increased frequency is called __________.

(696) **4.** Increased pressure in the chest and abdominal cavities caused by straining to have a bowel movement is called __________.

(694) **5.** A term used to describe a condition in which one or more nutrients are not digested or absorbed is __________.

A. Valsalva's maneuver
B. Diarrhea
C. Fecal impaction
D. Gluten
E. High-fiber foods
F. Steatorrhea
G. Anorexia
H. Sprue
I. Constipation
J. Malabsorption
K. Paralytic ileus
L. Milk and milk products
M. Clear liquids
N. Megacolon

Continued next page

Student Name ______________________________

(694) **6.** Celiac sprue is treated by avoiding products that contain __________.

(695) **7.** A condition in which a person has hard, dry, infrequent stools that are passed with difficulty is __________.

(697) **8.** The retention of a large mass of stool in the rectum that the patient is unable to pass is called __________.

(694) **9.** The diet recommended for acute diarrhea is __________.

(694) **10.** Two examples of malabsorption are lactase deficiency and __________.

(694) **11.** Lactase deficiency is treated by eliminating __________.

G. Complete the statements in the numbered column with the most appropriate term in the lettered column. Some terms may be used more than once, and some terms may not be used.

(701) **1.** The repair of the muscle defect in abdominal hernia by suturing is called __________.

(701) **2.** For patients who cannot tolerate the stress of surgical hernia repair, a pad called a(n) __________ is placed over the hernia to provide support for the weak muscles.

(700) **3.** The bulging portion of the large intestine pushing through the abdominal wall is __________.

(701) **4.** Factors that cause hernias include heavy lifting and __________.

(700) **5.** Weak locations where hernias occur include the lower inguinal areas of the abdomen and the __________.

(701) **6.** Nausea, vomiting, pain, fever, and tachycardia may be signs and symptoms of a hernia complication called __________.

(702) **7.** Following inguinal hernia repair, a common complication is __________.

(701) **8.** An irreducible hernia, sometimes called __________, may impair blood flow to the trapped loop of intestine.

A. Umbilicus
B. Hernia
C. Fecal incontinence
D. Scrotal swelling
E. Truss
F. Incarcerated
G. Coughing
H. Gangrene
I. Herniorrhaphy
J. Strangulation

H. Match the drugs in the numbered column with their actions in the lettered column.

(666)	**1.** _________ Anticholinergics	
(666)	**2.** _________ H_2-receptor antagonists	
(668)	**3.** _________ Antiemetics	
(666)	**4.** _________ Antacids	
(666)	**5.** _________ Mucosal barriers (Cytoprotective)	
(668)	**6.** _________ Antidiarrheals	
(659)	**7.** _________ Anti-infectives	
(669)	**8.** _________ Antifungals	

A. Treat ulcerative colitis and *H. pylori*
B. Neutralize gastric acid
C. Cling to the surface of the ulcer and protect it so that healing can take place
D. Treat yeast infections in the mouth
E. Decrease hydrochloric acid production by competing at receptor sites
F. Prevent and treat nausea
G. Decrease intestinal motility so liquid portion of feces is reabsorbed
H. Reduce gastrointestinal motility and secretions; block acetylcholine

I. List age-related changes in the seven areas of the digestive tract listed below.

(653) **1.** Gums (gingiva): ____________________

(653) **2.** Teeth: ____________________

(653) **3.** Taste buds: ____________________

(653) **4.** Walls of esophagus and stomach: ____________________

(653) **5.** Stomach secretions: ____________________

(653) **6.** Gastric motor activity: ____________________

(654) **7.** Large intestine muscle and mucosa: ____________________

J. Many experts believe that constipation is not a normal age-related change. List six factors that may cause constipation in the elderly.

(654) **1.** ____________________

(654) **2.** ____________________

(654) **3.** ____________________

(654) **4.** ____________________

(654) **5.** ____________________

(654) **6.** ____________________

Student Name____

K. Explain why auscultation is done before palpation.

(654)

L. List eight terms used to describe bowel sounds.

(655)	**1.**	__________	*(655)*	**5.**	__________
(655)	**2.**	__________	*(655)*	**6.**	__________
(655)	**3.**	__________	*(655)*	**7.**	__________
(655)	**4.**	__________	*(655)*	**8.**	__________

M. Identify the following two types of malignant tumors that develop in the mouth.

(673) **1.** Type that occurs on the buccal mucosa, gums, floor of the mouth, tonsils, and tongue: __________

(673) **2.** Type that most commonly occurs on the lip: __________

N. List three interventions to reduce pain in patients with peptic ulcer.

(689) **1.** __________

(689) **2.** __________

(689) **3.** __________

O. List three aspects of care that the nurse should teach the patient who experiences dumping syndrome.

(690) **1.** __________

(690) **2.** __________

(691) **3.** __________

P. In Figure 36-1, label the parts (A–W) of the digestive tract.

(652)

A. ______________________

B. ______________________

C. ______________________

D. ______________________

E. ______________________

F. ______________________

G. ______________________

H. ______________________

I. ______________________

J. ______________________

K. ______________________

L. ______________________

M. ______________________

N. ______________________

O. ______________________

P. ______________________

Q. ______________________

R. ______________________

S. ______________________

T. ______________________

U. ______________________

V. ______________________

W. ______________________

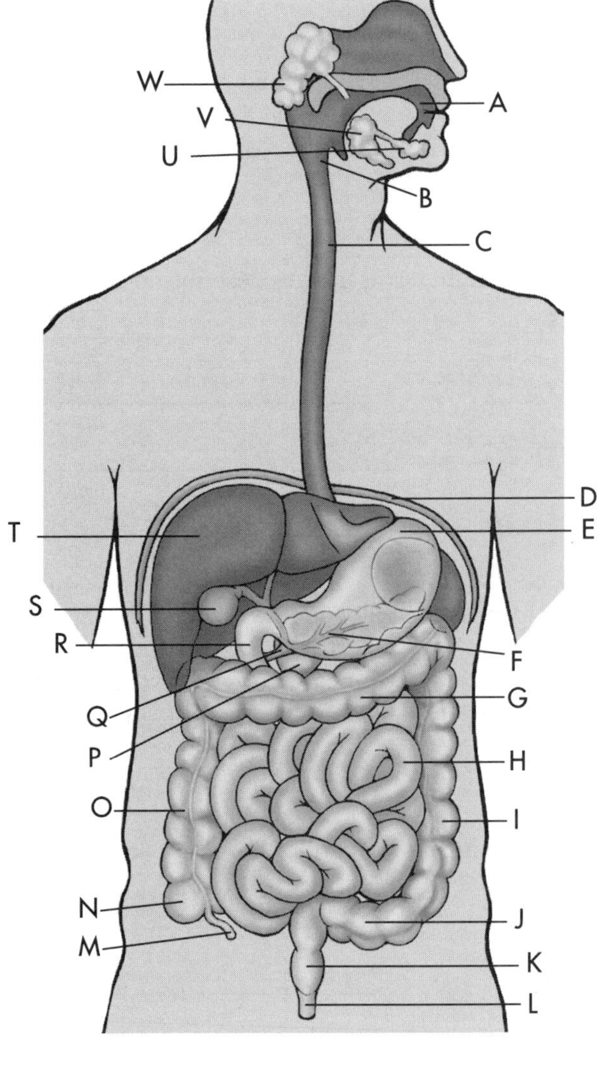

Student Name____

Q. Using Figure 36-5, label the gastrointestinal tubes using the following terms. *(661)*

Miller-Abbott tube	Weighted-flexible feeding tube	Salem sump tube
Sengstaken-Blakemore tube	Lavacuator tube (orogastric)	Cantor tube
Levin tube		

A. ____________________

B. ____________________

C. ____________________

D. ____________________

E. ____________________

F. ____________________

G. ____________________

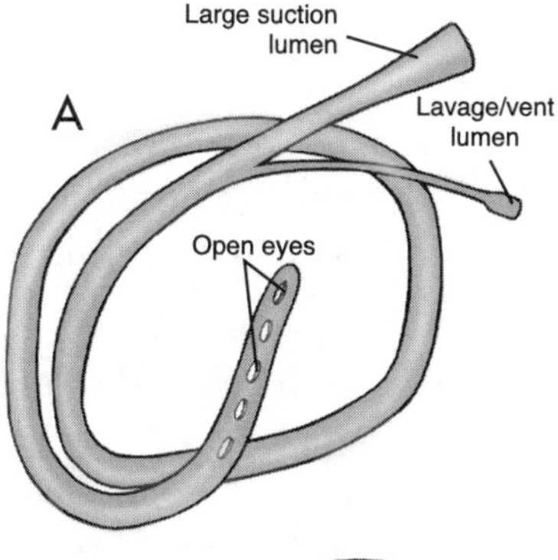

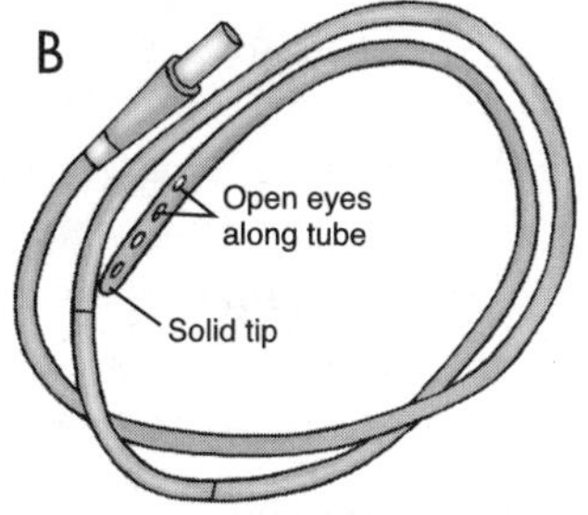

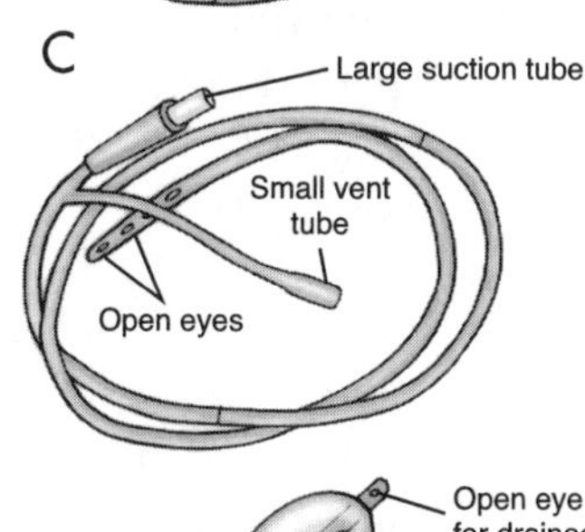

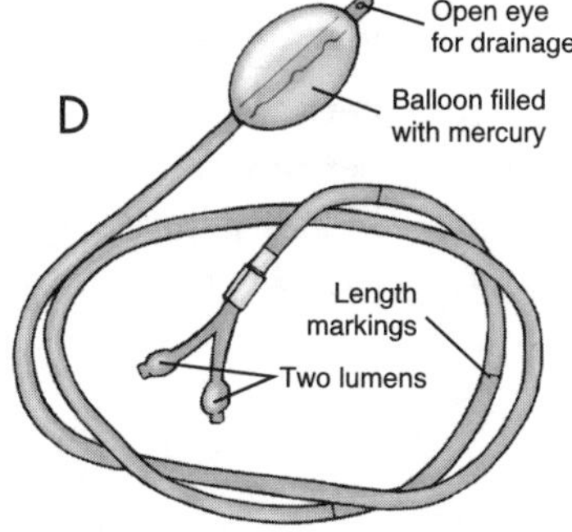

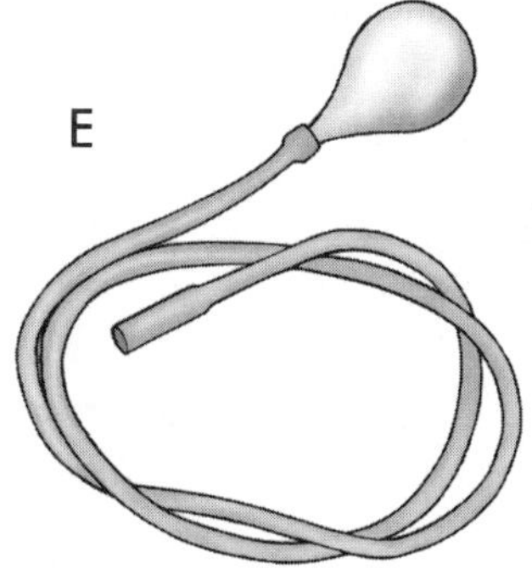

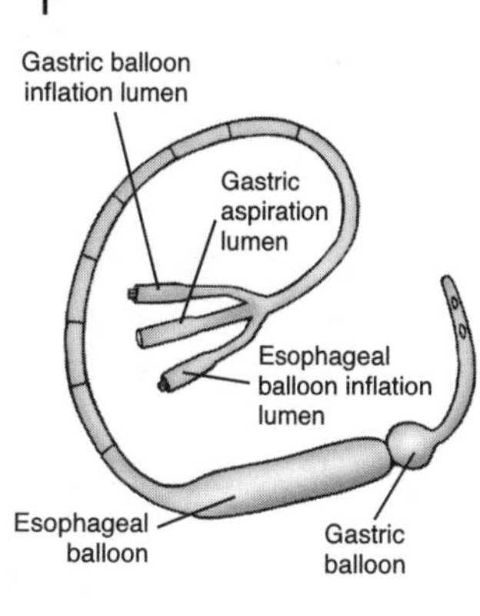

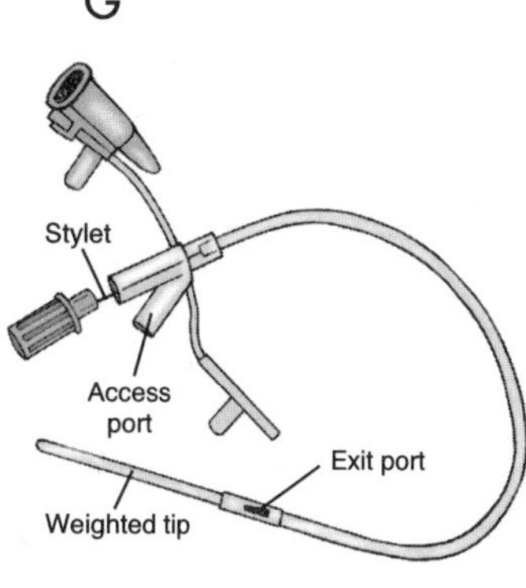

MULTIPLE-CHOICE QUESTIONS

R. Choose the most appropriate answer.

(678) **1.** The type of acid-base imbalance that results from prolonged vomiting is:

1. metabolic acidosis.
2. metabolic alkalosis.
3. respiratory acidosis.
4. respiratory alkalosis.

(655) **2.** Normal bowel sounds include:

1. minimal clicks and gurgles.
2. clicks and gurgles 5–30 times/minute.
3. steady, consistent gurgling sounds.
4. no sounds for 1 full minute.

(680) **3.** Which herb is effective in calming an upset stomach, reducing flatulence, and preventing motion sickness?

1. ginkgo 2. ginseng
3. ginger root 4. garlic

(660) **4.** After insertion of a gastric tube, feedings are not started until:

1. the patient requests food.
2. adequate oxygen levels are achieved on blood gases.
3. placement of tube is certain.
4. oral fluids are tolerated.

(678) **5.** Severe or prolonged vomiting puts the patient at risk for:

1. fluid volume deficit.
2. altered tissue perfusion.
3. hemorrhage.
4. infection.

(679) **6.** The vomiting patient who is also unconscious or who has impaired swallowing is at risk for aspiration and should be placed in which position?

1. lying flat in bed
2. with head of bed elevated at least 90 degrees
3. side-lying
4. with head of bed slightly elevated, for example, at 30 degrees

(682) **7.** To prevent nighttime reflux, the sleeping position for patients with hiatal hernia should be:

1. side-lying.
2. with head of bed at 90-degree angle.
3. flat.
4. with head of bed elevated 6 to 12 inches.

(686) **8.** Sudden, sharp pain starting in the midepigastric region and spreading across the entire abdomen in patients with peptic ulcer may indicate:

1. infection.
2. perforation.
3. dyspnea.
4. kidney failure.

(698) **9.** If the abdomen becomes rigid and tender and patients draw their knees up to their chest, this may indicate:

1. peritonitis.
2. perforation.
3. kidney failure.
4. pyloric obstruction.

Student Name______________________________

(685) **10.** The most prominent symptom of pyloric obstruction is persistent:

1. eructation.
2. heartburn.
3. vomiting.
4. hemorrhage.

(690) **11.** A complication of stomach surgery that occurs because the absence or decreased size of the stomach prevents the normal pacing of chyme moving into the intestine is:

1. malabsorption.
2. dumping syndrome.
3. coffee-ground emesis.
4. obstructed pyloric sphincter.

(697) **12.** Severe constipation accompanied by trickling of liquid stool suggests:

1. pyloric obstruction.
2. fecal impaction.
3. intestinal hemorrhage.
4. steatorrhea.

(698) **13.** A major complication of appendicitis is:

1. diarrhea.
2. constipation.
3. fluid volume deficit.
4. peritonitis.

(698) **14.** The classic symptom of appendicitis is pain at:

1. McBurney's point.
2. the xiphoid process.
3. right hypochondriac region.
4. inguinal node.

(698) **15.** When appendicitis is suspected, the patient is allowed:

1. clear liquids.
2. full liquids.
3. nothing by mouth.
4. soft foods.

(700) **16.** In addition to deficient fluid volume, patients with peritonitis may go into shock because of:

1. edema. 2. convulsions.
3. septicemia. 4. paralysis.

(706, 707) **17.** Pain is severe for several postoperative days following abdominoperineal resection. At first, the patient will probably be most comfortable in which position?

1. supine 2. side-lying
3. prone 4. Fowler's

(706, 707) **18.** Following abdominoperineal resection, a procedure that cleans, soothes, and increases circulation to the perineum is:

1. use of a TENS unit.
2. Kegel exercises.
3. the sitz bath.
4. débridement.

(684) **19.** What is the cause of most peptic ulcers?

1. *Helicobacter pylori*
2. *E. coli*
3. stress
4. infection

(693) **20.** A patient who should not use *Ephedra sinica* (Ma Huang) as an over-the-counter weight loss product is a person with:

1. a urinary tract infection.
2. arthritis.
3. dermatitis.
4. hypertension.

(694) **21.** Which natural substance can help control diarrhea?

1. garlic
2. rice water
3. kava kava
4. *Ephedra sinica*

(667) **22.** Which type of laxative may not be effective for several days?

1. bulk-producing laxative
2. intestinal stimulant
3. osmotic suppository
4. stool softener

(704) **23.** Which type of diet is prescribed for moderate inflammatory bowel disease?

1. low residue
2. high-fiber diet
3. low-potassium diet
4. low-salt diet

(709) **24.** The major nutritional goal of therapy for diarrhea is to replace:

1. potassium.
2. sodium.
3. calcium.
4. fluids.

CHAPTER 37

Student Name ______________________________

Disorders of the Liver, Gallbladder, and Pancreas

Answer Key: Textbook page references are provided as a guide for answering these questions. A complete answer key was provided for your instructor.

OBJECTIVES

1. Identify nursing assessment data related to the functions of the liver, gallbladder, and pancreas.
2. Identify the nurse's role in tests and procedures performed to diagnose disorders of the liver, gallbladder, and pancreas.
3. Describe the care of the patient who has an esophageal balloon tube in place.
4. Explain the pathology, signs and symptoms, diagnosis, complications, and medical treatment of selected disorders of the liver, gallbladder, and pancreas.
5. Assist in developing a nursing care plan care for the patient with liver, gallbladder, or pancreatic dysfunction.

LEARNING ACTIVITIES

A. Match the definition in the numbered column with the most appropriate term in the lettered column.

(723) **1.** __________ Chronic, progressive liver disease

(724) **2.** __________ Accumulation of excess fluid in the peritoneal cavity

(725) **3.** __________ Removal of ascitic fluid from the peritoneal cavity

(715) **4.** __________ Enlargement of the liver

(735) **5.** __________ Removal of the gallbladder

A. Paracentesis
B. Steatorrhea
C. Hepatomegaly
D. Icterus
E. Cirrhosis
F. Gynecomastia
G. Cholecystectomy
H. Cholangitis
I. Cholelithiasis
J. Ascites

Continued next page

(733) **6.** __________ Presence of gallstones in the gallbladder

(734) **7.** __________ Inflammation of the biliary ducts

(734) **8.** __________ Excess fat in stools

(715) **9.** __________ Jaundice

(724) **10.** __________ Enlargement of breast tissue in males

B. Complete the statements in the numbered column with the most appropriate term in the lettered column. Some terms may be used more than once, and some terms may not be used.

(712) **1.** Bile is produced in the __________.

(712) **2.** Specialized reticuloendothelial cells in the liver that ingest old red blood cells and bacteria are called __________.

(712) **3.** When fats pass into the duodenum, the gallbladder and the liver respond by delivering bile to the small intestine through the __________.

(712) **4.** A product of the normal breakdown of old red blood cells in the liver is __________.

(712) **5.** The vessel that delivers blood from the aorta to the liver is the __________.

(712) **6.** The vessel that delivers blood from the intestines to the liver is the __________.

(712) **7.** Bile produced in the liver passes into the gallbladder for storage through the ______.

(712) **8.** Bile is stored in the __________.

(715) **9.** When the sclera turns yellow in patients with liver disease, this condition is called scleral __________.

A. Bilirubin
B. Portal vein
C. Pancreas
D. Kupffer cells
E. Gallbladder
F. Hepatic artery
G. Pancreatic duct
H. Common bile duct
I. Icterus
J. Liver
K. Cystic duct
L. Jaundice

Student Name____

C. Complete the statements in the numbered column with the most appropriate term in the lettered column. Some terms may be used more than once, and some terms may not be used.

(716, 718) **1.** __________ A procedure in which a radioactive substance is injected into a vein and visualized in a radiograph to reveal tumors and abscesses

(716, 719) **2.** __________ The use of sound waves to create an image of the liver, spleen, pancreas, gallbladder, and biliary system that is noninvasive and painless

(716, 719) **3.** __________ A procedure that involves removal of a small specimen of liver tissue for examination

(720) **4.** __________ A primary complication of liver biopsy that occurs because of the liver's rich blood supply and potential for impaired coagulation

(720) **5.** __________ A primary complication of liver biopsy that occurs if the lung is accidentally punctured during the biopsy

A. Liver biopsy
B. Pneumothorax
C. Ultrasonography
D. Hemothorax
E. Liver scan
F. Hemorrhage
G. PET scan

D. Match the statements in the numbered column with the most appropriate term in the lettered column. Some terms may be used more than once, and some terms may not be used.

(721) **1.** __________ The second phase of hepatitis, which lasts from 2–4 weeks, characterized by jaundice and clay-colored stools

(720) **2.** __________ Serum hepatitis transmitted in body fluids

(720) **3.** __________ Elevation in serum bilirubin when bile channels are compressed due to inflammation in the liver

A. Hepatitis B
B. Preicteric phase
C. Angioedema
D. Jaundice
E. Icteric phase
F. Anorexia
G. Posticteric phase
H. Hepatitis A

Continued next page

(721) **4.** __________ The third phase of hepatitis, in which fatigue, malaise, and liver enlargement last for several months

(720) **5.** __________ Infectious hepatitis or epidemic hepatitis, transmitted by water, food, or contaminated medical equipment

(721) **6.** __________ The first phase of hepatitis, which lasts from 1–21 days, when the patient is most infectious

(720) **7.** __________ The most common type of hepatitis

E. Match the definition or description in the numbered column with the most appropriate term in the lettered column. Some terms may be used more than once, and some terms may not be used.

(724) **1.** __________ A symptom common in cirrhosis that is characterized by tingling or numbness in the extremities thought to be caused by vitamin B deficiencies

(724) **2.** __________ Obstructive cirrhosis that develops as a result of obstruction to bile flow

(724) **3.** __________ Results from venous congestion and hypoxia

(724) **4.** __________ A chronic, progressive disease of the liver that is characterized by degeneration and destruction of liver cells

(724) **5.** __________ Liver enlarges, becomes "knobby," and shrinks later

A. Alcoholic cirrhosis (Laennec's disease)
B. Peripheral neuropathy
C. Cirrhosis
D. Postnecrotic cirrhosis
E. Biliary cirrhosis
F. Dyspepsia
G. Cardiac cirrhosis

Student Name____

F. Match the effects of cirrhosis complications in the numbered column with the most appropriate complication of cirrhosis in the lettered column. Some terms may be used more than once, and some may not be used.

(724) **1.** __________ Results in leaking of lymph fluid and albumin-rich fluid from the diseased liver

(725) **2.** __________ Renal failure following diuretic therapy, paracentesis, or GI hemorrhage

(724) **3.** __________ Caused by excessive ammonia in the blood, resulting in cognitive disturbances

(724) **4.** __________ May cause fatal hemorrhage

(724) **5.** __________ Development of collateral vessels

A. Hepatic encephalopathy
B. Esophageal varices
C. Portal hypertension
D. Epistaxis
E. Hepatorenal syndrome
F. Peripheral neuropathy
G. Ascites

G. When patients with cholelithiasis are discharged from the hospital, the nurse should advise them to report the four signs of bile duct obstruction; list the signs below.

(733) **1.** ____

(733) **2.** ____

(733) **3.** ____

(733) **4.** ____

H. In Figure 37-10 below, label the anatomic parts (A–G).

(733)

A. ______________________

B. ______________________

C. ______________________

D. ______________________

E. ______________________

F. ______________________

G. ______________________

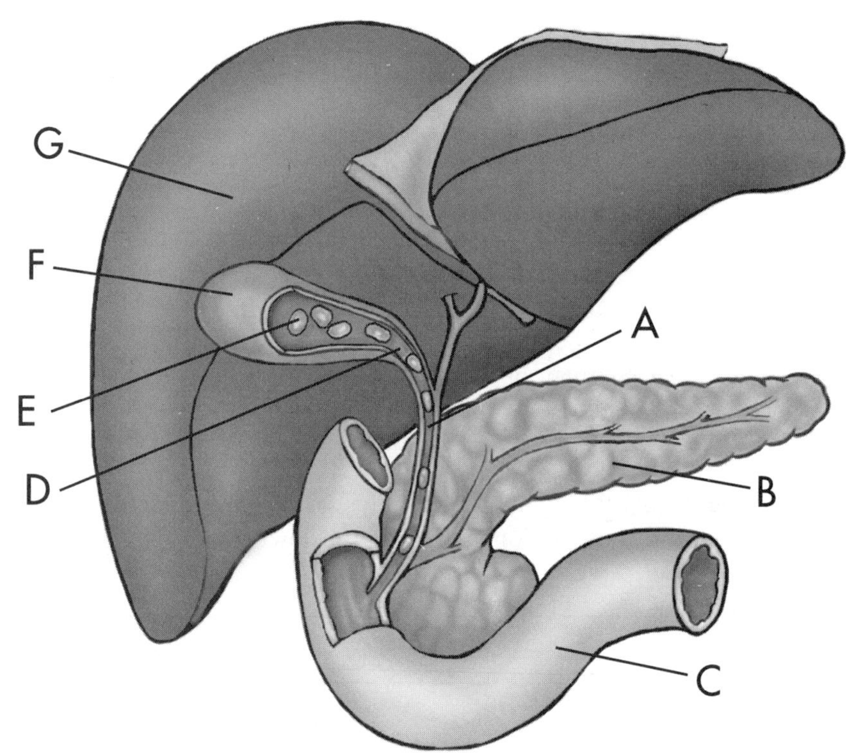

Student Name____

I. Using Figure 37-5, list the five areas of clinical manifestations of cirrhosis.

(716)

A. ____________________________

B. ____________________________

C. ____________________________

D. ____________________________

E. ____________________________

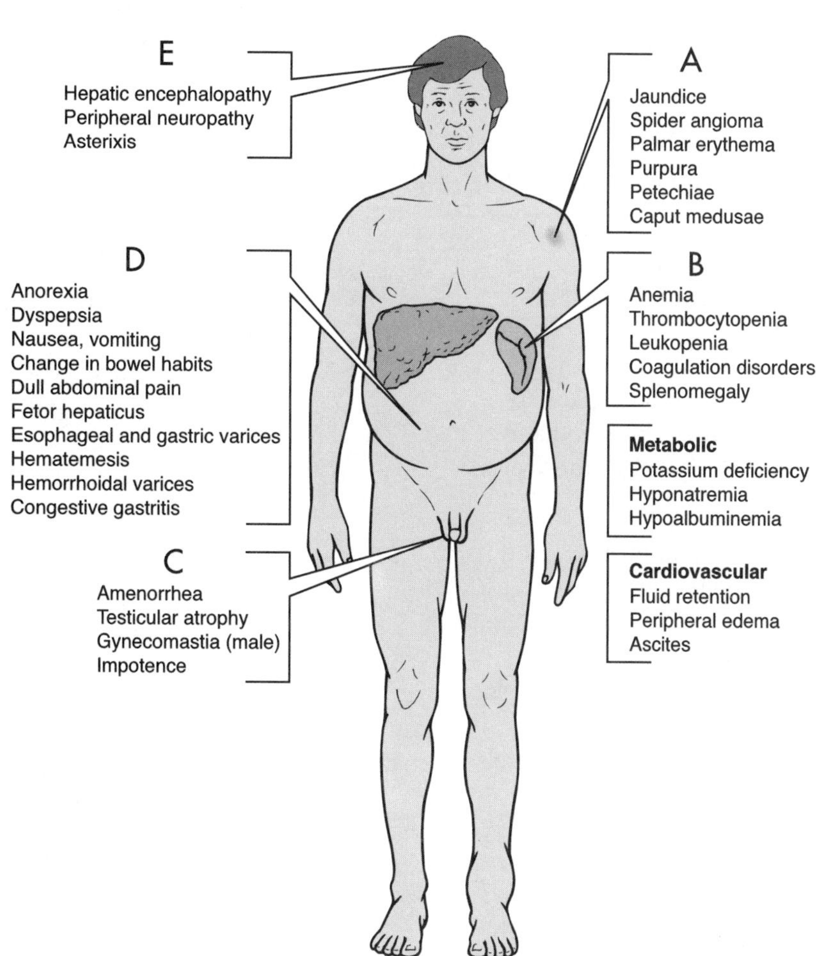

MULTIPLE-CHOICE QUESTIONS

J. Choose the most appropriate answer.

(714) **1.** Patients with liver disease are at increased risk for drug:

1 incompatibilities.
2. toxicities.
3. idiosyncrasies.
4. synthesis.

(733) **2.** Clay-colored stools are characteristic of:

1. bile obstruction.
2. pancreatitis.
3. gastritis.
4. Crohn's disease.

(722) **3.** The prescribed diet for patients with hepatitis usually contains:

1. high carbohydrates and vitamins, low protein, low to moderate fat.
2. low carbohydrates, moderate to high protein, high fat.
3. high carbohydrates and vitamins, moderate to high protein, low to moderate fat.
4. low carbohydrates, low protein, low to moderate fat.

(723) **4.** Patients with hepatitis may have impaired skin integrity due to:

1. jaundice.
2. pruritus or scratching.
3. nausea and vomiting.
4. fluid volume deficit.

(722) **5.** The nurse should explain to patients with hepatitis that rest is necessary to allow the liver to heal by:

1. producing more white blood cells to fight infection.
2. producing more platelets to assist in clotting.
3. regenerating new cells to replace damaged cells.
4. regenerating new blood vessels to replace damaged ones.

(723) **6.** The nurse should be alert for signs of fluid retention in patients with hepatitis, which include increasing abdominal girth, rising blood pressure, and:

1. dry mucous membranes.
2. tachycardia.
3. edema.
4. concentrated urine.

(723) **7.** Which drugs may be ordered for pruritus, which occurs with hepatitis?

1. antihistamines
2. antiemetics
3. antibiotics
4. analgesics

(723) **8.** The patient with hepatitis may be self-conscious about appearance because of:

1. cyanosis. 2. redness.
3. ulcerations. 4. jaundice.

(723) **9.** Health care workers who work with hospitalized patients should receive:

1. hepatitis B vaccinations.
2. RhoGAM.
3. influenza virus vaccine.
4. immune globulin.

(722) **10.** A frequent problem in cirrhosis for which small, semisolid meals are recommended is:

1. peripheral neuropathy.
2. jaundice.
3. anorexia.
4. ascites.

(725) **11.** The medical management of ascites aims to promote reabsorption and elimination of the fluid by means of salt restriction and:

1. antihistamines.
2. analgesics.
3. diuretics.
4. antibiotics.

Student Name____

(725) **12.** Potential complications of peritoneal-venous shunts used to allow ascitic fluid to drain from the abdomen and return to the bloodstream are tubing obstruction and:

1. jaundice.
2. peripheral neuropathy.
3. pruritus.
4. peritonitis.

(730) **13.** The best position for patients with ascites to help them breathe more easily is:

1. side-lying.
2. prone.
3. supine.
4. with the head of the bed elevated.

(730) **14.** The patient with cirrhosis is at great risk for injury or hemorrhage due to impaired:

1. coagulation.
2. immunity.
3. skin integrity.
4. breathing patterns.

(730) **15.** Since the esophagus and the trachea are adjacent to each other, upward movement of the esophageal balloon in the patient with cirrhosis may cause:

1. impaired circulation.
2. airway obstruction.
3. cardiac shock.
4. perforated intestine.

(733) **16.** Bile ducts respond to obstruction (such as gallstones) with spasms in an effort to move the stone; the intense spasmodic pain is called:

1. hepatic encephalopathy.
2. renal colic.
3. biliary colic.
4. peripheral neuropathy.

(733) **17.** A common symptom of cholecystitis is right upper quadrant pain that radiates to the:

1. sternum. 2. shoulder.
3. umbilicus. 4. jaw.

(735) **18.** When the cholecystectomy patient first returns from surgery, the drainage from the T tube may be bloody, but it should soon become:

1. dark amber.
2. clay-colored.
3. bright red.
4. greenish brown.

(736) **19.** What type of diet is recommended for patients with cholecystitis to decrease attacks of biliary colic?

1. low-protein
2. low-fat
3. low-carbohydrate
4. low-salt

(736) **20.** Patients with obstructed bile flow may have a deficiency of vitamin:

1. A. 2. C.
3. D. 4. K.

(739) **21.** A complication of endoscopic sphincterotomy is pancreatitis caused by accidental entry of the endoscope into the pancreatic duct; early signs of pancreatitis are:

1. jaundice and confusion.
2. nausea and vomiting.
3. ascites and hypertension.
4. pain and fever.

(738) **22.** A gland that has both endocrine and exocrine functions is the:

1. pancreas.
2. adrenal gland.
3. thyroid gland.
4. sebaceous gland.

(736) **23.** Vitamin K is needed for the production of:

1. bile.
2. calcium.
3. prothrombin.
4. thyroxine.

(739) **24.** Specific blood studies used to assess pancreatic function include serum:

1. bilirubin.
2. amylase.
3. prothrombin.
4. albumin.

(739) **25.** The most prominent symptom of pancreatitis is:

1. jaundice.
2. abdominal pain.
3. hypertension.
4. diarrhea.

(742) **26.** To remove the stimulus for secretion of pancreatic fluid in acute pancreatitis, the patient is usually allowed:

1. nothing by mouth.
2. a low-fat diet.
3. a clear-liquid diet.
4. a low-sodium diet.

(742) **27.** Which drugs do patients with chronic pancreatitis need to take in order to digest food?

1. analgesics
2. anticholinergics
3. antiemetics
4. pancreatic enzymes

(739) **28.** Early signs of shock that may occur in patients with pancreatitis include:

1. restlessness.
2. bradycardia.
3. hypotension.
4. easy bruising.

(744) **29.** When patients with pancreatitis are on TPN in order to restrict oral intake and reduce pancreatic fluid secretion, the nurse must monitor for:

1. hyperkalemia.
2. hypernatremia.
3. hyperchloremia.
4. hyperglycemia.

(714) **30.** Which herb can harm the liver?

1. garlic
2. ginkgo
3. comfrey
4. ginseng

(720) **31.** The bile channels in the liver are compressed in patients with hepatitis, resulting in elevated:

1. serum creatinine.
2. BUN.
3. bilirubin.
4. hemoglobin.

(721) **32.** Which is a finding that supports the diagnosis of hepatitis?

1. increased serum bilirubin
2. decreased prothrombin time
3. increased albumin
4. decreased urinary bilirubin

(722) **33.** What is the prescribed diet for hepatitis?

1. increased protein
2. increased fat
3. decreased carbohydrate
4. decreased calories

(723) **34.** Which cultural group has the highest rate of death from cirrhosis of the liver?

1. Hispanics
2. African-Americans
3. Caucasians
4. Asians

Student Name______________________________

(729) **35.** The medical treatment of hepatic encephalopathy is directed toward:

1. raising hemoglobin.
2. reducing ammonia formation.
3. decreasing urea.
4. increasing prothrombin time.

(722, 725) **36.** In patients with hepatitis and in patients with cirrhosis, most of the calories should come from:

1. carbohydrates.
2. protein.
3. saturated fats.
4. unsaturated fats.

CHAPTER 38

Student Name ______________________________

Urologic Disorders

Answer Key: Textbook page references are provided as a guide for answering these questions. A complete answer key was provided for your instructor.

OBJECTIVES

1. List the data to be collected when assessing a patient who has a urologic disorder.
2. Describe the diagnostic tests and procedures for patients with urologic disorders.
3. Explain the nursing responsibilities for patients having tests and procedures to diagnose urologic disorders.
4. Describe the nursing responsibilities for common therapeutic measures used to treat urologic disorders.
5. Explain the pathophysiology, signs and symptoms, complications, and treatment of disorders of the kidney, ureters, bladder, and urethra.
6. Assist in developing a nursing care plan for patients with urologic disorders.

LEARNING ACTIVITIES

A. Complete the statement in the numbered column with the most appropriate term in the lettered column. Some terms may be used more than once, and some terms may not be used.

(753) **1.** Some nonelectrolyte substances that are reabsorbed by the tubules include uric acid, urea, and __________.

(753) **2.** Reabsorption of water by the tubules occurs through the process of __________.

(753) **3.** The end product of glomerular filtration and tubular reabsorption is __________.

(753) **4.** Aldosterone is secreted by the adrenal glands in response to __________.

A. Aldosterone
B. Glucose
C. Ions
D. Peristalsis
E. Concentrated urine
F. Urethra
G. Urine
H. Creatinine
I. Osmosis
J. Sodium
K. Dilute urine

Continued next page

(754) **5.** Aldosterone causes the reabsorption of water and __________.

(753) **6.** Substances secreted by the tubules are called __________.

(753) **7.** The amount of water reabsorbed in the kidneys is influenced by antidiuretic hormone and __________.

(753) **8.** Urine is moved from the kidney to the bladder by means of __________.

B. Match the description or definition in the numbered column with the most appropriate term in the lettered column. Some terms may be used more than once, and some terms may not be used.

(754) **1.** __________ Causes reabsorption of water in the renal tubules, decreasing urine volume

(754) **2.** __________ Is released in response to inadequate renal blood flow or low arterial pressure

(754) **3.** __________ The hormone secreted in the kidneys that stimulates the bone marrow to produce red blood cells

(754) **4.** __________ The hormone that is released from the pituitary gland when stimulated by hypertonic plasma

(754) **5.** __________ Used to describe very concentrated plasma

(754) **6.** __________ A common condition that leads to hypertonic plasma

A. Erythropoietin
B. Angiotensin II
C. Hypertonic
D. Calcium
E. Renin
F. Hypotonic
G. Antidiuretic hormone
H. Dehydration

Student Name____

C. Complete the statements in the numbered column with the most appropriate term in the lettered column. Some terms may be used more than once, and some terms may not be used.

(756) **1.** With normally functioning kidneys, the serum creatinine level is __________.

(756) **2.** __________ is a general indicator of the kidneys' ability to excrete urea; values are raised by high-protein diets, gastrointestinal bleeding, dehydration, and some drugs.

(756) **3.** A better measurement of kidney functioning than the BUN because it is elevated only in kidney disorders is the __________.

(756) **4.** With normally functioning kidneys, the urine creatinine level is __________.

(756) **5.** The best test of overall kidney function is __________.

(756) **6.** Two tests that are compared to each other and that should be opposite each other if kidneys are functioning normally are the creatinine clearance and the __________.

A. Blood urea nitrogen (BUN)
B. High
C. Serum electrolytes
D. Urine culture
E. Very low
F. Serum creatinine
G. Creatinine clearance

D. Match the definition or description in the numbered column with the most appropriate term in the lettered column. Some terms may be used more than once, and some terms may not be used.

(761) **1.** __________ A catheter is inserted into the bladder, and fluid is instilled until the patient reports the urge to void

(761) **2.** __________ Measures the rate of urine flow during voiding

A. Reflux
B. Urodynamic study
C. Ultrasonography
D. Flat plate
E. Cystometrogram
F. Cystogram
G. Intravenous pyelogram

Continued next page

(761) **3.** __________ Outlines the contour of the bladder and shows reflux of urine

(761) **4.** __________ The backward movement of urine from the bladder into the ureters

(760) **5.** __________ Dye is injected IV, radiographs of kidney, ureters, and bladder are taken; used to assess kidney function

(761) **6.** __________ A catheter is inserted into the bladder, dye is injected, and radiographs are taken

(761) **7.** __________ Used to evaluate bladder tone in the patient with incontinence or with a neurogenic bladder

E. Complete the statement in the numbered column with the most appropriate term in the lettered column. Some terms may be used more than once, and some terms may not be used.

(771) **1.** __________ is the condition in which calculi are formed in the kidneys.

(772) **2.** Three diagnostic tests to confirm the presence and location of calculi in the urinary tract include ultrasound, IVP, and the __________.

(769) **3.** __________ is inflammation of the renal pelvis.

(770) **4.** A hereditary disorder in which grapelike cysts replace normal kidney tissue is __________.

(772) **5.** __________ is the removal of a calculus.

(772) **6.** The removal of a calculus from the renal pelvis is __________.

(767) **7.** Inflammation of the urinary bladder is __________.

A. Polycystic kidney disease
B. Anticholinergics
C. Pyelolithotomy
D. Hemorrhage
E. Nephrolithiasis
F. KUB
G. MRI
H. Proteinuria
I. Glomerulonephritis
J. Lithotomy
K. Antispasmodics
L. Urolithiasis
M. Cystitis
N. Platelets
O. Nephrolithiasis
P. Pyelonephritis

Continued next page

Student Name ____________________

(770) **8.** A urinalysis is done in patients with glomerulonephritis to detect red blood cell casts and __________.

(771) **9.** The formation of calculi in the urinary tract is called __________.

(771) **10.** The formation of calculi in the kidneys is called __________.

(772) **11.** The intense, colicky pain of renal calculi may be relieved by narcotic analgesics and __________.

(772) **12.** Possible complications of lithotripsy include bruising and __________.

(770) **13.** Inflammation of the capillary loops in the glomeruli is __________.

F. Match the definition or description in the numbered column with the most appropriate term in the lettered column. Some terms may be used more than once, and some terms may not be used.

(762) **1.** __________ Removal of a kidney

(762) **2.** __________ A noninvasive procedure to break up calculi

(762) **3.** __________ Removal of the bladder

(762) **4.** __________ An incision made to open the bladder

(762) **5.** __________ A surgical procedure that reroutes the flow of urine

A. Urinary diversion
B. Lithotripsy
C. Cystoscopy
D. Cystectomy
E. Nephrectomy
F. Cystotomy

G. Complete the statement in the numbered column with the most appropriate term in the lettered column. Some terms may be used more than once, and some terms may not be used.

(784) **1.** ________ can be caused by the accumulation of calcium phosphate crystals and urea in the skin.

(777) **2.** Following the removal of a kidney, the condition in which peristalsis does not return within 3 to 4 days is called ________.

(775) **3.** When a calculus obstructs urine flow, the urine may back up into the kidney, causing ________.

A. Hydronephrosis
B. Red blood cells
C. Nephrectomy
D. Cystectomy
E. Calculi
F. Paralytic ileus
G. Nephrostomy
H. Itching

Continued next page

(775) **4.** The placement of a tube in the kidney so that urine may drain through the tube into an external collection device is called ________.

(775) **5.** In patients with hydronephrosis, urine is usually strained and examined for ________.

(775) **6.** Distention of the kidney with urine is called ________.

H. Complete the statement in the numbered column with the most appropriate term in the lettered column. Some terms may be used more than once, and some terms may not be used.

(784) **1.** __________, which is most often noted around the mouth, is a very late sign in chronic renal failure.

(783) **2.** Most patients with chronic renal failure retain water and __________

(787) **3.** Emotional responses to chronic renal failure include depression, disturbed body image, and __________.

(784) **4.** Ovulation and __________ usually cease in females with chronic renal failure.

(784) **5.** The skeletal changes characteristic of chronic renal failure are known as __________.

(784) **6.** A diet high in carbohydrates and low in protein is prescribed to reduce the accumulation of __________.

(784) **7.** __________ is the condition in which calcium is lost from bones and replaced with fibrous tissue.

(784) **8.** Related to endocrine function, patients with chronic renal failure usually have __________.

(784) **9.** The effects of chronic renal failure on the male reproductive system typically include low sperm counts and __________.

A. Anxiety
B. Impotence
C. Osteitis fibrosa
D. Hypothyroidism
E. Osteomalacia
F. Sodium
G. Cholesterol
H. Uremic frost
I. Urea
J. Menstruation
K. Renal osteodystrophy

Student Name____

I. Complete the statement in the numbered column with the most appropriate term in the lettered column. Some terms may be used more than once, and some terms may not be used.

(784) **1.** __________ is the passage of molecules through a semipermeable membrane into a special solution.

(784) **2.** A "__________" is a rippling sensation palpable on the venous side of the cannula or fistula.

(785) **3.** A leading cause of death in hemodialysis patients is __________.

(785) **4.** Vascular access for hemodialysis may be accomplished by temporary catheter, cannula, graft, or __________.

(785) **5.** A process by which blood is removed from the body and circulated through an artificial kidney is called __________.

(787) **6.** The major complication of peritoneal dialysis is __________.

(787) **7.** Vascular access sites must be assessed for __________.

(787) **8.** __________ allows a patient to have dialysis performed at night by a machine, giving the patient freedom during the day and reducing the risk of infection.

(785) **9.** A rushing, roaring, or "swoosh" noise heard through a stethoscope with each heartbeat is known as a __________.

(787) **10.** __________ allows the patient freedom from a machine and the independence to perform dialysis alone.

A. Thrill
B. Peritonitis
C. Cerebrovascular accident
D. Nausea
E. Dialysis
F. Bruit
G. Continuous ambulatory peritoneal dialysis
H. Hemodialysis
I. Murmur
J. Fistula
K. Patency
L. Trocar
M. Automated peritoneal dialysis

J. Match the description or definition in the numbered column with the appropriate diagnostic test in the lettered column. Some tests may be used more than once, and some tests may not be used.

(756) **1.** __________ Examination of voided urine (or from catheter) specimen for pH, blood, glucose, and protein

(756) **2.** __________ Clean-catch or midstream urine specimen is collected to determine which antibiotics will be effective against the specific organisms found in the culture

(756) **3.** __________ Collection of urine for 12 or 24 hours, which is an estimate of the glomerular filtration rate

(756) **4.** __________ A blood test that is a general indicator of the kidneys' ability to excrete urea

(756) **5.** __________ A blood test that is indicative of the kidney's ability to excrete wastes

(756) **6.** __________ A blood test that may show elevated sodium and potassium levels and decreased calcium levels, which indicate renal failure

A. Creatinine clearance
B. Osmolality
C. Serum creatinine
D. Urinalysis
E. Serum electrolytes
F. Blood urea nitrogen (BUN)
G. Urine sensitivity

Student Name____

K. Match the description of pain in the numbered column with the location of pain in the lettered column. Some locations may be used more than once, and some locations may not be used.

(772) **1.** __________ Dull flank pain

(772) **2.** __________ Excruciating abdominal pain that radiates to the groin or perineum

A. Calculus in urethra
B. Calculus in renal pelvis
C. Calculus in ureter

L. Match the characteristics of acute renal failure in the numbered column with the stage in which it occurs in the lettered column. Some stages may be used more than once, and some stages may not be used.

(781) **1.** __________ Urine output exceeds 400 ml/day and may rise above 4 liters/day

(781) **2.** __________ Serum electrolytes, BUN, and creatinine return to normal

(781) **3.** __________ Urine specific gravity becomes fixed at 1.010

(781) **4.** __________ Primary treatment goal is reversal of failing renal function to prevent further damage

(781) **5.** __________ Urine output decreased to 400 ml/day or less

(781) **6.** __________ Lasts 1–12 months

(781) **7.** __________ Lasts up to 14 days

(781) **8.** __________ Few waste products are excreted despite the production of large quantities of urine

(781) **9.** __________ Lasts 1–3 days

A. Onset stage
B. Oliguric stage
C. Diuretic stage
D. Recovery stage

M. For the following drugs, indicate whether it is used to treat oliguria or hyperkalemia.

A. Oliguria
B. Hyperkalemia

(781) **1.** ________ Hypertonic glucose and insulin

(781) **2.** ________ Furosemide (Lasix)

(781) **3.** ________ Sodium bicarbonate

(781) **4.** ________ Calcium gluconate

(781) **5.** ________ Ethacrynic acid (Edecrin)

(781) **6.** ________ Sodium polystyrene sulfonate (Kayexalate)

N. Describe the age-related changes in the kidneys that occur with respect to the areas listed below.

(754) **1.** Function of kidneys: ________

(754) **2.** Adaptation of kidneys under stress: ________

(754) **3.** Number of nephrons: ________

(754) **4.** Renal blood vessels: ________

(754) **5.** Renal blood flow: ________

(754) **6.** Glomerular filtration rate: ________

(754) **7.** Plasma renin and aldosterone levels: ________

(754) **8.** Antidiuretic hormone's effect on tubules: ________

(754) **9.** Kidney's ability to concentrate and dilute urine: ________

(754) **10.** Creatinine clearance rate: ________

(754) **11.** Incidence of nocturia: ________

O. Describe the age-related changes of the bladder that occur in the areas listed below.

(754) **1.** Bladder muscles: ________

(754) **2.** Connective tissue in the bladder: ________

(754) **3.** Capacity of bladder: ________

(754) **4.** Emptying function of bladder: ________

Student Name____

P. Describe what the following color or appearance of urine may indicate in patients with urinary disorders.

(760) **1.** Straw-colored: ____________________

(760) **2.** Bright red: ____________________

(760) **3.** Tea-colored: ____________________

(760) **4.** Cloudy or hazy appearance: ____________________

(760) **5.** Colorless: ____________________

Q. List four symptoms of an allergic reaction to iodine dye used for NP procedures.

(758) **1.** ____________________

(758) **2.** ____________________

(758) **3.** ____________________

(758) **4.** ____________________

R. List four signs of blood loss for which the nurse observes when a patient with kidney disease returns from undergoing angiography.

(758) **1.** ____________________

(758) **2.** ____________________

(758) **3.** ____________________

(758) **4.** ____________________

S. List eight factors that influence the development of renal calculi.

(771) **1.** ____________________

(771) **2.** ____________________

(771) **3.** ____________________

(771) **4.** ____________________

(771) **5.** ____________________

(771) **6.** ____________________

(771) **7.** ____________________

(771) **8.** ____________________

T. In Figure 38-1 below, label the parts (A–I) of the urinary system.

(751)

A. ______________________________ F. ______________________________

B. ______________________________ G. ______________________________

C. ______________________________ H. ______________________________

D. ______________________________ I. ______________________________

E. ______________________________

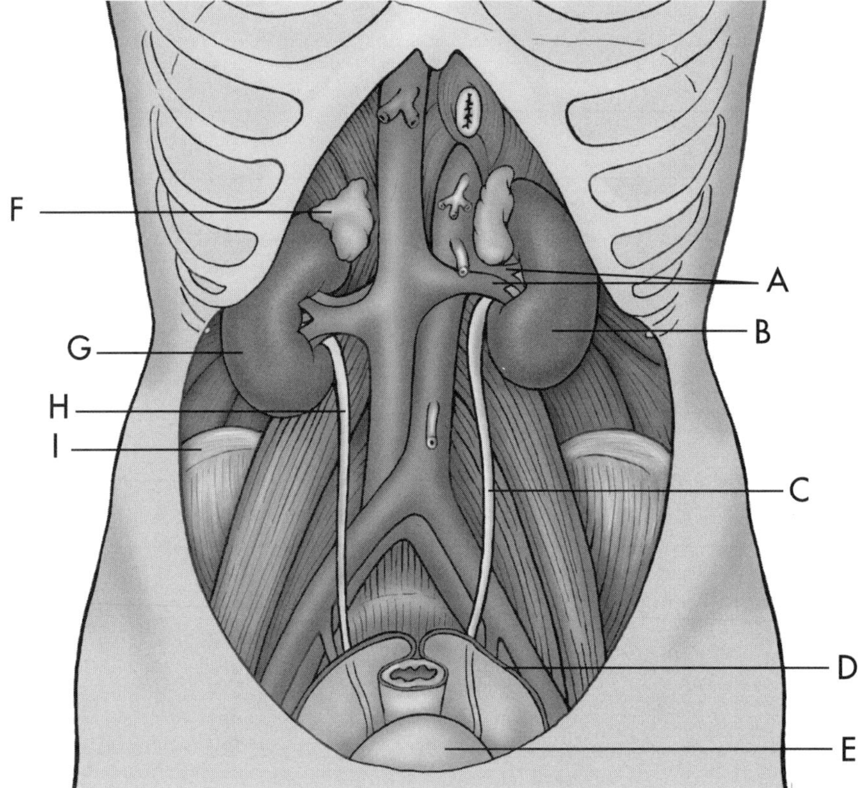

Student Name____

U. In Figure 38-3 below, label the parts (A–K) of the kidney.

(752)

A.	____________________	**G.**	____________________
B.	____________________	**H.**	____________________
C.	____________________	**I.**	____________________
D.	____________________	**J.**	____________________
E.	____________________	**K.**	____________________
F.	____________________		

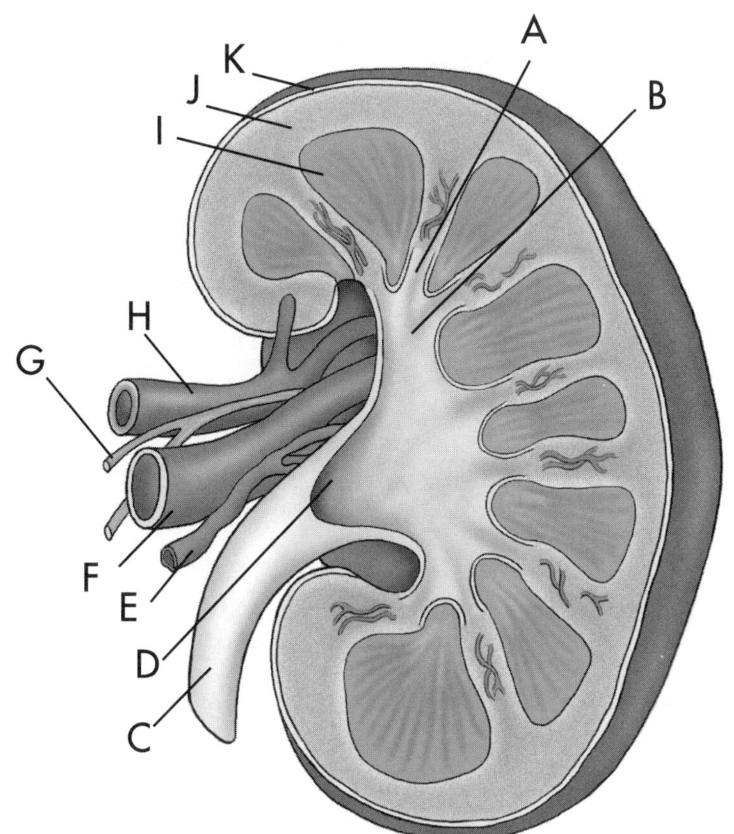

V. In Figure 38-4, label the parts (A–L) of the nephron.

(752)

A.	____________________	**G.**	____________________
B.	____________________	**H.**	____________________
C.	____________________	**I.**	____________________
D.	____________________	**J.**	____________________
E.	____________________	**K.**	____________________
F.	____________________	**L.**	____________________

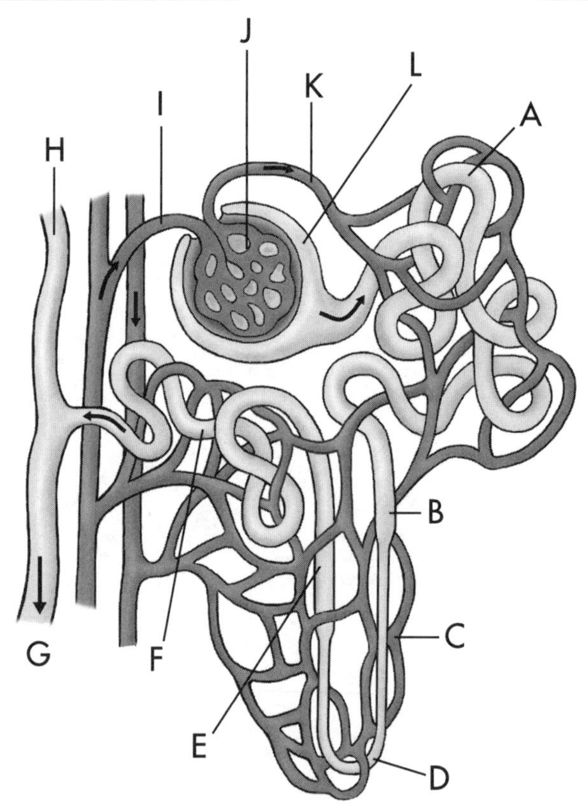

MULTIPLE-CHOICE QUESTIONS

W. Choose the most appropriate answer.

(753) **1.** Glomerular filtrate and blood plasma are essentially the same, except that the filtrate does not have:

1. water.
2. sodium.
3. potassium.
4. proteins.

(753) **2.** As the blood passes through the glomerulus, which element is too large to pass through the semipermeable membrane?

1. serum sodium
2. serum potassium
3. plasma protein
4. glucose

Student Name____

(753) **3.** The normal pH of urine is:

1. 1.0–3.0.
2. 4.5–8.0.
3. 8.5–10.0.
4. 10.5–3.0.

(753) **4.** The body normally excretes how many liters of urine per day?

1. 0.5 liter
2. 1–2 liters
3. 5 liters
4. 7–10 liters

(753) **5.** Two substances that are present in blood but not normally present in urine are:

1. sodium and chloride.
2. glucose and protein.
3. calcium and magnesium.
4. potassium and bicarbonate.

(753) **6.** Glomerular damage may be indicated by the presence of which of the following in the urine?

1. sodium
2. chloride
3. protein
4. potassium

(753) **7.** The presence of how much urine usually causes the urge to urinate?

1. 100–150 ml
2. 200–400 ml
3. 500–600 ml
4. 800–1000 ml

(753) **8.** Voiding is primarily controlled by:

1. involuntary reflex.
2. voluntary muscles.
3. peristalsis.
4. tubular secretion.

(754) **9.** A hormone that helps maintain normal serum calcium and phosphate levels is:

1. antidiuretic hormone.
2. epinephrine.
3. parathormone.
4. aldosterone.

(754) **10.** Blood pressure is regulated through fluid volume maintenance and release of the hormone:

1. aldosterone.
2. renin.
3. antidiuretic hormone.
4. parathormone.

(754) **11.** A change in blood volume will result in a change in:

1. body temperature.
2. heart rate.
3. blood pressure.
4. respiratory rate.

(754) **12.** Decreased oxygen in renal blood triggers the secretion of:

1. aldosterone.
2. antidiuretic hormone.
3. epinephrine.
4. erythropoietin.

(754) **13.** Patients in renal failure have a deficiency of erythropoietin, which causes them to have:

1. pneumonia.
2. anemia.
3. seizures.
4. hypertension.

(754) **14.** A common age-related problem in males related to the urinary system is:

1. urethral obstruction.
2. incontinence.
3. relaxed pelvic musculature.
4. lack of testosterone.

(755) **15.** If crystals on the skin are observed during the examination of patients with urinary disorders, this is recorded as:

1. ashen skin.
2. edema.
3. uremic frost.
4. scaly skin.

(755) **16.** Tissue turgor is evaluated in patients with urinary disorders to detect:

1. uremic frost.
2. Kussmaul's respirations.
3. infection.
4. dehydration.

(755) **17.** The eyes of patients with urinary disorders are examined for periorbital edema, the presence of which suggests:

1. dehydration.
2. fluid retention.
3. uremic frost.
4. Kussmaul's respirations.

(755) **18.** If patients with urinary disorders have dyspnea, this may be a sign of:

1. dehydration.
2. uremic frost.
3. potassium imbalance.
4. fluid overload.

(755) **19.** If patients with urinary disorders have an odor of urine on their breath, this may indicate:

1. urinary tract infection.
2. kidney failure.
3. cardiac failure.
4. diabetes mellitus.

(755) **20.** Patients with urinary disorders who have potassium imbalances may have:

1. uremic frost.
2. heart irregularities.
3. hypertension.
4. rapid respirations.

(755) **21.** Swishing sounds caused by the turbulence of blood are called:

1. bruits.
2. uremic frost.
3. crackles.
4. rhonchi.

(755) **22.** An indication of renal artery stenosis (narrowing) is:

1. urinary tract infection.
2. crackles.
3. bruits.
4. uremic frost.

(755) **23.** The edema found in renal failure is described as:

1. dependent.
2. peripheral.
3. pitting.
4. generalized.

(755) **24.** In patients with renal failure, the skin over edematous areas is apt to be described as:

1. warm and moist.
2. dry and flushed.
3. pink and intact.
4. pale and thick.

(755) **25.** Inspection of the genitalia during the examination of patients with urinary disorders must always be done utilizing:

1. auscultation.
2. palpation.
3. standard precautions.
4. aseptic technique.

(756) **26.** Normal urine is:

1. bright red.
2. straw-colored.
3. tea-colored.
4. smoke-colored.

(760) **27.** Urine with a cloudy appearance may be indicative of:

1. bacterial infection.
2. excessive fluid intake.
3. dehydration.
4. diabetes mellitus.

Student Name ______________________

(756) **28.** Normally, urine is sterile and slightly:

1. alkaline. 2. acidic.
3. pyuric. 4. hematuric.

(756) **29.** A diagnostic test for the identification of microorganisms present in urine is:

1. blood urea nitrogen.
2. urinalysis.
3. urine culture.
4. creatinine clearance.

(756) **30.** The best test of overall kidney function, which is an estimate of glomerular filtration rate, is:

1. blood urea nitrogen.
2. urinalysis.
3. urine culture.
4. creatinine clearance.

(759) **31.** Which blood test needs to be within normal limits before a renal biopsy is performed?

1. electrolytes
2. blood urea nitrogen
3. serum creatinine
4. clotting studies

(761) **32.** After a renal biopsy, what is the most important side effect to watch for?

1. infection 2. dyspnea
3. bleeding 4. fatigue

(759) **33.** Following cystoscopy, at first the urine will be:

1. colorless.
2. pink-tinged.
3. tea-colored.
4. orange.

(759) **34.** Following cystoscopy, urine should lighten to its usual color within:

1. 4–6 hours.
2. 8–10 hours.
3. 24–48 hours.
4. 60–72 hours.

(761) **35.** Following cystoscopy, belladonna and opium suppositories may be ordered to reduce:

1. bladder spasm.
2. hematuria.
3. infection.
4. back pain.

(761) **36.** Bladder perforation is rare following cystoscopy, but it may be indicated by severe:

1. hematuria.
2. abdominal pain.
3. tachycardia.
4. hypotension.

(761) **37.** The major concern with catheterization is the potential for:

1. hemorrhage.
2. shock.
3. kidney failure.
4. infection.

(761) **38.** To measure residual volume, the patient must be catheterized immediately after voiding; which of the following is an abnormal finding?

1. 5 ml 2. 10 ml
3. 25 ml 4. 75 ml

(762) **39.** Following urologic surgery, which of the following outputs should be reported to the physician?

1. less than 30 ml/hour
2. less than 50 ml/hour
3. less than 70 ml/hour
4. less than 100 ml/hour

(767) **40.** The most common nosocomial infections are:

1. skin infections.
2. wound infections.
3. urinary tract infections.
4. blood infections.

(767) **41.** Most urinary tract infections are caused by:

1. viruses.
2. bacteria.
3. yeasts.
4. fungi.

(767) **42.** Dysuria, frequency, urgency, and bladder spasms are common symptoms of:

1. pyelonephritis.
2. kidney failure.
3. vaginitis.
4. urethritis.

(772) **43.** The passage of renal calculi is facilitated by:

1. bed rest.
2. opiates.
3. restricted fluids.
4. ambulation.

(767) **44.** The pain of urethritis may be reduced by:

1. antiemetics.
2. back massage.
3. sitz baths.
4. bubble baths.

(769) **45.** A common symptom of pyelonephritis is:

1. polyuria.
2. hypotension.
3. bradycardia.
4. flank pain.

(769) **46.** When forcing fluids on patients with pyelonephritis, the nurse needs to be careful to prevent:

1. infection.
2. hemorrhage.
3. kidney failure.
4. circulatory overload.

(769) **47.** An elderly patient with pyelonephritis who experiences a suddenly increased fluid volume may develop:

1. hypotension.
2. congestive heart failure.
3. seizures.
4. thrombophlebitis.

(770) **48.** The most common type of glomerulonephritis follows a respiratory tract infection caused by:

1. *Staphylococcus.*
2. a virus.
3. a fungus.
4. *Streptococcus.*

(770) **49.** In addition to antibiotics, acute glomerulonephritis is treated medically with:

1. diuretics and antihypertensives.
2. antihistamines and antiemetics.
3. anticholinergics and analgesics.
4. narcotics and anticonvulsants.

Student Name________________________________

(770) **50.** In the acute phase of glomerulonephritis, bed rest is ordered to prevent or treat heart failure and severe hypertension that result from:

1. fluid volume deficit.
2. fluid overload.
3. altered renal tissue perfusion.
4. respiratory distress.

(771) **51.** A common nursing diagnosis for patients with acute glomerulonephritis is:

1. fluid volume deficit.
2. excess fluid volume.
3. altered renal tissue perfusion.
4. high risk for injury.

(771) **52.** The incidence of uric acid stones is high among:

1. Caucasian females.
2. Jewish males.
3. African-American females.
4. Hispanic males.

(753) **53.** When a person is dehydrated, the kidneys conserve water, causing urine to be:

1. dilute.
2. cloudy.
3. alkaline.
4. concentrated.

(771) **54.** A diet that can contribute to calculus formation is one that is high in purines and:

1. sodium. 2. potassium.
3. calcium. 4. fat.

(775) **55.** In order to prevent renal calculi, the nurse should teach patients to:

1. follow a high-calcium diet.
2. follow a high-purine diet.
3. have a high fluid intake.
4. limit physical activity.

(773) **56.** A major nursing concern for patients with renal calculi is:

1. frequent ambulation.
2. emotional support.
3. range-of-motion exercises.
4. pain relief.

(776) **57.** The treatment of choice for renal cancer is:

1. lithotripsy.
2. radical nephrectomy.
3. cystectomy.
4. nephrostomy.

(777) **58.** The location of the flank incision following nephrectomy causes pain with expansion of the:

1. abdomen. 2. pelvis.
3. cerebrum. 4. thorax.

(777) **59.** When patients after nephrectomy protect the chest by not breathing deeply, this leads to the development of:

1. hemorrhage.
2. infection.
3. atelectasis.
4. shock.

(778) **60.** The most common malignancy of the urinary tract is:

1. cancer of the kidney.
2. cervical cancer.
3. bladder cancer.
4. liver cancer.

(778) **61.** The most frequent symptom of bladder cancer is intermittent:

1. glycosuria.
2. proteinuria.
3. pyuria.
4. hematuria.

(778) **62.** When the bladder is removed completely, urinary diversion is sometimes provided, which allows urine to be excreted through the:

1. urethra.
2. ileal conduit.
3. ureter.
4. cystoscopy.

(779) **63.** Preoperative care for an ileal or sigmoid conduit includes thorough preparation of the intestinal tract, which includes administration of an antibiotic that is not absorbed from the intestinal tract, called:

1. Keflex.
2. penicillin.
3. neomycin.
4. tetracycline.

(782) **64.** An effective means of assessing changes in fluid status of patients in acute renal failure is:

1. monitoring edema.
2. recording intake and output.
3. weighing daily.
4. taking signs.

(782) **65.** When 90–95% of kidney function is lost, the patient is considered to be in:

1. acute renal failure.
2. chronic renal failure.
3. renal shock.
4. renal oliguria.

(783) **66.** The most life-threatening effect of renal failure is:

1. hypernatremia.
2. hyponatremia.
3. hyperkalemia.
4. hypokalemia.

(789) **67.** When a kidney is obtained from a living related donor, the 1-year survival rate for transplantation is about:

1. 30–33%. 2. 65–70%.
3. 75–80%. 4. 95–97%.

(790) **68.** To control the body's response to foreign tissue, the transplant recipient is given:

1. analgesics.
2. immunosuppressants.
3. anticholinergics.
4. antihistamines.

(791) **69.** Specific nursing diagnoses related to possibility of organ rejection after renal transplantation may include:

1. Risk for injury.
2. Altered role performance.
3. Anxiety.
4. Diarrhea.

(791) **70.** Signs of dehydration in the patient who has had a renal transplant may include thready pulse, poor tissue turgor, and:

1. low blood pressure.
2. high blood pressure.
3. high fever.
4. abnormally low body temperature.

(791) **71.** Complications of lithotripsy include:

1. bruising.
2. congestive heart failure.
3. dyspnea.
4. thrombus.

Student Name ______________________________

(778) **72.** Risk factors for bladder cancer include:

1. obesity.
2. cigarette smoking.
3. a high-purine diet.
4. a sedentary lifestyle.

(760) **73.** Which procedure is contraindicated in patients with known renal insufficiency or diabetes mellitus?

1. Intravenous pyelogram (IVP)
2. Flat plate
3. Renal scan
4. Ultrasonography

CHAPTER 39

Student Name ______________________________

Connective Tissue Disorders

Answer Key: Textbook page references are provided as a guide for answering these questions. A complete answer key was provided for your instructor.

OBJECTIVES

1. Define connective tissue.
2. Describe the function of connective tissue.
3. Describe the characteristics and prevalence of connective tissue diseases.
4. Describe the diagnostic tests and procedures used for assessing connective tissue diseases.
5. Discuss the drugs used to treat connective tissue diseases.
6. Describe the pathologic basis for osteoarthritis (degenerative joint disease), rheumatoid arthritis, osteoporosis, gout, progressive systemic sclerosis, polymyositis, bursitis, carpal tunnel syndrome, ankylosing spondylitis, polymyalgia rheumatica, Reiter's syndrome, Behçet's syndrome, and Sjögren's syndrome.
7. Identify the data to be collected in the nursing assessment of a patient with a connective tissue disorder.
8. Assist in developing a nursing care plan for a patient whose life has been affected by a connective tissue disease.

LEARNING ACTIVITIES

A. Match the definition in the numbered column with the most appropriate term in the lettered column.

(796)	**1.**	________	Instrument used to measure joint range of motion
(803)	**2.**	________	Within the joint
(814)	**3.**	________	Elevated level of uric acid in the blood
(818)	**4.**	________	Muscle pain
(814)	**5.**	________	Deposit of sodium urate crystals under the skin
(803)	**6.**	________	Protrusions of the distal interphalangeal finger joints; associated with osteoarthritis
(803)	**7.**	________	Enlarged proximal interphalangeal joints of the fingers
(819)	**8.**	________	Chronic musculoskeletal pain disorder
(810)	**9.**	________	Granulation of tissue surrounding cores of fibrous debris
(804)	**10.**	________	Plastic repair of a joint
(810)	**11.**	________	Inflammation of blood vessels
(796)	**12.**	________	Crackling sound or sensation
(809)	**13.**	________	Joint immobility

A. Hyperuricemia
B. Ankylosis
C. Fibromyalgia
D. Tophus
E. Vasculitis
F. Intra-articular
G. Heberden's nodes
H. Crepitus
I. Goniometer
J. Myalgia
K. rheumatoid nodules
L. Bouchard's nodes
M. Arthroplasty

Student Name____

B. Complete the statement in the numbered column with the most appropriate term in the lettered column. Some terms may be used more than once, and some terms may not be used.

(808) **1.** A device that is used after joint replacement surgery to move the joints through a set range of motions at a set rate of movements per minute is the __________.

(802) **2.** The most common form of arthritis, which is also called degenerative joint disease, is __________.

(804) **3.** The surgical treatment of choice for OA is __________.

(802) **4.** Joint activities are compromised because the basic structure of the cartilage is altered in __________.

(804) **5.** The primary indication for total joint replacement in patients with OA is __________.

(802) **6.** A condition that generally affects joints under pressure (such as the spine and knees) is __________.

A. Total joint replacement
B. Physical therapy
C. Continuous passive movement machine
D. Osteoarthritis (OA)
E. Ankylosing spondylitis
F. Intractable pain

C. Complete the statement in the numbered column with the most appropriate term in the lettered column. Some terms may be used more than once, and some terms may not be used.

(809) **1.** The synovium thickens and fluid accumulates in the joint space of patients with __________.

(809) **2.** A loss of joint mobility occurring in RA is called __________.

(810) **3.** Morning stiffness lasting more than 1 hour is a common symptom of ________.

(810) **4.** If blood vessels are affected by RA, they become inflamed, a condition called __________.

(810) **5.** Subcutaneous nodules over bony prominences, which are often present in RA, are called __________.

A. Rheumatoid arthritis (RA)
B. Osteoarthritis
C. Rheumatoid nodules
D. Bursitis
E. Vasculitis
F. Polymyositis
G. Ankylosis
H. Carpal tunnel syndrome

Continued next page

(818) **6.** Inflammation of sacs at joints treated by lidocaine injections for temporary relief is _________.

(818) **7.** Compression of the median nerve in the wrist, causing pain and tenderness, is _________.

(809) **8.** A chronic, progressive inflammatory disease is _________.

D. Complete the statements in the numbered column with the most appropriate term in the lettered column. Some terms may be used more than once, and some terms may not be used.

(810) **1.** A disease characterized by dry mouth, dry eyes, and dry vagina is called _________.

(810) **2.** An uncommon disease that consists of an enlarged liver and spleen and neutropenia is called _________.

(810) **3.** A disease marked by rheumatoid nodules in the lungs that occurs most often in coal miners and asbestos workers is called _________.

(812) **4.** A condition in which there is loss of bone mass, making the patient susceptible to fractures, is _________.

(812) **5.** Common sites of fractures due to osteoporosis are the wrist, vertebrae, and _________.

(812) **6.** Bone mass can be measured using a technique called _________.

(814) **7.** A systemic disease characterized by the deposition of urate crystals in the joints and other body tissues is _________.

(814) **8.** An excessive rate of uric acid production or decreased uric acid excretion by the kidneys results in _________.

(814) **9.** The joint commonly affected by gout is that of the _________.

(815) **10.** A diet low in _________ is recommended for patients with gout.

A. Caplan's syndrome
B. Absorptiometry
C. Great toe
D. Felty's syndrome
E. Periarteritis nodosa
F. Hyperuricemia
G. Purines
H. Hip
I. Systemic lupus erythematosus
J. Tophi
K. Sjögren's syndrome
L. Doppler ultrasound
M. Osteoporosis
N. Gout
O. Ankle
P. Milk and milk products

Student Name____

E. Complete the statement in the numbered column with the most appropriate term in the lettered column. Some terms may be used more than once, and some terms may not be used.

(816) **1.** Decreased elasticity, stenosis, and occlusion of vessels are manifestations of __________.

(818) **2.** __________ is an inflammatory disease that primarily affects the vertebral column, causing spinal deformities.

(816) **3.** The management of Raynaud's phenomenon is aimed at elimination of anything that causes __________.

(816) **4.** Scleroderma may be brought into remission with high doses of immunosuppressants or __________.

(810) **5.** __________ is a condition characterized by inflammation and damage to blood vessels that is present in nearly all connective tissue diseases.

(818) **6.** A chronic inflammatory disease of unknown cause, which is classified as an autoimmune disease, is __________.

(819) **7.** The primary symptom of polymyositis is __________.

(818) **8.** __________ is a disease that is a form of systemic necrotizing vasculitis.

(816) **9.** A chronic multisystem disease that draws its name from the characteristic hardening of the skin is __________.

(816) **10.** Patients with scleroderma who have esophageal involvement may be given drugs to decrease acidity of __________.

A. Periarteritis nodosa
B. Furosemide (Lasix)
C. Muscle weakness
D. Probenecid (Benemid)
E. Systemic lupus erythematosus
F. Polymyositis
G. Vasculitis
H. Steroids
I. Sjögren's syndrome
J. Progressive systemic sclerosis (scleroderma)
K. Ankylosing spondylitis
L. Antihypertensives
M. Gastric acid
N. Vasospasm
O. Allopurinol (Zyloprim)
P. Shoulder pain

Continued next page

(819) **11.** A relatively rare inflammatory disease that primarily affects the skeletal muscles is __________.

(801) **12.** The antigout agent that inhibits the synthesis of uric acid is __________.

(801) **13.** __________ is the antigout agent that increases urinary excretion of uric acid.

F. Match the purpose or description in the numbered column with the appropriate diagnostic test in the lettered column. Some tests may be used more than once, and some tests may not be used.

(797) **1.** __________ Results of this test are elevated in any inflammatory process, especially RA

(797) **2.** __________ Detection of blood dyscrasias; differentiation of anemias, leukemia; decreased values in RA and SLE

(797) **3.** __________ Increased values with infection, tissue necrosis, and inflammation; sometimes decreased values in SLE

(797) **4.** __________ Determines the presence of antibodies; present in about 80% of persons with RA

(797) **5.** __________ Assesses renal function; elevated values in SLE, scleroderma, and polyarteritis

A. C-reactive protein
B. Rheumatoid factor (RF)
C. Erythrocyte sedimentation rate (ESR)
D. White blood cell count (WBC)
E. Antinuclear antibodies (ANA)
F. Red blood cell count (RBC)
G. Platelet count
H. Creatinine

Continued next page

Student Name____

(797) **6.** __________ Positive reading in active inflammation, often positive for RA and SLE

(797) **7.** __________ Measures presence of antibodies that react with a variety of nuclear antibodies; positive in SLE, RA, scleroderma, Raynaud's disease, Sjögren's syndrome

G. Match the purpose or description in the numbered column with the appropriate radiologic test in the lettered column. Some tests may be used more than once, and some may not be used.

(798) **1.** __________ Intravenous radioactive material that is taken up by bone is injected for visualization of entire skeletal system; procedure detects malignancies, osteoporosis, osteomyelitis, and some fractures

(798) **2.** __________ Determines density, texture, and alignment of bones; assesses soft tissue involvement

(798) **3.** __________ Scans the soft tissues and bones by use of both radiographs and computers; determines presence of tumors or some spinal fractures

A. Ultrasound
B. Magnetic resonance imaging (MRI)
C. Radiography
D. Diskography
E. Bone scan
F. PET
G. Computed tomography (CT) scan
H. Arthrography

Continued next page

(798) **4.** __________ Examines soft tissue joint structures; performed most commonly on shoulder or knee when a traumatic injury is suspected and determines presence of bone chips, torn ligaments, or other loose bodies

(798) **5.** __________ Contrast medium injected directly into vertebral disk being examined

(798) **6.** __________ Visualization of soft tissue produced by sound waves

(798) **7.** __________ A noninvasive procedure that makes use of magnetic energy sources to view soft tissue

H. When mobility is severely impaired following hip replacement surgery, list four complications for which the patient is at risk.

(807) **1.** ______________________________

(807) **2.** ______________________________

(807) **3.** ______________________________

(807) **4.** ______________________________

I. In Figure 39-1 below, label the major structures (A–H) of the normal synovial joint.

(802) **A.** ______________________________

(802) **B.** ______________________________

(802) **C.** ______________________________

(802) **D.** ______________________________

(802) **E.** ______________________________

(802) **F.** ______________________________

(802) **G.** ______________________________

(802) **H.** ______________________________

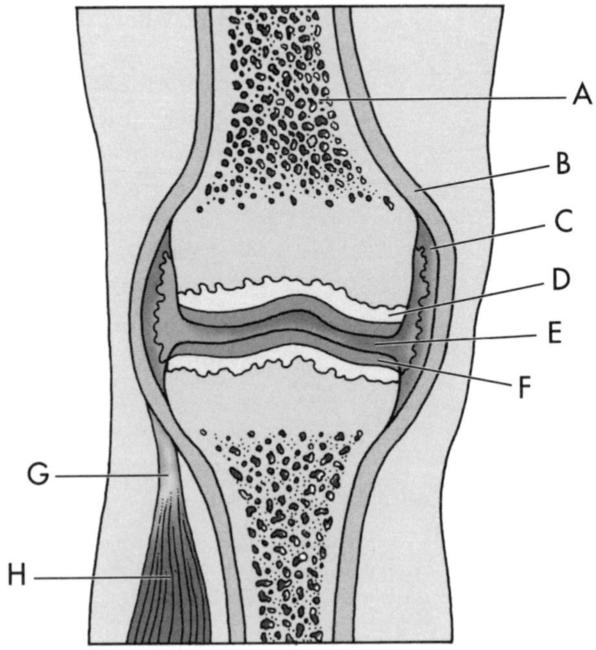

Student Name____

MULTIPLE-CHOICE QUESTIONS

J. Choose the most appropriate answer.

(795) **1.** Important changes in the connective tissue of the body that occur with aging include loss of bone strength and:

1. nutrients. 2. mass.
3. vitamins. 4. minerals.

(795) **2.** Which of the following connective tissue components remains unchanged with aging?

1. joint cartilage
2. bone strength
3. bone mass
4. blood volume

(796) **3.** During the physical examination of persons with connective tissue disorders, what is assessed by asking the patient to move each extremity through the normal range of motion?

1. joint pain and range of motion
2. fever and tachycardia
3. weight loss and nutritional deficiencies
4. tachypnea and bone function

(796) **4.** When assessing patients for joint pain and range of motion, the nurse watches for signs of pain and listens for the crackling sound called:

1. bursitis. 2. grinding.
3. crepitus. 4. scraping.

(796) **5.** Besides a complete blood count, the routine blood studies for evaluation of musculoskeletal disorders should include the:

1. prothrombin time.
2. BUN.
3. electrolyte count.
4. erythrocyte sedimentation rate.

(799) **6.** Anti-inflammatory drugs used for musculoskeletal disorders include NSAIDs and:

1. prednisone.
2. morphine.
3. furosemide.
4. digoxin.

(802) **7.** Following joint replacement surgery, a continuous passive motion (CPM) machine may be used to prevent formation of scar tissue and promote:

1. phagocytosis.
2. clotting.
3. flexibility.
4. circulation.

(803) **8.** Often the pain in osteoarthritis (OA) can be controlled with:

1. beta blockers.
2. salicylates.
3. anticholinergics.
4. narcotics.

(803) **9.** Symptoms of salicylate toxicity in the elderly may be atypical; instead of the common symptoms of gastrointestinal complaints or ototoxicity, the older person may exhibit:

1. drowsiness. 2. confusion.
3. malaise. 4. hypotension.

(805) **10.** A nursing diagnosis that patients with OA may have related to pain and limited range of motion is:

1. Knowledge deficit.
2. Altered self-esteem.
3. Impaired tissue perfusion.
4. Impaired physical mobility.

(806) **11.** Bathroom grab bars, a seat in the shower, and a raised toilet seat may promote independence and safety for the patient with poor:

1. shoulder mobility.
2. ankle mobility.
3. upper arm mobility.
4. hip mobility.

(806) **12.** A nursing diagnosis following total joint replacement that is related to improper alignment, dislocated prosthesis, and/or weakness is:

1. Altered peripheral tissue perfusion.
2. Risk for injury.
3. Risk for infection.
4. Knowledge deficit.

(807) **13.** Uncontrolled pain may make the patient reluctant to participate in rehabilitation measures following total joint replacement surgery; an intervention to improve patient participation is:

1. assess nerve and circulatory status before exercises.
2. check vital signs at least every 4 hours.
3. assist patient in and out of bed.
4. administer analgesics 30 minutes to 1 hour before exercises.

(807) **14.** Prosthetic joints can become dislocated if they are not maintained in proper alignment; after hip replacement, the affected leg must be kept in a position of:

1. abduction.
2. adduction.
3. slight elevation.
4. supination.

(808) **15.** Body areas distal to the operative joint are monitored for circulatory adequacy by assessing warmth, color, and:

1. peripheral pulses.
2. ulceration.
3. skin necrosis.
4. wound drainage.

(808) **16.** Pillows and pads should not be placed under the legs of patients with joint replacements in order to reduce the risk of:

1. ulceration.
2. gangrene.
3. deep vein thrombosis.
4. infection.

(808) **17.** A positive Homans' signs in patients who have had joint replacement surgery is indicative of:

1. wound infection.
2. deep vein thrombosis.
3. septicemia.
4. cardiac shock.

(808) **18.** After joint replacement, the patient has altered tissue perfusion and is at risk for:

1. headache.
2. hemorrhage.
3. seizure.
4. pneumonia.

(809) **19.** If a patient shows signs of cerebral blood vessel occlusion, headache, confusion, or loss of consciousness, the patient may have:

1. deep vein thrombosis.
2. hemorrhage.
3. fat embolus.
4. neuropathy.

Student Name______________________________

(809) **20.** Pressure caused by edema or constrictive dressings following joint replacement surgery can cause nerve damage, which may be manifested as:

1. paresthesia.
2. infection.
3. positive Homans' sign.
4. hemorrhage.

(809) **21.** If the nurse suspects that a dressing is too tight and is causing nerve damage, the nurse monitors sensations:

1. at the wound site.
2. proximal to the joint.
3. distal to the joint.
4. within the joint.

(809) **22.** A nursing intervention related to the patient's high risk for infection is that the nurse will:

1. place the call light in easy reach.
2. instruct patient to keep legs slightly abducted.
3. use strict sterile technique for dressing changes.
4. assess nerve and circulatory status.

(809) **23.** Drugs that are administered to patients with joint replacements who are at risk for infection are:

1. antihistamines.
2. antimicrobials.
3. antiemetics.
4. anticoagulants.

(811) **24.** A measure to control morning pain and stiffness in patients with RA is to:

1. take a warm shower.
2. increase intake of fluids.
3. eat foods low in purines.
4. use aseptic technique.

(813) **25.** A factor that slows bone loss and improves strength, balance, and reaction time (reducing the risk of falls and fractures) is:

1. vitamin C.
2. increased fluid intake.
3. regular exercise.
4. protein.

(815) **26.** Patients with gout may have altered urinary elimination related to:

1. dehydration.
2. restricted fluid intake.
3. kidney stones.
4. edema.

(815) **27.** To prevent the complication of kidney stones in patients with gout, patients are advised to:

1. protect affected joints from trauma.
2. keep walking pathways lighted and free of obstacles.
3. obtain assistance with activities of daily living.
4. drink at least eight glasses of fluid daily.

(819) **28.** Polymyalgia rheumatica, Reiter's syndrome, Behçet's syndrome, and Sjögren's syndrome all involve:

1. urinary tract disorders.
2. connective tissue disorders.
3. central nervous system disorders.
4. cardiac disorders.

(812) **29.** When a patient has pain from rheumatoid arthritis, which group is most likely to face pain stoically?

1. Dominican Republican
2. Germans
3. Caucasian Americans
4. Italians

(803) **30.** When a patient is taking NSAIDs for rheumatoid arthritis, the nurse monitors the patient for:

1. fatigue.
2. edema.
3. bruising.
4. infection.

(815) **31.** An important teaching point for patients taking antigout medications is to:

1. increase potassium intake.
2. avoid foods high in vitamin K.
3. rise slowly from a sitting position.
4. increase fluids.

(815) **32.** Which food should be avoided in patients with acute gout?

1. sardines
2. aged cheese
3. bananas
4. orange juice

(802) **33.** Which antiinflammatory drugs work much like older NSAIDs but are less likely to cause stomach ulcers and bleeding?

1. COX-2 inhibitors
2. disease-modifying antirheumatic drugs (DMARDs)
3. biologic response modifiers (BRMs)
4. glucocorticoids

(819) **34.** Fatigue, morning stiffness, sleep disturbance, and specific tender points are symptoms of:

1. fibromyalgia.
2. Sjögren's syndrome.
3. ankylosing spondylitis.
4. bursitis.

CHAPTER 40

Student Name ____________________

Fractures

Answer Key: Textbook page references are provided as a guide for answering these questions. A complete answer key was provided for your instructor.

OBJECTIVES

1. Identify the types of fractures.
2. Describe the five stages of the healing process.
3. Discuss the major complications of fractures, their signs and symptoms, and their management.
4. Compare the types of medical treatment for fractures, particularly reduction and fixation.
5. Describe common therapeutic measures for fractures, including casts, traction, crutches, walkers, and canes.
6. Discuss the nursing care of a patient with a fracture.
7. Describe specific types of fractures, including hip fractures, Colles' fractures, and pelvic fractures.

LEARNING ACTIVITIES

A. Match the definition in the numbered column with the most appropriate term in the lettered column.

(823) 1. ________ Condition in which fat globules are released from the marrow of the broken bone into the bloodstream, migrate to the lungs, and cause pulmonary hypertension

(821) 2. ________ Fracture in which the broken bone does not break through the skin

(821) 3. ________ Fracture in which the fragments of the broken bone break through the skin

(823) 4. ________ Serious complication of a fracture caused by internal or external pressure to the affected area, resulting in decreased blood flow, pain, and tissue damage

(824) 5. ________ Failure of a fracture to heal

(821) 6. ________ Fracture in which the break extends across the entire bone, dividing it into two separate pieces

A. Compartmental syndrome
B. Open reduction
C. Fixation
D. Closed or simple fracture
E. Delayed union
F. Incomplete fracture
G. Fracture
H. Nonunion
I. Bone remodeling
J. Closed reduction or manipulation
K. Fat embolism
L. Complete fracture
M. Stress fracture
N. Open or compound fracture
O. Reduction
P. Comminuted fracture
Q. Greenstick fracture
R. Malunion

Continued next page

Student Name____

(825) **7.** __________ Procedure done during the open reduction surgical procedure to attach the fragments of the broken bone together when reduction alone is not feasible

(825) **8.** __________ Process of bringing the ends of the broken bone into proper alignment

(821) **9.** __________ Fracture in which the bone breaks only part way across, leaving some portion of the bone intact

(825) **10.** __________ Nonsurgical realignment of the bones to their previous anatomic position using traction, angulation, rotation, or a combination of these

(825) **11.** __________ Surgical procedure in which an incision is made at the fracture site, usually on patients with open (compound) or comminuted fractures, to cleanse the area of fragments and debris

(821) **12.** __________ Fracture caused by either sudden force or prolonged stress

(822) **13.** __________ Process in which immature bone cells are gradually replaced by mature bone cells

(824) **14.** __________ Healing of fracture does not occur in the normally expected time

(821) **15.** __________ Break or disruption in the continuity of a bone

(825) **16.** __________ Improper alignment of a fracture resulting in deformity

(821) **17.** __________ Fracture in which the bone is broken or crushed into small pieces

(824) **18.** __________ Fracture in which the bone is broken on one side but only bent on the other; most common in children

B. Complete the statements in the numbered column with the most appropriate term in the lettered column. Some terms may be used more than once, and some terms may not be used.

(826) **1.** Pins in the bone are attached to an external frame in __________.

(823) **2.** The first sign of a fat embolism is __________.

(824) **3.** __________ can cause irreversible muscle damage within 4–6 hours following fractures.

(824) **4.** A primary symptom of compartmental syndrome is __________.

(826) **5.** The use of rods, pins, nails, screws, or metal plates to align bone fragments and keep them in place for healing is called __________.

(823) **6.** A condition in which fat globules are released from the marrow of the broken bone is called __________.

(821) **7.** A fracture that occurs because of a pathologic condition in the bone, such as a tumor or disease process that causes a spontaneous break, is called __________.

(824) **8.** The goal of treatment for compartmental syndrome is to relieve __________.

(824) **9.** Infections associated with fractures result from indwelling hardware used to repair the broken bone or from __________.

(824) **10.** In deep, grossly contaminated fracture wounds, __________ is likely to develop.

(824) **11.** __________ is infection of the bone.

A. Internal fixation
B. Petechiae
C. Pathologic fracture
D. Respiratory distress
E. Pressure
F. Stress fracture
G. Pain
H. Gangrene
I. External fixation
J. Osteomyelitis
K. Fat embolism
L. Compartmental syndrome
M. Wound contamination

Student Name____

C. Complete the statements in the numbered column with the most appropriate term in the lettered column. Some terms may be used more than once, and some terms may not be used.

(829) **1.** __________ A cast used for breaks in the forearm, elbow, or humerus

(828) **2.** __________ A cast used for fracture of the distal femur, knee, or lower leg

(828) **3.** __________ A cast that encircles the trunk; used for stable spine injuries of thoracic or lumbar spine

(828) **4.** __________ A cast that encases the trunk plus two extremities used for fractures of the femur, acetabulum, or pelvis

(828) **5.** __________ Used for fractures of the foot, ankle, or distal tibia or fibula

(828) **6.** __________ Used for injury to the knee or knee dislocation

(827) **7.** __________ Used for injury to knee, allowing knee to bend

(829) **8.** __________ Used for postoperative immobilization following open reduction and internal fixation

(829) **9.** __________ Used for fracture of the hand or wrist

A. Body jacket cast
B. Short arm cast
C. Leg cylinder cast
D. Spica cast
E. Short leg cast
F. Bilateral long leg hip spica cast
G. Long leg cast
H. Long arm cast
I. Cast brace

D. Complete the statements in the numbered column with the most appropriate term in the lettered column. Some terms may be used more than once, and some terms may not be used.

(827) **1.** A pulling force on a fractured extremity to provide alignment of the broken bone fragments is called __________.

(827) **2.** Traction applied directly to a bone is called __________.

(827) **3.** Traction applied directly to the skin is called __________.

(830) **4.** A type of traction used for immobilization of fractures of the cervical vertebrae is called __________.

(827) **5.** A type of traction used for hip and knee contractures, muscle spasms, and alignment of hip fractures is called __________.

(827) **6.** Crutchfield's traction and halo vest are examples of __________.

(827) **7.** A type of traction in which tongs are inserted into either side of the skull is called __________.

A. Plastic traction
B. Skin traction
C. Buck's traction
D. Contracture traction
E. Traction
F. Vest traction
G. Crutchfield's traction
H. Skeletal traction

Student Name____

E. Match the definition or description in the numbered column with the most appropriate stage of healing in the lettered column. Some stages may be used more than once, and some may not be used.

(822) **1.** __________ Granulation tissue forms a collar around each end of the broken bone, gradually becoming firm

(822) **2.** __________ Within 2–3 weeks after the break, a permanent bone callus forms; ends of the broken bone begin to "knit"

(822) **3.** __________ Formation of a clot between the two broken ends of the bones in 48–72 hours

(822) **4.** __________ The distance between bone fragments closes, and immature bone cells are replaced by mature bone cells

(822) **5.** __________ Formation of a temporary splint by the end of the first week; granulation tissue turns into formation of cartilage, osteoblasts, calcium, and phosphorus

A. Fibrocartilage formation
B. Consolidation and remodeling
C. Callus formation
D. Cellular proliferation
E. Ossification
F. Hematoma formation

F. Match the cause of the signs and symptoms of fracture in the numbered column with the most appropriate sign or symptom in the lettered column. Some signs and symptoms may be used more than once, and some may not be used.

(825) **1.** _________ Strong muscle pull may cause bone fragments to override

(825) **2.** _________ Edema may appear rapidly from localization of serous fluid at the fracture site and extravasation of blood into adjacent tissues

(825) **3.** _________ Caused by subcutaneous bleeding

(825) **4.** _________ Involuntary muscle contraction near the fracture

(825) **5.** _________ Occurs over fracture site due to underlying injuries

(825) **6.** _________ Severe at the time of injury; following injury, this symptom may result from muscle spasm or damage to adjacent structures

(825) **7.** _________ Results from nerve damage

(825) **8.** _________ Grating sensations or sounds felt or heard if the injured part is moved; results from broken bone ends rubbing together

(825) **9.** _________ Results from blood loss or other injuries

A. Muscle spasm
B. Crepitus
C. Pain
D. Hypovolemic shock
E. Swelling
F. Impaired sensation (numbness)
G. Abnormal mobility
H. Bruising (ecchymosis)
I. Fever
J. Deformity
K. Tenderness

Student Name ____________________

G. Match the proper positioning in the numbered column with the fracture in the lettered column.

(834) **1.** __________ Before medical treatment, keep patient supine and immobilize patient's neck; after treatment, turn with head well supported

(834) **2.** __________ Avoid high sitting positions; log roll

(834) **3.** __________ When fracture is stable or after fixation, turn to side opposite fracture

(834) **4.** __________ Elevate head of bed to comfort; turn to side opposite fracture

(834) **5.** __________ Elevate distal portion of extremity higher than heart

A. Pelvis fracture
B. Forearm or foreleg fracture
C. Cervical spine fracture
D. Lumbar spine fracture
E. Shoulder or humerus fracture

H. In Figure 40-1 below, label each type of fracture (A–L) with numbers from the following list.

(822)

1. greenstick
2. oblique
3. transverse
4. displaced
5. longitudinal
6. stress
7. comminuted (fragmented)
8. interarticular
9. spiral
10. avulsion
11. impacted
12. pathologic

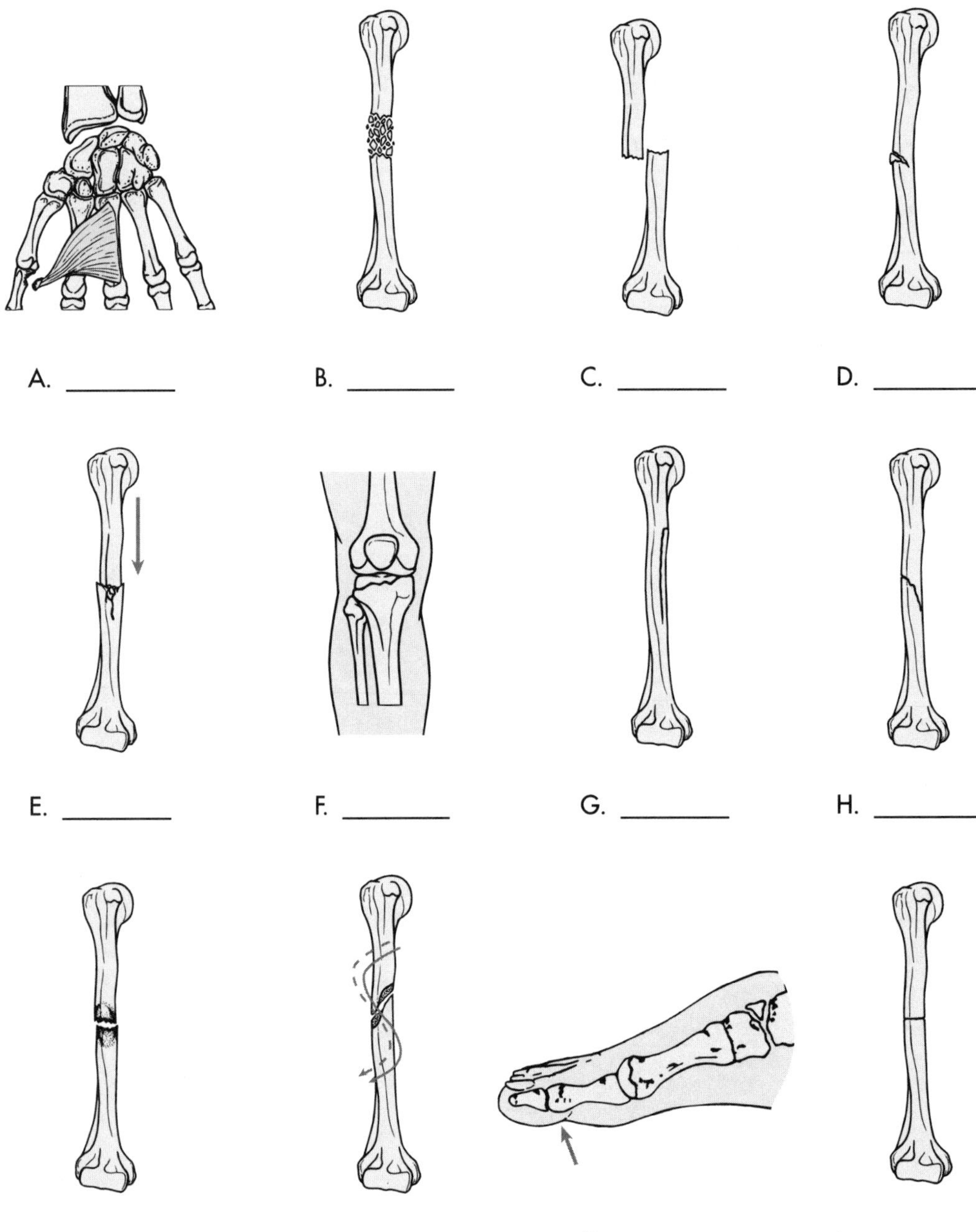

Student Name____

I. Using Figure 40-10, label the anatomic regions in A and the type of fractures in B–E.

(831)

A. Anatomic Regions

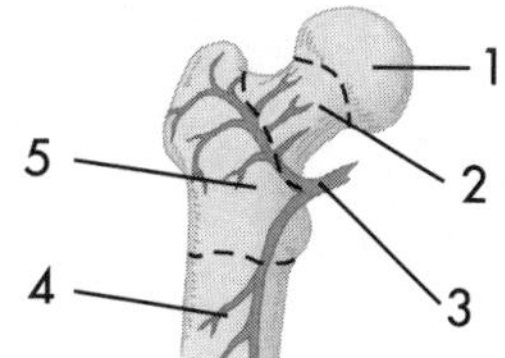

A.

1. ____________________

2. ____________________

3. ____________________

4. ____________________

5. ____________________

B. ____________________

C. ____________________

D. ____________________

E. ____________________

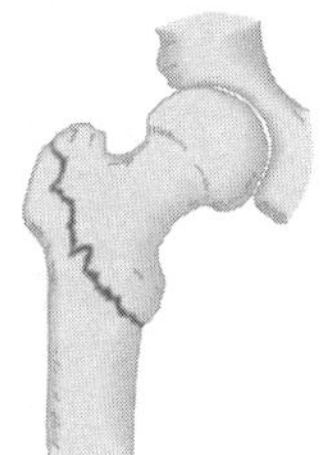

B

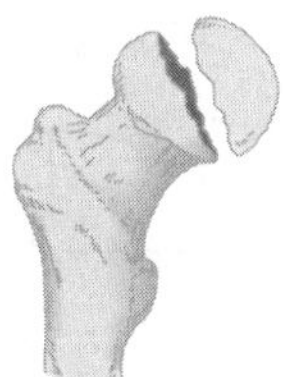

C

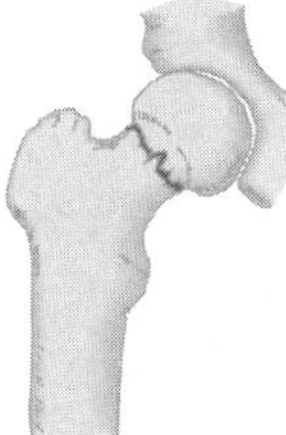

D

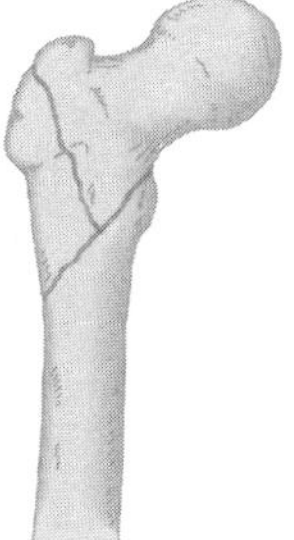

E

J. In Figure 40-7 below, label each type of traction (A–E) using the following list.

(829)

1. head halter traction __________
2. pelvic traction __________
3. Russell's traction __________
4. Buck's traction __________
5. balanced suspension traction __________

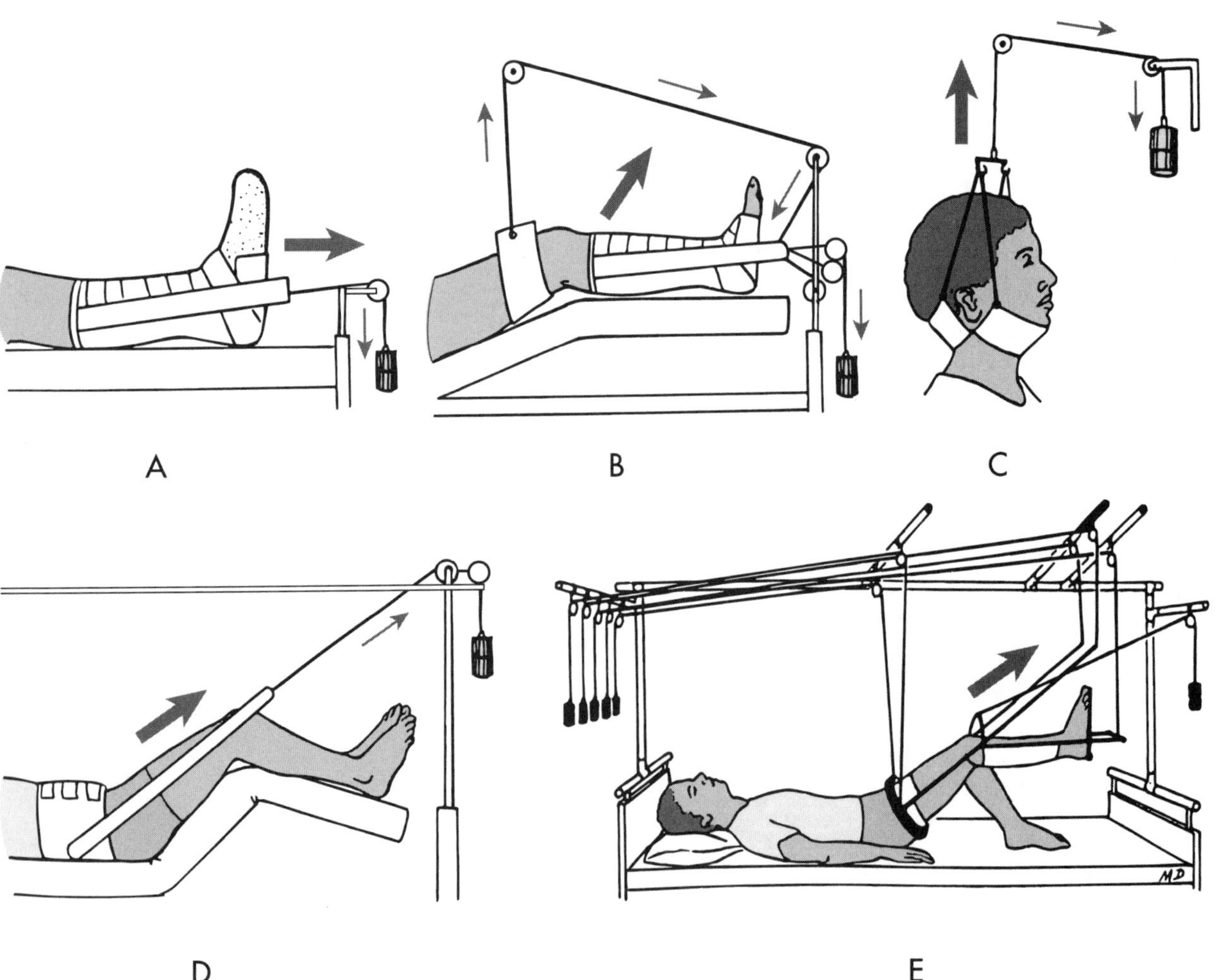

Student Name____________________________________

MULTIPLE-CHOICE QUESTIONS

J. Choose the most appropriate answer.

(821) **1.** In adults, the bones most commonly fractured are:

1. femurs.
2. ribs.
3. pelvic bones.
4. wrists.

(821) **2.** In young and middle-aged adults, the most common fractures are those of the:

1. femur. 2. rib.
3. wrist. 4. pelvis.

(821) **3.** The most common fractures in the elderly are fractures of the wrist and:

1. femur. 2. rib.
3. hip. 4. shoulder.

(823) **4.** Which is a characteristic of fat embolism following a fracture?

1. bradycardia
2. decreased respirations
3. oliguria
4. petechiae

(825) **5.** The most common diagnostic test used to reveal bone disruption, deformity, or malignancy following a fracture is:

1. myelography.
2. standard radiography.
3. ultrasonography.
4. bone scan.

(826) **6.** The use of rods, pins, nails, screws, or metal plates to align bone fragments is called:

1. external fixation.
2. closed reduction.
3. internal fixation.
4. mechanical reduction.

(826) **7.** Which is used for external fixation of extensive fractures and fractures of the extremities?

1. casts
2. rods
3. pins
4. metal plates

(827) **8.** A condition in which a patient in a body cast may have feelings of claustrophobia is called:

1. compartmental syndrome.
2. cardiac shock.
3. cast syndrome.
4. fat embolus.

(830) **9.** After a fracture of the lower extremity, crutches are used to assist with ambulation and to increase:

1. pain relief.
2. deep breathing.
3. mobility.
4. circulation.

(830) **10.** Crutch use requires good:

1. lower extremity function.
2. cardiac function.
3. lung expansion.
4. upper body strength.

(830) **11.** When walking with crutches, patients should put their weight on the:

1. top of the crutches.
2. hand grips.
3. lower extremities.
4. shoulders.

(830) **12.** The type of gait pattern used with bilateral lower extremity prostheses is called:

1. four-point.
2. swing-to.
3. swing-through.
4. two-point.

(830) **13.** When a patient is climbing stairs using crutches, which body part goes up the step first while the body is supported by the crutches?

1. unaffected leg
2. affected leg
3. upper extremities
4. spine

(831) **14.** Which gait is used with a walker?

1. two-point
2. four-point
3. modified swing-to
4. modified swing-through

(831) **15.** Canes should be held close to the body on the:

1. left side.
2. right side.
3. affected side.
4. unaffected side.

(832) **16.** When the nurse is assessing the patient with a fracture, the affected extremity is compared with the:

1. proximal body parts.
2. distal body parts.
3. unaffected extremity.
4. normal skeleton.

(832) **17.** In order to assess circulation and sensation in the affected and unaffected extremity, the nurse should perform neurovascular checks in the areas:

1. distal to the wound.
2. proximal to the wound.
3. surrounding the wound.
4. inside the wound.

(832) **18.** A good indication of circulation to the extremity in patients with a fracture is:

1. size of the wound.
2. edema.
3. skin color.
4. infection.

(832) **19.** If pallor is observed in the extremity of patients with fractures, this may be an indication of:

1. infection.
2. poor circulation.
3. hemorrhage.
4. skin breakdown.

(832) **20.** The primary method of pain relief for patients with fractures is:

1. application of cold to the affected part.
2. application of heat to the affected part.
3. wrapping the affected part with a blanket.
4. immobilization of the affected part.

(833) **21.** An appropriate intervention for patients with fractures who have impaired physical mobility is:

1. strict aseptic technique.
2. monitor for fever.
3. isolation precautions.
4. gait training.

Student Name________________________________

(833) **22.** An appropriate intervention for patients with fractures who have ineffective tissue perfusion is:

1. strict aseptic technique.
2. gait training.
3. elevation of the affected part above the heart.
4. rest periods to preserve strength.

(834) **23.** Patients with fractures are at risk for impaired skin integrity; treatment measures such as casts or traction to immobilize parts may result in:

1. pressure sores.
2. petechiae.
3. palmar erythema.
4. paralysis.

(835) **24.** For older patients with hip fractures, the treatment of choice is:

1. immobilization.
2. antibiotic therapy.
3. surgical repair.
4. traction.

(835) **25.** Colles' fracture is a break in the distal:

1. humerus. 2. tibia.
3. radius. 4. fibula.

(835) **26.** Colles' fractures frequently occur in older adults when they use their hands to:

1. sew or knit.
2. break a fall.
3. write letters.
4. reach for objects above their heads.

(836) **27.** Interventions for Colles' fractures are aimed at relieving pain and preventing edema; for the first few days, the extremity should be:

1. below the heart.
2. exercised.
3. elevated.
4. flat.

(836) **28.** Patients with Colles' fractures are encouraged to move their fingers and thumb to promote circulation and reduce:

1. temperature.
2. swelling.
3. infection.
4. dyspnea.

(836) **29.** Patients with Colles' fractures are encouraged to move their shoulder to prevent:

1. infection. 2. circulation.
3. cyanosis. 4. stiffness.

(836) **30.** The most common cause of pelvic fractures in young adults is:

1. head injury.
2. motor vehicle accidents.
3. falls.
4. myocardial infarction.

(836) **31.** The main cause of pelvic fractures in older adults is:

1. motor vehicle accidents.
2. head injury.
3. falls.
4. heart attacks.

(836) **32.** The nurse needs to observe the patient with a pelvic fracture closely for signs of:

1. internal trauma.
2. bone infection.
3. kidney failure.
4. dyspnea.

(836) **33.** Which is restricted in patients with pelvic fractures until healing is complete?

1. use of a trapeze while in bed
2. range-of-motion exercises
3. coughing and deep-breathing exercises
4. weight bearing

(835) **34.** Following total hip replacement, which patient teaching is incorrect?

1. Avoid crossing the legs.
2. Use an elevated toilet seat.
3. Sit in supportive chairs.
3. Do not extend the affected hip more than 90 degrees.

CHAPTER 41

Student Name ______________________________

Amputations

Answer Key: Textbook page references are provided as a guide for answering these questions. A complete answer key was provided for your instructor.

OBJECTIVES

1. Identify the clinical indications for amputations.
2. Describe the different types of amputations.
3. Discuss the medical and surgical management of the amputation patient.
4. Identify appropriate nursing interventions during the preoperative and postoperative phases of care.
5. Assist in developing a nursing process to plan care for the amputation patient.

LEARNING ACTIVITIES

A. Match the definition in the numbered column with the most appropriate term in the lettered column.

(840) **1.** __________ Type of amputation in which a limb or portion of a limb is severed from the body and the wound is left open; a type of open amputation

(1197) **2.** __________ Amputation that is done over the course of several surgeries; usually done to control the spread of infection or necrosis

A. Phantom limb
B. Amputee
C. Guillotine amputation
D. Staged amputation
E. Gangrene
F. Open amputation
G. Replantation
H. Closed amputation
I. Congenital amputation
J. Stump
K. Amputation
L. Residual limb

Continued next page

(840) 3. __________ Amputation in which a limb or part of a limb is removed and the wound is surgically closed

(832) 4. __________ Individual who has undergone an amputation

(841) 5. __________ Necrosis, or death of tissue, usually due to a deficient or absent blood supply; may result from inflammatory processes, injury, arteriosclerosis, frostbite, or diabetes mellitus

(838, 839) 6. __________ Deformity or absence of a limb or limbs occurring during fetal development in the uterus

(840) 7. __________ Following an amputation of a limb; the sensation that the limb still exists

(840) 8. __________ Amputation in which the wound is left open; usually done in cases of infection or necrosis

(840) 9. __________ Partial limb remaining after amputation

(838) 10. __________ Removal of a limb, part of a limb, or an organ; may be done by surgical means or may be the result of an accident

(838) 11. __________ Surgical reattachment of an organ to its original site; reimplantation

(1197) 12. __________ Refers to the distal portion of an amputated limb

B. List three examples of diseases leading to impaired circulation that may result in the need for an amputation.

(838) 1. ______________________________

(838) 2. ______________________________

(838) 3. ______________________________

C. Two types of amputations are called closed and open. List one reason for performing each type.

(840) 1. Closed: ______________________________

(840) 2. Open: ______________________________

Student Name ______________________________

D. List eight complications associated with amputations.

(840)	**1.**	________	*(840)*	**5.**	________
(840)	**2.**	________	*(840)*	**6.**	________
(840)	**3.**	________	*(840)*	**7.**	________
(840)	**4.**	________	*(840)*	**8.**	________

E. What is the significance of a capillary refill of 6 seconds? *(842)*

F. Patient instruction for stump and prosthesis care is extremely important. Describe teaching for each of the eight topics listed below.

(848) **1.** Residual limb:

(848) **2.** Prosthetic socket and residual limb sock:

(848) **3.** Shoes:

(848) **4.** Lotions, ointments, and powders:

(848) **5.** Care of prosthesis if redness or irritation develops on the residual limb :

(848) **6.** Size of residual limb:

(848) **7.** Care of prosthesis:

(848) **8.** Problems with prosthesis:

G. List findings in the four areas below that are signs of arterial occlusion and venous congestion following replantation. *(849)*

	Arterial Occlusion	Venous Congestion
1. Color		
2. Capillary refill		
3. Appearance		
4. Temperature		

H. Complete the statement in the numbered column with the most appropriate term in the lettered column. Some terms may be used more than once, and some terms may not be used.

(838) **1.** The removal of the lower leg at the middle of the shin is called a __________.

(838) **2.** Removal of part or all of a limb during a serious accident is called __________.

(838) **3.** Conditions that lead to the need for an amputation include trauma, disease, and __________.

(838) **4.** An amputation through the joint is called __________.

A. Tumors
B. Open amputation
C. Traumatic amputation
D. Disarticulation
E. Below-knee amputation

Student Name____

I. Match the indication in the numbered column with the name of the appropriate diagnostic test relating to amputation in the lettered column.

(839) **1.** __________ Record heat present to measure amount of blood flow to certain part of body

(840) **2.** __________ After imaging reveals suspicious lesions

(840) **3.** __________ Infection

(839) **4.** __________ Nature of tumor

(840) **5.** __________ Volume of blood flow to extremity

(840) **6.** __________ Pulses in extremities

(839) **7.** __________ Compromised circulation

A. Bone biopsy
B. Pulse volume recording (plethysmography)
C. Doppler ultrasound
D. WBC
E. Transcutaneous PO_2
F. Vascular studies (angiography)
G. Thermography

J. Match the postoperative nursing diagnosis for patients with amputations in the numbered column with the "related to" statement in the lettered column.

(845) **1.** __________ Ineffective coping

(845) **2.** __________ Acute pain

(845) **3.** __________ Self-care deficit

(845) **4.** __________ Disturbed sensory perception

(845) **5.** __________ Risk for infection

(845) **6.** __________ Decreased cardiac output

(845) **7.** __________ Impaired skin integrity

(845) **8.** __________ Disturbed body image

(845) **9.** __________ Anxiety or fear

A. Blood loss
B. Surgical incision, scar formation on a severed nerve
C. Surgical wound
D. Loss of a body part
E. Surgical disruption of skin integrity
F. Inability to carry out ADLs
G. Perceived threat of disability
H. Inadequate support system
I. Incision
J. Phantom limb
K. Loss of limb, weakness, debilitation
L. Loss of limb
M. Prolonged bed rest, weakness

Continued next page

(845) **10.** ________ Activity intolerance

(845) **11.** ________ Impaired physical mobility

(845) **12.** ________ Risk for injury

K. Match the postoperative nursing diagnosis in the numbered column with the appropriate nursing intervention in the lettered column.

(847) **1.** ________ Risk for injury

(845) **2.** ________ Decreased cardiac output

(848) **3.** ________ Disturbed body image

(846) **4.** ________ Impaired skin integrity

(847) **5.** ________ Impaired physical mobility

(846) **6.** ________ Risk for infection

(846) **7.** ________ Pain

(847) **8.** ________ Disturbed sensory perception

A. Active and passive range-of-motion exercises; use of overbed trapeze, if indicated; prosthesis fitting
B. Check temperature; watch for foul or unpleasant odor from stump; check lab work (WBC)
C. Encourage patient to do exercises as ordered; keep environment free of clutter
D. Whirlpool, massage, or TENS stimulation if ordered
E. Check vital signs; observe for excessive bleeding
F. Use of imagery, acupuncture, analgesics
G. Wrap bandage smoothly; inspect residual limb for irritation and edema; elevate residual limb
H. Encourage patient to talk about changes and effects of amputation

L. Match the nursing goal in the numbered column relating to the postoperative patient following amputation with the appropriate outcome criterion in the lettered column.

(845) **1.** ________ Positive body image

(845) **2.** ________ Absence of infection

(845) **3.** ________ Absence of new skin lesions

(845) **4.** ________ Pain relief

(845) **5.** ________ Healed wound

(845) **6.** ________ Normal cardiac output

A. Patient accepts limb loss, demonstrates proper care of residual limb
B. Patient states relief of phantom limb sensation
C. Pulse and blood pressure are consistent with patient norms
D. Body temperature returns to normal; drainage decreases
E. Patient states pain relief; has relaxed expression
F. Skin intact; no redness due to pressure
G. Patient demonstrates residual limb care within limits
H. Incision margins intact
I. No falls result from weakness or problems with balance
J. Patient carries out daily activities without excessive fatigue

Continued next page

Student Name ______________________________

(845) **7.** __________ Resumed self care

(845) **8.** __________ Absence of injury

(845) **9.** __________ Patient states understanding of phantom limb sensation

(845) **10.** __________ Improved activity tolerance results

M. Match the characteristics of the elderly amputee in the numbered column with the nursing interventions in the lettered column.

(848) **1.** __________ May have one or more chronic health problems

(848) **2.** __________ Sometimes easily distracted

(848) **3.** __________ May have decreased appetite and poor nutritional status

(848) **4.** __________ May feel foolish in describing phantom sensations

A. Emphasize high-calorie and high-protein diet
B. Remind patient that phantom sensations are not unusual or bizarre
C. Skip unnecessary details when teaching; make sure that patients with glasses or hearing aids have them in place
D. Provide a prosthesis with extra padding and support to patients with diabetes; recognize that poor vision and decreased sensation may keep older people from recognizing complications

N. Match the nursing goal in the numbered column with the appropriate outcome criterion in the lettered column for postoperative replantation patients.

(850) **1.** __________ Improved body image

(849) **2.** __________ Adequate circulation in the replanted limb

(850) **3.** __________ Pain relief

A. Patient touches and looks at affected part
B. Patient states less pain; has relaxed expression
C. Warmth, normal skin color, and arterial pulses are present in the replanted limb

O. List four complementary therapies that are used with analgesics to control pain in patients after surgical amputation.

(846) **1.** ______________________________

(846) **2.** ______________________________

(846) **3.** ______________________________

(846) **4.** ______________________________

MULTIPLE-CHOICE QUESTIONS

P. Choose the most appropriate answer.

(849) **1.** Replantation surgery is most likely to be performed on the:

1. shoulder.
2. hand.
3. forearm.
4. upper arm.

(850) **2.** The purpose of giving heparin to a postoperative replantation patient is to reduce the risk of:

1. thrombosis.
2. edema.
3. infection.
4. hypersensitivity.

(841) **3.** A complication of amputation due to inadequate hemostasis is:

1. necrosis.
2. hemorrhage.
3. gangrene.
4. contracture.

(841) **4.** A complication of amputation manifested by redness, warmth, swelling, and exudate formation at the residual limb site due to invasion of tissues by pathogens is called:

1. contracture.
2. infection.
3. edema.
4. necrosis.

(841) **5.** Which may be prevented by frequent position changes and range-of-motion exercises?

1. infection
2. hemorrhage
3. necrosis
4. contractures

(841) **6.** Which is an opening of the suture line (caused by early removal of sutures or falling) that requires reclosure?

1. gangrene
2. necrosis
3. wound dehiscence
4. contracture

(842) **7.** Which person will request that an amputated body part be present for burial?

1. Roman Catholic
2. Mormon
3. Orthodox Jew
4. Muslim

(845) **8.** Which diagnosis is a priority in the postoperative period for a patient after surgical amputation?

1. Disturbed body image
2. Impaired skin integrity
3. Pain
4. Disturbed sensory perception

CHAPTER 42

Student Name ______________________________

Pituitary and Adrenal Disorders

Answer Key: Textbook page references are provided as a guide for answering these questions. A complete answer key was provided for your instructor.

OBJECTIVES

1. Identify nursing assessment data relevant to the function of the adrenal and pituitary glands.
2. Describe the tests and procedures used to diagnose disorders of the adrenal and pituitary glands including relevant nursing considerations.
3. Describe the pathophysiology and medical treatment of adrenocortical insufficiency, excess adrenocortical hormones, hypopituitarism, diabetes insipidus, and pituitary tumors.
4. Assist in developing nursing care plans for patients with selected disorders of the adrenal and pituitary glands.

LEARNING ACTIVITIES

A. Match the definition in the numbered column with the most appropriate term in the lettered column..

(852) **1.** ________ Ductless gland that produces an internal secretion discharged into the lymph or bloodstream and circulated to all parts of the body; hormones, the active substances of these glands, cause an effect on certain organs or tissues

A. Acromegaly
B. Addison's disease
C. Adrenaline
D. Androgens
E. Catecholamines
F. Cushing's disease
G. Cushing's syndrome
H. Diabetes insipidus
I. Endocrine gland
J. Estrogens
K. Gigantism
L. Glucocorticoids
M. Hypophysectomy
N. Mineralocorticoids
O. Syndrome of inappropriate antidiuretic hormone (SIADH)

Continued next page

(868) **2.** __________ Disease resulting from a deficiency of adrenocorticotropic hormone (ACTH) caused by destruction or dysfunction of the adrenal glands; characterized by increased pigmentation of the skin and mucous membranes, weakness, fatigue, hypotension, nausea, weight loss, and hypoglycemia

(864) **3.** __________ Disease caused by inadequate secretion of antidiuretic hormone (ADH) by the posterior pituitary gland; symptoms include excessive urination, thirst, and dehydration

(857) **4.** __________ Disease of middle-aged adults resulting from overproduction of growth hormone (GH) by the anterior pituitary gland; characterized by enlargement of the facial bones, nose, lips, and jaw; also associated with decreased libido, moodiness, fatigue, muscle pains, sweating, and headache

(867) **5.** __________ Type of hormone secreted by the adrenal cortex and involved in the regulation of fluid and electrolyte levels in the body

(865) **6.** __________ Disorder caused by excess antidiuretic hormone production; symptoms include decreased urination, edema, and fluid overload

(874) **7.** __________ Disorder resulting from excessive glucocorticoids in the body as a result of tumor or hypersecretion of the pituitary; may also be caused by prolonged administration of large doses of exogenous steroids; symptoms include fat deposits in the neck and abdomen, fatigue, weakness, edema, excess hair growth, glucose intolerances, skin discoloration, and mood swings

(867) **8.** __________ Class of adrenocortical hormones that affects protein and carbohydrate metabolism and helps protect the body against stress

Continued next page

Student Name ____________________

(866) **9.** __________ Chemical (dopamine, epinephrine, norepinephrine) released at sympathetic nerve endings in response to stress

(868) **10.** __________ Hormones produced by the ovaries, adrenal glands, and fetoplacental unit in females that are responsible for the development and maturation of females

(857) **11.** __________ Disease caused by excessive growth hormone in children and young adolescents, resulting in excessive proportional growth

(874) **12.** __________ Disease caused by the hypersecretion of glucocorticoids as a result of excessive release of adrenocorticotropic hormone by the pituitary gland

(868) **13.** __________ Hormones produced by the adrenal cortex, testes, and ovaries that stimulate the development of male characteristics

(860) **14.** __________ Surgical removal of all or part of the pituitary gland

(857) **15.** __________ Epinephrine; a powerful vasoactive substance produced by the medulla or adrenal gland in times of stress or danger, allowing the body to react by fighting or fleeing

B. Complete the statements in the numbered column with the most appropriate term in the lettered column. Some terms may be used more than once, and some terms may not be used.

(857) **1.** The first symptom of a problem in hyperpituitarism is often __________.

(857) **2.** Radiographic films of the skull of persons with hyperpituitarism may show a large sella turcica and increased __________.

(860) **3.** For patients with a diagnosis of pituitary tumors, the treatment of choice is __________.

(857) **4.** A disease that occurs in early childhood or puberty in which the diaphysis of the long bones grows to great lengths stimulated by excess GH is __________.

(857) **5.** A disease that appears when adults are in their 30s and 40s in which bones increase in thickness and width after epiphyseal closure is __________.

A. Gigantism
B. Hypothalamus
C. Cushing's syndrome
D. Hypophysectomy
E. Bone density
F. Parathyroid gland
G. Acromegaly
H. Visual deficit

C. Complete the statements in the numbered column with the most appropriate term in the lettered column. Some terms may be used more than once, and some terms may not be used.

(865) **1.** A syndrome characterized by a water imbalance related to an increase in ADH secretion is called __________.

(865) **2.** Kidneys retain fluid due to the elevation of __________.

(865) **3.** Plasma volume expands when ADH is elevated in SIADH, causing an increased __________.

(865) **4.** When the ADH level is elevated, the patient experiences water intoxication and the body's sodium is diluted, resulting in __________.

A. Blood pressure
B. Potassium
C. Excess water
D. SIADH
E. Hyponatremia
F. Heart rate
G. ADH
H. Diabetes insipidus
I. Sodium chloride

Continued next page

Student Name____

(865) **5.** Weight gain without edema is one of the main symptoms of __________.

(866) **6.** The treatment of SIADH promotes the elimination of __________.

(866) **7.** In patients with SIADH, fluids are restricted and patients are given __________.

(866) **8.** Patients with SIADH have fluid volume excess related to excess secretion of __________.

D. Complete the statements in the numbered column with the most appropriate term in the lettered column. Some terms may be used more than once, and some terms may not be used.

(868) **1.** Addison's disease results in the loss of aldosterone and __________.

(870) **2.** A test that is necessary for a definitive diagnosis of hypo-adrenalism, such as Addison's disease, is __________.

(871) **3.** The mainstay of treatment of patients with Addison's disease is replacement therapy with mineralocorticoids and __________.

(869) **4.** Potassium excretion is decreased when cortisol is not secreted, resulting in __________.

(869) **5.** Secondary adrenal insufficiency is a result of dysfunction of the hypothalamus or the __________.

(869) **6.** Decreased levels of aldosterone alter the clearance of potassium, water, and __________.

(869) **7.** When sodium and water excretion rates accelerate, problems such as hyponatremia and __________ can result.

(869) **8.** Acute adrenal crisis is also called __________.

(869) **9.** Impaired secretion of cortisol results in decreased liver and muscle glycogen and decreased __________.

A. Hypovolemia
B. Pituitary gland
C. Addison's disease
D. Gluconeogenesis
E. Norepinephrine
F. Glucocorticoids
G. Tachycardia
H. ACTH stimulation test
I. SIADH
J. Hypoglycemia
K. Hyperkalemia
L. Metabolic acidosis
M. Sodium
N. Androgen
O. Cortisol
P. Addisonian crisis
Q. Androgens

Continued next page

(869) **10.** Secondary adrenal insufficiency leads to decreased production of cortisol and __________.

(868) **11.** Primary adrenal insufficiency is also called __________.

(869) **12.** Decreased supplies of available glucose, which occurs as a result of impaired secretion of cortisol, is called __________.

(869) **13.** Patients with either primary or secondary adrenal insufficiency are at risk for episodes of __________.

(869) **14.** A condition that occurs because hyperkalemia promotes hydrogen ion retention is __________.

E. Complete the statements in the numbered column with the most appropriate term in the lettered column. Some terms may be used more than once, and some terms may not be used.

(874) **1.** Prolonged administration of high doses of corticosteroids may cause Cushing's syndrome; this is an example of a(n) __________ cause.

(875) **2.** An initial screening for Cushing's syndrome is the overnight __________ test.

(877) **3.** In the immediate postoperative period of adrenalectomy patients, __________ may be needed to maintain blood pressure.

(874) **4.** The most common cause of Cushing's syndrome is long-term exogenous __________ use.

(874) **5.** Corticotropin-secreting pituitary tumors may cause Cushing's syndrome; this is an example of a(n) __________ cause.

(877) **6.** Patients with a pheochromocytoma exhibit episodes of hypertension, hypermetabolism, and __________.

(874) **7.** Excessive production of ACTH resulting from a pituitary tumor is called __________.

A. Cushing's disease
B. SIADH
C. Exogenous
D. Pheochromocytoma
E. Steroid
F. Cushing's syndrome
G. Hyperglycemia
H. Corticosteroids
I. Diabetes insipidus
J. Dexamethasone
K. Endogenous
L. Adrenal crisis
M. Vasopressors
N. Asepsis

Continued next page

Student Name____

(874) **8.** Hypersecretion of the adrenal cortex may result in the production of excess amounts of __________.

(877) **9.** The prevention of infections in adrenalectomy patients is maintained through observance of __________.

(877) **10.** A tumor of the adrenal medulla that causes secretion of excessive catecholamines is a(n) __________.

(874) **11.** The condition that results from excessive cortisol is called __________.

(875) **12.** Patients who take drugs that suppress adrenal function are at risk of acute __________.

F. Match the definition or description in the numbered column with the most appropriate term in the lettered column. Some terms may be used more than once, and some may not be used.

(854) **1.** __________ Stimulates the growth and development of bone, muscles, or organs

(854) **2.** __________ Controls ovulation or egg release in the female and testosterone production in the male

(854) **3.** __________ Controls the release of glucocorticoids and adrenal androgens

(854) **4.** __________ Stimulates the development of eggs in the ovary of the female and the production of sperm in the testes of the male

(854) **5.** __________ Another name for the somatotrophic hormone

(854) **6.** __________ Stimulates breast milk production in the female

A. Luteinizing hormone
B. Thyroid-stimulating hormone
C. Oxytocin
D. Melanocyte-stimulating hormone
E. Growth hormone
F. Norepinephrine
G. Antidiuretic hormone
H. Adrenocorticotropic hormone
I. Prolactin
J. Follicle-stimulating hormone

Continued next page

(854) **7.** __________ Promotes pigmentation

(854) **8.** __________ Another name for the lactogenic hormone

(854) **9.** __________ Causes the reabsorption of water from the renal tubules of the kidney

(854) **10.** __________ Causes contractions of the uterus in labor and the release of breast milk

(854) **11.** __________ Another name for vasopressin

(854) **12.** __________ Controls the secretory activities of the thyroid gland

G. Complete the statements in the numbered column with the most appropriate term in the lettered column. Some terms may be used more than once, and some terms may not be used.

(864) **1.** Increased plasma osmolarity stimulates the osmoreceptors, which in turn relay information to the cerebral cortex, causing the person to experience __________.

(864) **2.** Massive dehydration leads to severe __________ imbalances.

(864) **3.** With ADH deficiency, massive dehydration occurs, which leads to decreased intravascular volume, circulatory collapse, and __________.

(864) **4.** Electrolyte imbalances contribute to circulatory collapse by causing arrhythmias and impaired contractility of the __________.

(864) **5.** Massive diuresis results in increased plasma __________.

A. Thirst
B. Skeletal muscles
C. Heart
D. Electrolyte
E. Osmolarity
F. Hypotension

Student Name____

H. Indicate whether the following laboratory study results would be expected to (A) increase or (B) decrease in patients with Addison's disease.

(870)	**1.** __________	Serum cortisol level	A.	Increase
			B.	Decrease
(870)	**2.** __________	Fasting glucose		
(870)	**3.** __________	Sodium		
(870)	**4.** __________	Potassium		
(870)	**5.** __________	Blood urea nitrogen		

I. Match the nursing diagnoses for patients with Cushing's syndrome in the numbered column with the most appropriate "related to" statements in the lettered column.

(876)	**1.** __________	Risk for infection	A.	Changes in skin and connective tissue and edema
(876)	**2.** __________	Disturbed thought processes	B.	Changes in physical appearance and function
			C.	Fluid and electrolyte imbalance
			D.	Osteoporosis
(876)	**3.** __________	Risk for impaired skin integrity	E.	High serum cortisol levels
(876)	**4.** __________	Risk for injury (fracture)		
(876)	**5.** __________	Disturbed body image		

J. Match the interventions in the numbered column with the nursing diagnoses for patients with Cushing's syndrome in the lettered column. Some nursing diagnoses may be used more than once, and some may not be used.

(876)	**1.** __________	Avoid exposure to infections	A.	Risk for injury
			B.	Risk for impaired skin integrity
			C.	Sexual dysfunction
(876)	**2.** __________	Report minor signs, such as low-grade fever, sore throat, or aches to the physician	D.	Disturbed body image
			E.	Risk for infection
			F.	Ineffective management of therapeutic regimen
			G.	Disturbed thought processes
(876)	**3.** __________	Seek a psychiatric referral if mood swings continue to be a problem		

Continued next page

(876) 4. ______ Assist patient to change positions at least every 2 hours

(876) 5. ______ Protect patient from falls or trauma

(876) 6. ______ Discuss bruises, abnormal fat distribution, and hirsutism with the patient if they cause embarrassment

(876) 7. ______ Teach patient about the importance of continuing drug therapy under medical supervision

K. Indicate age-related changes in the healthy older person regarding pituitary function.

(855) 1. Pituitary function: ______

(855) 2. ADH secretion: ______

(855) 3. Ability to concentrate urine: ______

(855) 4. Risk for dehydration: ______

L. Monitoring the postoperative hypophysectomy patient for signs and symptoms of infection is important; list four signs and symptoms that may be indications of meningitis.

(861) 1. ______

(861) 2. ______

(861) 3. ______

(861) 4. ______

M. List two medications that will be given as hormone replacement therapy following a complete hypophysectomy.

(861) 1. ______

(861) 2. ______

N. The postoperative hypophysectomy patient is instructed to avoid any activities that can cause Valsalva's maneuver; list four activities that may create enough intracranial pressure to disrupt the surgical site and cause CSF leakage.

(861) 1. ______

(861) 2. ______

(861) 3. ______

(861) 4. ______

Student Name____________________________

O. List three signs of decreased gonadotropins (when gonads become atrophied) that occur in both males and females with hypopituitarism.

(862) **1.** ____________________________

(862) **2.** ____________________________

(862) **3.** ____________________________

P. List three measures that the nurse can take to help enforce fluid restrictions in patients with SIADH, which may be as little as 500 ml per 24 hours.

(866) **1.** ____________________________

(866) **2.** ____________________________

(866) **3.** ____________________________

Q. List eight manifestations of an addisonian crisis related to the areas listed below.

(870) **1.** Blood pressure: ____________________________

(870) **2.** Heart rate: ____________________________

(870) **3.** Fluid balance: ____________________________

(870) **4.** Mental status: ____________________________

(870) **5.** Sodium level: ____________________________

(870) **6.** Potassium level: ____________________________

(870) **7.** Calcium level: ____________________________

(870) **8.** Glucose level: ____________________________

R. Using Figure 42-1 below, label the organs of the endocrine system (A–G).

(853)

A. ______________________

B. ______________________

C. ______________________

D. ______________________

E. ______________________

F. ______________________

G. ______________________

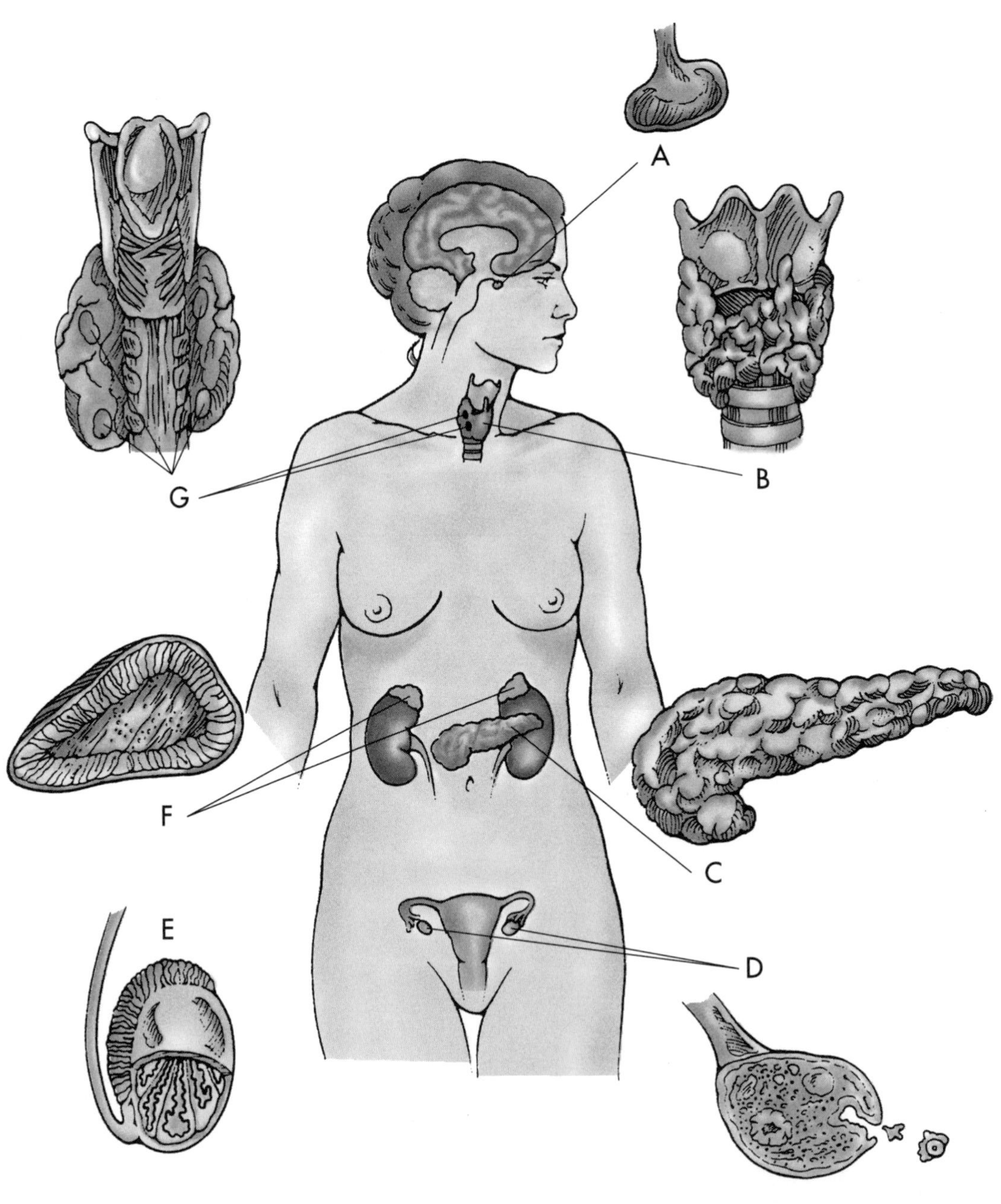

Student Name____

MULTIPLE-CHOICE QUESTIONS

S. Choose the most appropriate answer.

(855) **1.** In the healthy older person, there may be increased secretion of ADH, which may lead to:

1. fluid imbalance.
2. dyspnea.
3. hypertension.
4. hypopituitarism.

(857) **2.** The production of excess GH may lead to the development of:

1. atherosclerosis and hyperglycemia.
2. edema and congestive heart failure.
3. dyspnea and pneumonia.
4. oliguria and kidney failure.

(857) **3.** Growth hormone antagonizes insulin and interferes with its effects, thus leading to:

1. hyperkalemia.
2. hypokalemia.
3. hyperglycemia.
4. hypoglycemia.

(857) **4.** Because growth hormone mobilizes stored fat for energy, levels of free fatty acids are elevated in the bloodstream, leading to the development of:

1. pneumonia.
2. kidney failure.
3. hypotension.
4. atherosclerosis.

(857) **5.** Visual problems occur in hyperpituitarism due to pressure on the:

1. occipital lobe.
2. optic nerves.
3. frontal lobe.
4. oculomotor nerves.

(857) **6.** Patients with gigantism and acromegaly initially present with increased strength, progressing rapidly to complaints of:

1. hypotension and syncope.
2. weakness and fatigue.
3. edema and dry skin.
4. dehydration and bradycardia.

(858) **7.** One drug commonly prescribed for patients with hyperpituitarism is:

1. bromocriptine (Parlodel).
2. furosemide (Lasix).
3. levothyroxine (Synthroid).
4. digoxin.

(860) **8.** A common nursing diagnosis for patients with hyperpituitarism is:

1. Altered tissue perfusion.
2. Altered skin integrity.
3. High risk for infection.
4. Disturbed body image.

(859) **9.** Bromocriptine (Parlodel) inhibits the release of prolactin and GH by activating:

1. antidiuretic hormone.
2. the thyroid gland.
3. the adrenal gland.
4. dopamine receptors.

(861) **10.** Following hypophysectomy, the nurse asks the patient to place the chin to the chest to assess for nuchal rigidity, which is associated with:

1. bone density.
2. meningeal irritation.
3. cerebral edema.
4. impaired circulation.

(861) **11.** Changes in assessment findings following hypophysectomy that may reflect edema due to the manipulation of tissues or bleeding intracranially include:

1. unequal pupil size.
2. decreasing alertness.
3. decreasing blood pressure.
4. rising body temperature.

(861) **12.** Strict documentation of intake and output and measurement of specific gravity are important because postoperative hypophysectomy patients are at risk for:

1. congestive heart failure.
2. kidney failure.
3. pneumonia.
4. diabetes insipidus.

(861) **13.** Because CSF leaks sometimes occur in postoperative hypophysectomy patients, the nurse should check:

1. intake and output.
2. pupil reactivity.
3. nasal packing.
4. vital signs.

(861) **14.** A bedside test can be done with a chemical strip to detect whether drainage in a postoperative hypophysectomy patient is CSF, since CSF has a high content of:

1. glucose.
2. protein.
3. white blood cells.
4. red blood cells.

(862) **15.** Decreased pigmentation of the skin results in:

1. edema.
2. pallor.
3. pruritus.
4. erythema.

(862) **16.** The patient who has a complete hypophysectomy requires hormone replacement:

1. preoperatively.
2. during the postoperative recovery period.
3. for 6 months to 1 year.
4. for a lifetime.

(862) **17.** In patients with hypopituitarism, insufficient thyroid hormone is available for normal metabolism and:

1. visual acuity.
2. muscle tone.
3. heat production.
4. bone growth.

(862) **18.** If there is a lack of melanocyte-stimulating hormone, the skin exhibits decreased:

1. sensory perception.
2. immunity.
3. pigmentation.
4. thermoregulation.

(863) **19.** Deficiency of thyroid-stimulating hormones necessitates thyroid replacement with a drug such as:

1. octreotide acetate (Sandostatin).
2. bromocriptine (Parlodel).
3. levothyroxine (Synthroid).
4. vasopressin (Pitressin Synthetic).

(863) **20.** To produce or maintain libido, secondary sexual characteristics, and well-being, males with hypopituitarism should receive:

1. testosterone.
2. estrogen.
3. levothyroxine (Synthroid).
4. bromocriptine (Parlodel).

Student Name____

(864) **21.** Drug-related diabetes insipidus is often caused by:

1. bromocriptine (Parlodel).
2. lithium carbonate (Eskalith).
3. levothyroxine (Synthroid).
4. digitalis.

(864) **22.** A 24-hour urine output of greater than 4 liters of fluid suggests a diagnosis of:

1. hypertension.
2. kidney infection.
3. congestive heart failure.
4. diabetes insipidus.

(864) **23.** In order to maintain adequate blood volume in patients with diabetes insipidus, two measures that are required include intravenous fluid volume replacement and:

1. diuretics.
2. vasopressors.
3. anticholinergics.
4. antihistamines.

(865) **24.** The level of consciousness deteriorates and the patient may have seizures or lapse into a coma when water intoxication affects the:

1. respiratory system.
2. urinary system.
3. cardiovascular system.
4. central nervous system.

(866) **25.** A nursing diagnosis for patients with SIADH is Risk for injury related to confusion associated with:

1. acute adrenal insufficiency.
2. impaired physiologic response to stress.
3. water intoxication.
4. decreased ADH secretion.

(866) **26.** To prevent progressive cerebral edema in patients with SIADH, patients are placed in which position in bed?

1. flat
2. semi-Fowler's
3. Fowler's
4. side-lying

(868) **27.** In postmenopausal women, the primary source of endogenous estrogen is the:

1. hypothalamus.
2. thyroid gland.
3. adrenal cortex.
4. ovarian follicle.

(868) **28.** A common skin finding in patients with adrenal dysfunction is:

1. protruding bones.
2. erythema.
3. bronze pigmentation.
4. pruritus.

(868) **29.** An age-related change that affects the adrenal glands is that adrenal function:

1. decreases in epinephrine.
2. remains adequate.
3. becomes hyperactive.
4. increases in metabolism.

(868) **30.** The response to sodium restriction and to position changes is less efficient in the elderly because of declines in the secretion of plasma renin and:

1. thyroxine.
2. aldosterone.
3. estrogen.
4. androgens.

(871) **31.** Signs and symptoms of hyperkalemia that should be reported to the physician by patients with Addison's disease include:

1. dyspnea and coughing.
2. oliguria and flank pain.
3. constipation and fatty stools.
4. weakness and paresthesia.

(872) **32.** Which substance may be used liberally in the diet of patients with Addison's disease?

1. carbohydrates.
2. salt.
3. saturated fats.
4. caffeine.

(864) **33.** What is a common sign of diabetes insipidus?

1. massive diuresis
2. edema
3. hyperglycemia
4. oliguria

CHAPTER 43

Student Name ______________________________

Thyroid and Parathyroid Disorders

Answer Key: Textbook page references are provided as a guide for answering these questions. A complete answer key was provided for your instructor.

OBJECTIVES

1. Identify nursing assessment data related to the functions of the thyroid and parathyroid glands.
2. Describe tests and procedures used to diagnose disorders of the thyroid and parathyroid glands and identify nursing responsibilities relevant for each.
3. Describe the pathophysiology, signs and symptoms, complications, and treatment of hyperthyroidism, hypothyroidism, hyperparathyroidism, and hypoparathyroidism.
4. Assist in the development of nursing care plans for patients with disorders of the thyroid or parathyroid glands, including assessment, nursing diagnoses, goals, interventions, and outcome criteria.

LEARNING ACTIVITIES

A. Match the definition in the numbered column with the most appropriate term in the lettered column.

(887) **1.** __________ Facial edema that develops with severe, long-term hypothyroidism; sometimes used as a synonym for hypothyroidism

(882, 891) **2.** __________ Enlargement of the thyroid gland, causing the neck to appear swollen

(896) **3.** __________ Steady muscle contraction caused by hypocalcemia

A. Goiter
B. Goitrogen
C. Exophthalmos
D. Myxedema
E. Nodule
F. Cretinism
G. Parotiditis
H. Tetany
I. Laryngospasm
J. Thyroiditis
K. Thyrotoxicosis

Continued next page

(892) **4.** __________ Small mass of tissue that can be palpated

(886) **5.** __________ Spasmodic closure of the larynx

(887) **6.** __________ Permanent mental and physical retardation caused by congenital deficiency of thyroid hormones

(882) **7.** __________ Excessive metabolic stimulation caused by elevated thyroid hormone level

(883) **8.** __________ Inflammation of the parotid (salivary) gland

(883) **9.** __________ Inflammation of the thyroid gland

(891) **10.** __________ Substance that suppresses thyroid function

(882) **11.** __________ Protrusion of the eyeballs associated with hyperthyroidism

B. For each of the following signs or symptoms, indicate whether it is characteristic of (A) hyperthyroidism or (B) hypothyroidism.

(882) **1.** __________ Heat intolerance

(889) **2.** __________ Apathy

(889) **3.** __________ Increased appetite

(882) **4.** __________ Tachycardia

(889) **5.** __________ Cold intolerance

(882) **6.** __________ Weight loss

(889) **7.** __________ Anorexia

(888) **8.** __________ Bradycardia

(882) **9.** __________ Nervousness and restlessness

(888) **10.** __________ Weight gain

A. Hyperthyroidism
B. Hypothyroidism

C. List two things that should be placed at the bedside before the patient who is having a thyroidectomy returns from surgery.

(886) **1.** ______________________________

(886) **2.** ______________________________

Student Name____

D. List two reasons why respiratory distress can result following thyroidectomy.

(886) **1.** ____

(886) **2.** ____

E. Following thyroidectomy surgery, where should the nurse check for bleeding? *(887)*

F. If thyroid enlargement is mild and thyroid hormone production is normal, what treatment is required? *(892)*

G. Explain why thyroidectomy surgery may be followed with radioactive iodine treatment. *(892)*

H. Explain why an electrocardiogram may be ordered for patients with parathyroid disorders. *(893)*

I. Under what conditions will demineralization be apparent on radiographs of patients with a parathyroid disorder? *(893)*

J. Complete the statements below with either (A) increase(s) or (B) decrease(s).

(882) **1.** When thyroid hormones are elevated, the pulse rate __________.

(882) **2.** Excess thyroxine __________ the body's metabolic rate.

(893) **3.** High levels of PTH __________ retention of calcium.

(882) **4.** When thyroid hormones are elevated, blood pressure __________.

(893) **5.** High levels of PTH __________ loss of phosphates by the kidneys.

A. Increase(s)
B. Decrease(s)

K. Complete the statement in the numbered column with the most appropriate term in the lettered column. Some terms may be used more than once, and some terms may not be used.

(882) **1.** The most common forms of hyperthyroidism are Graves' disease and __________.

(882) **2.** If untreated, hyperthyroidism may lead to __________.

(882) **3.** Symptoms of thyrotoxicosis include tachycardia, heart failure, and __________.

(882) **4.** Drugs that block the synthesis, release, or activity of thyroid hormones are __________.

(882) **5.** The two classes of drugs commonly used as antithyroid drugs are thioamides and __________.

(882) **6.** When a patient is taking drugs that interfere with thyroxine secretion, the nurse should monitor for edema, weight gain, and __________.

(882) **7.** Examples of thioamides are methimazole (Tapazole) and __________.

(882) **8.** One main disadvantage of the thioamides is that they can cause __________.

A. Antithyroids
B. Cold intolerance
C. Agranulocytosis
D. Heat intolerance
E. Hyperthermia
F. Iodides
G. Propylthiouracil (PTU)
H. Multinodular goiter
I. Hypothermia
J. Thyrotoxicosis

Student Name____

L. Complete the statements in the numbered column with the most appropriate term in the lettered column. Some terms may be used more than once, and some terms may not be used.

(882) **1.** A condition in which deposits of fat and fluid behind the eyeballs make them bulge forward is called __________.

(883) **2.** A complication in patients undergoing thyroidectomies that can be prevented by preoperative treatment with antithyroid drugs is __________.

(886) **3.** Signs and symptoms of poor oxygenation due to airway obstruction that may occur after thyroidectomy include restlessness, increased pulse, and __________.

(886) **4.** Signs of laryngeal nerve damage include inability to speak and __________.

(886) **5.** A complication of thyroidectomies includes injury to the parathyroid glands, which results in __________.

(886) **6.** The most serious side effect of hypocalcemia is __________.

(887) **7.** Signs of severe hyperthyroidism include fever, confusion, and __________.

(887) **8.** Symptoms of infection that should be reported after thyroidectomy include fever, wound swelling, and __________.

(887) **9.** The result of inadequate secretion of thyroid hormones is called __________.

A. Hyperthyroidism
B. Dyspnea
C. Laryngospasm
D. Bradycardia
E. Tetany
F. Hypothyroidism
G. Calcium salts
H. Foul discharge
I. Hoarseness
J. Exophthalmos
K. Tachycardia
L. Thyroid crisis
M. Tetany

M. Complete the statement in the numbered column with the most appropriate term in the lettered column. Some terms may be used more than once, and some terms may not be used.

(892) **1.** Parathyroid hormone (parathormone, PTH) plays a critical role in regulating __________.

(893) **2.** The most notable effect of hyperparathyroidism is __________.

(893) **3.** People who undergo kidney transplantation after being on dialysis for a long time may experience __________.

(893) **4.** When the serum calcium level falls, __________ is secreted.

(893) **5.** Generally, calcium retention by the kidney is balanced by the loss of __________.

(886) **6.** A spasm of the facial muscle when the face is tapped over the facial nerve is __________.

(886) **7.** A carpopedal spasm that occurs when a blood pressure cuff is inflated beyond a patient's systolic blood pressure and is left in place for several minutes is __________.

(892) **8.** __________ is an element that is an important component of strong bones and that plays a vital role in the functions of nerve and tissue cells.

(893) **9.** The secretion of excess PTH is called __________.

A. Trousseau's sign
B. Phosphates
C. Hypoparathyroidism
D. Chvostek's sign
E. Calcium
F. PTH
G. Hyperparathyroidism
H. TSH
I. Hypercalcemia
J. Sodium

Student Name____

MULTIPLE-CHOICE QUESTIONS

N. Choose the most appropriate answer.

(879) **1.** Which is secreted when serum calcium levels are high to limit the shift of calcium from the bones into the blood?

1. calcitonin
2. thyroxine
3. thymine
4. phosphorus

(882) **2.** Hyperthyroid patients often experience sleep disturbances and:

1. sedation.
2. bradycardia.
3. restlessness.
4. hypotension.

(882) **3.** Poor tolerance of heat and excessive perspiration are symptoms of:

1. hyperparathyroidism.
2. hypoparathyroidism.
3. hyperthyroidism.
4. hypothyroidism.

(882) **4.** If untreated, hyperthyroidism may lead to:

1. thyrotoxicosis.
2. hypotension.
3. bradycardia.
4. decreased metabolism.

(883) **5.** Signs of iodine toxicity include:

1. bradycardia and hypotension.
2. urinary retention and oliguria.
3. esophageal ulcers and pyloric sphincter spasms.
4. swelling and irritation of mucous membranes and increased salivation.

(882) **6.** Elevated thyroid hormones result in:

1. decreased pulse and blood pressure.
2. increased pulse and blood pressure.
3. decreased temperature and infection.
4. increased temperature and infection.

(885) **7.** An important nursing diagnosis for the patient with exophthalmos is:

1. Risk for infection.
2. Knowledge deficit (of disease process).
3. Decreased cardiac output.
4. Altered body image.

(886) **8.** A complication of thyroidectomies includes injury to the parathyroid glands, which results in:

1. bradycardia.
2. cyanosis.
3. tetany.
4. headache.

(886) **9.** Results of two tests that are indicative of hypocalcemia are:

1. positive Chvostek's and Trousseau's signs.
2. increased blood urea nitrogen and potassium levels.
3. increased WBC and decreased RBC levels.
4. increased phosphorus and decreased iodine levels.

(886) **10.** An early symptom of tetany is:

1. flank pain with hematuria.
2. difficulty breathing.
3. a tingling sensation around the mouth and fingers.
4. muscle cramps in leg and arm muscles.

(882) **11.** Graves' disease (toxic diffuse goiter) is characterized by:

1. increased secretion of thyroid hormones.
2. a decreased metabolic rate.
3. intolerance to cold.
4. constipation.

(883) **12.** Which drug stains the teeth and should be sipped through a straw?

1. iron
2. saturated solution of potassium iodide (SSKI)
3. levothyroxine (Synthroid)
4. propylthiouracil

(883) **13.** In patients with toxic diffuse goiter, there is a risk for injury related to:

1. increased metabolic energy production.
2. exophthalmos.
3. increased thyroid hormone stimulation.
4. intolerance to heat.

(888) **14.** Lack of iodine is associated with:

1. goiter.
2. hypoparathyroidism.
3. tetany.
4. thyrotoxicosis.

(879) **15.** Thyroxine (T_4), triiodothyronine (T_3) and calcitonin are hormones produced by the:

1. adrenal gland.
2. thymus gland.
3. thyroid gland.
4. parathyroid gland.

(888) **16.** Which drug is used to treat hypothyroidism?

1. SSKI
2. Synthroid
3. methimazole (Tapazole)
4. Lugol's solution

CHAPTER 44

Student Name ____________________

Diabetes Mellitus and Hypoglycemia

Answer Key: Textbook page references are provided as a guide for answering these questions. A complete answer key was provided for your instructor.

OBJECTIVES

1. Describe the role of insulin in the body.
2. Explain the pathophysiology of diabetes mellitus and hypoglycemia.
3. Describe the signs and symptoms of diabetes mellitus and hypoglycemia.
4. Explain tests and procedures used to diagnose diabetes mellitus and hypoglycemia.
5. Discuss treatment of diabetes mellitus and hypoglycemia.
6. Explain the difference between type 1 and type 2 diabetes mellitus.
7. Differentiate between acute hypoglycemia and diabetic ketoacidosis.
8. Describe the treatment of a patient experiencing acute hypoglycemia or diabetic ketoacidosis.
9. Describe the complications of diabetes mellitus.
10. Identify nursing interventions for a patient diagnosed with diabetes mellitus or hypoglycemia.
11. Identify nursing interventions for a patient diagnosed with ketoacidosis.

LEARNING ACTIVITIES

A. Complete the statement in the numbered column with the most appropriate term in the lettered column. Some terms may be used more than once, and some terms may not be used.

(899) **1.** An inadequate amount of insulin to meet daily requirements characterizes __________.

(899) **2.** Insulin is released in the body in response to the ingestion of __________.

(899) **3.** The absence of endogenous insulin characterizes __________.

(900) **4.** When insulin is absent, the blood becomes thick with glucose, causing the patient to experience __________.

(900) **5.** Tissue breakdown and burning of lean body mass send hunger signals to the hypothalamus; consequently, the patient experiences __________.

(900) **6.** The hormone that stimulates the active transport of glucose into the cells of muscle and adipose tissue is __________.

(900) **7.** A precursor to diabetes mellitus is thought to be __________.

A. Weight loss
B. Insulin
C. Type 1 diabetes mellitus
D. Type 2 diabetes mellitus
E. Glycogen
F. Polydipsia
G. Carbohydrates
H. Polyphagia
I. Insulin resistance

B. Complete the statement in the numbered column with the most appropriate term in the lettered column. Some terms may be used more than once, and some terms may not be used.

(902) **1.** Diabetes is the leading cause of __________.

(902) **2.** With diabetic retinopathy, the vitreous becomes cloudy and vision is lost as a result of __________.

A. "Floaters"
B. Neuropathy
C. Polyuria
D. Hemorrhage
E. Atherosclerosis
F. Capillary permeability
G. "Cobwebs"
H. Nephropathy
I. End-stage renal disease (ESRD)

Continued next page

Student Name______________________________

(902) **3.** A symptom of eye problems for patients with diabetes is the presence of spots, which are called __________.

(902) **4.** Persons with diabetes account for a large percentage of patients with renal disease, which is called __________.

(902) **5.** Elevated insulin levels circulating in the blood of patients with diabetes contribute to the premature development of __________.

C. Complete the statement in the numbered column with the most appropriate term in the lettered column. Some terms may be used more than once, and some terms may not be used.

(905) **1.** Treatment of ketoacidosis is aimed at correction of three main problems, which are acidosis, dehydration, and __________.

(905) **2.** The patient with ketoacidosis may have lost a large volume of fluid as the result of vomiting, hyperventilation, and __________.

(905) **3.** Replacement of potassium is vital in patients with ketoacidosis because hypokalemia can lead to severe __________.

(904) **4.** A life-threatening emergency caused by lack of insulin or inadequate amounts of insulin is called diabetic __________.

(905) **5.** Air hunger, seen in patients with ketoacidosis, is observed as __________.

(905) **6.** The movement of potassium from the extracellular compartment into the cells is enhanced by __________.

(904) **7.** Ketoacidosis results in disorders in the metabolism of carbohydrate, fat, and __________.

(905) **8.** The electrolyte of primary concern in ketoacidosis is __________.

A. Glucose
B. Ketoacidosis
C. Insulin
D. Electrolyte imbalance
E. Potassium
F. Cardiac dysrhythmias
G. Kussmaul's respirations
H. Protein
I. Sodium
J. Polyuria

D. Indicate for each of the following actions or conditions whether insulin (A) increases or (B) decreases it.

A. Increases
B. Decreases

(900) **1.** __________ Rate of metabolism of carbohydrates

(900) **2.** __________ Conversion of glucose to glycogen

(900) **3.** __________ Conversion of glycogen to glucose

(900) **4.** __________ Fatty acid synthesis and conversion of fatty acids into fat

(900) **5.** __________ Breakdown of adipose tissue

(900) **6.** __________ Rate of glucose utilization

(900) **7.** __________ Mobilization of fat

(900) **8.** __________ Conversion of fats to glucose

(900) **9.** __________ Protein synthesis in tissue

(900) **10.** __________ Conversion of protein into glucose

E. List four organs of the body that do not depend on insulin for the transport of glucose into them.

(900) **1.** ______________________________

(900) **2.** ______________________________

(900) **3.** ______________________________

(900) **4.** ______________________________

Student Name ________________________________

F. List six groups of people who are at risk for diabetes.

(901)	**1.**	____________	*(901)*	**4.**	____________
(901)	**2.**	____________	*(901)*	**5.**	____________
(901)	**3.**	____________	*(901)*	**6.**	____________

G. List two causes of foot problems in the person with diabetes.

(903) **1.** ________________________________

(903) **2.** ________________________________

H. Explain why the patient with diabetes may have an ulcer or necrotic area in the foot and may be unaware of the problem. *(903)*

I. List changes that occur in the three items below when the foot's nerve supply is impaired and when the foot's blood supply is impaired. *(903)*

	Impaired Nerve Supply	**Impaired Blood Supply**
1. Color and temperature		
2. Pulses		
3. Sensation		

J. List four situations that put the patient with diabetes at risk for ketoacidosis.

(905) **1.** ________________________________

(905) **2.** ________________________________

(905) **3.** ________________________________

(905) **4.** ________________________________

K. Explain why patients receiving total parenteral nutrition or dialysis are apt to have hyperosmolar nonketotic coma. *(906)*

L. List three areas of injection sites for insulin.

(910) **1.** ________________________________

(910) **2.** ________________________________

(910) **3.** ________________________________

M. Indicate whether (A) too much or (B) not enough of the following factors causes serum glucose levels to drop.

(903) **1.** __________ Insulin

(903) **2.** __________ Food

(903) **3.** __________ Exercise

A. Too much
B. Not enough

N. List nine initial signs and symptoms of hypoglycemia.

(903) **1.** ____________________

(903) **2.** ____________________

(903) **3.** ____________________

(903) **4.** ____________________

(903) **5.** ____________________

(903) **6.** ____________________

(903) **7.** ____________________

(903) **8.** ____________________

(903) **9.** ____________________

MULTIPLE-CHOICE QUESTIONS

O. Choose the most appropriate answer.

(900) **1.** Which of the following inhibits the conversion of glycogen to glucose?

1. fatty acids
2. insulin
3. triglycerides
4. ketones

(904) **2.** Which herbal supplement can lower blood glucose?

1. ginseng
2. ginkgo
3. kava kava
4. Ephedra

Student Name____

(906) **3.** The diagnosis of diabetes is based on serum:

1. amylase levels.
2. red blood cell count.
3. hemoglobin.
4. glucose levels.

(906) **4.** Which of the following represents normal fasting serum glucose levels?

1. 30–50 mg/dl
2 80–120 mg/dl
3. 150–200 mg/dl
4. 205–300 mg/dl

(907) **5.** The American Diabetes Association recommends that 60–70% of the total daily calories should come from:

1. protein.
2. saturated fats.
3. carbohydrates and monounsaturated fats.
4. polyunsaturated fats.

(909) **6.** The most commonly used insulin concentration is:

1. U-40. 2. U-80.
3. U-100. 4. U-500.

(909) **7.** The prescription for insulin, including schedule for dosages, type, and amount, is written to mimic the action of a normal:

1. stomach. 2. liver.
3. gallbladder. 4. pancreas.

(909) **8.** Regular insulin should be given:

1. at bedtime.
2. before meals.
3. during meals.
4. after meals.

(910) **9.** Which injection site has the fastest rate of absorption for insulin?

1. upper arm
2. upper buttocks
3. abdomen
4. thighs

(912) **10.** The two oral sulfonylurea hypoglycemic agents that are recommended for elderly patients are glipizide (Glucotrol) and:

1. chlorpropamide (Diabinese).
2. glyburide (DiaBeta, Micronase).
3. tolbutamide (Orinase).
4. acetohexamide (Dymelor).

(910) **11.** When mixing regular and longer-acting insulins, which should be drawn into the syringe first?

1. regular insulin
2. protamine zinc insulin
3. Ultralente U insulin
4. Lente L insulin

(912) **12.** A reason for avoiding long-acting oral sulfonylurea hypoglycemic agents in the elderly is that decreased renal function in older adultsmakes them more prone to:

1. hyponatremia.
2. hypernatremia.
3. hypoglycemia.
4. hyperglycemia.

(911) **13.** Which is a side effect of sulfonylureas used in the treatment of diabetes mellitus?

1. hyperglycemia
2. hypoglycemia
3. hyperkalemia
4. hypokalemia

(909) **14.** Patients who require insulin injections need to self-monitor levels of:

1. serum cholesterol.
2. red blood cells.
3. amylase.
4. blood glucose.

(904) **15.** Late signs of hypoglycemia include:

1. palpitations and dyspnea.
2. oliguria and hypotension.
3. peripheral edema and tachypnea.
4. confusion and unconsciousness.

(914) **16.** To detect possible changes in the eyes associated with diabetes mellitus, the nurse inquires whether the patient has had floaters, blurred vision, or:

1. hemorrhage.
2. infection.
3. diplopia.
4. conjunctivitis.

(914) **17.** During the physical assessment of the diabetic patient, the nurse inspects the feet carefully for lesions, discoloration, and:

1. edema.
2. ability to dorsiflex.
3. ability to evert.
4. dehydration.

(915) **18.** A nursing diagnosis for patients with diabetes is Chronic pain related to:

1. abnormal blood glucose levels.
2. adverse effects of drugs.
3. neuropathy.
4. alterations in urine output.

(915) **19.** Patients with diabetes may have sensory/perceptual alterations related to:

1. dietary restrictions.
2. anxiety and fear.
3. imbalance between food intake and activity expenditure.
4. neurologic and circulatory changes.

(916) **20.** Alterations in tactile sensations in diabetic patients may result in:

1. burns or frostbite.
2. floaters or diplopia.
3. altered urine output or oliguria.
4. abnormal blood glucose levels.

(916) **21.** Altered thought processes in diabetic patients, including confusion, anger, and decreased level of consciousness, may be due to:

1. neuropathy.
2. nephropathy.
3. ketoacidosis.
4. hyperglycemia.

(919) **22.** Hypoglycemia is defined as a syndrome that develops when the blood glucose level falls to less than:

1. 10–15 mg/dl.
2. 45–50 mg/dl.
3. 80–120 mg/dl.
4. 200–300 mg/dl.

(920) **23.** Endogenous hypoglycemia occurs when internal factors cause an excessive secretion of insulin or an increase in the metabolism of:

1. protein.
2. fats.
3. calcium.
4. glucose.

Student Name____

(921) **24.** When blood glucose levels fall rapidly, the four substances that are secreted by the body in an attempt to increase glucose levels are cortisol, glucagon, growth hormone, and:

1. antidiuretic hormone.
2. epinephrine.
3. aldosterone.
4. thyroxine.

(921) **25.** Early signs of hypoglycemia include:

1. bradycardia and edema.
2. oliguria and constipation.
3. infection and red skin.
4. weakness and hunger.

(912) **26.** Which group of oral antidiabetic agents does not cause hypoglycemia as a side effect?

1. biguanides (metformin)
2. alpha-glucosidase inhibitors (Precose)
3. sulfonylureas
4. thiazolidinediones (Avandia)

(921) **27.** Patients with hypoglycemia are at risk for injury related to:

1. oliguria and nephropathy.
2. polydipsia and polyphagia.
3. dizziness and weakness.
4. retinopathy and hypotension.

(905) **28.** Hyperosmolar nonketotic coma is loss of consciousness caused by extremely high serum:

1. ketones. 2. glucose.
3. calcium. 4. potassium.

(905) **29.** When a patient is given insulin for diabetic ketoacidosis, the nurse should monitor the patient for:

1. hyperglycemia.
2. hypoglycemia.
3. hypokalemia.
4. thrombocytopenia.

(908) **30.** When a patient's serum glucose is 260 mg/dl, the patient should:

1. administer glucagon.
2. drink 8 ounces of skim milk.
3. drink 4 ounces of concentrated orange juice.
4. avoid exercise.

(908) **31.** Your patient has taken NPH insulin at 8:00 AM. At what time of day should he avoid exercise in order to prevent hypoglycemia?

1. 9:00 AM. 2. 10:00 AM.
3. 12:00 PM. 4. 4:00 PM.

(908) **32.** Which type of insulin is a clear solution?

1. Ultralente
2. NPH insulin
3. Lente insulin
4. Insulin glargine (Lantus)

(906) **33.** The goal of the diabetic diet is to:

1. limit carbohydrate intake.
2. increase protein intake.
3. limit total calorie intake.
4. maintain normal plasma glucose levels.

CHAPTER 45

Student Name ____________________

Female Reproductive Disorders

Answer Key: Textbook page references are provided as a guide for answering these questions. A complete answer key was provided for your instructor.

OBJECTIVES

1. List data to be collected when assessing the female reproductive system.
2. Describe the nursing interventions for women who are undergoing diagnostic tests and procedures for reproductive system disorders.
3. Identify the nursing interventions associated with douche, cauterization, heat therapy, and topical medications used to treat disorders of the female reproductive system.
4. Explain the pathophysiology, signs and symptoms, complications, diagnostic procedures, and medical or surgical treatment for selected disorders of the female reproductive system.
5. Assist in developing a nursing care plan for the patient with common disorders of the female reproductive system.
6. Describe the nursing interventions for the patient who is menopausal.

LEARNING ACTIVITIES

A. Match the definition in the numbered column with the most appropriate term in the lettered column.

(946) **1.** ________ Surgical excision of a fallopian tube and ovary

(943) **2.** ________ Difficult or painful sexual intercourse in women

(944) **3.** ________ A condition in which endometrial tissue is located, abnormally, outside the uterus

(942) **4.** ________ Inflammation of breast tissue

A. Cystocele
B. Menopause
C. Dysmenorrhea
D. Endometriosis
E. Menorrhagia
F. Metrorrhagia
G. Rectocele
H. Dyspareunia
I. Hysterectomy
J. Dysplasia
K. Mastitis
L. Menarche
M. Salpingo-oophorectomy

Continued next page

(938, 966) **5.** ________ Menstrual periods characterized by profuse or prolonged bleeding

(950) **6.** ________ Herniation of the urinary bladder into the vagina

(938, 966) **7.** ________ Bleeding or spotting between menstrual periods

(946) **8.** ________ Surgical removal of the uterus

(929) **9.** ________ Abnormal cells

(927) **10.** ________ Cessation of menstruation

(950) **11.** ________ Herniation of part of the rectum into the vagina

(927) **12.** ________ Age at which the first menstrual period occurs

(945) **13.** ________ Painful menstruation

B. Match the definition or description in the numbered column with the most appropriate term in the lettered column. Some terms may be used more than once, and some terms may not be used.

(929) **1.** ________ A type of invasive surgery procedure in which a large amount of cervical tissue is removed to treat cancer

(929) **2.** ________ An invasive surgical procedure that provides direct visualization of the female pelvic cavity

(929) **3.** ________ A test for which specimens are collected routinely to detect cervical cancer and dysplasia

(929) **4.** ________ A procedure that is commonly done before cervical biopsies

(929) **5.** ________ A type of biopsy done in a physician's office or an outpatient clinic to diagnose cervical cancer

A. Multiple-punch biopsy
B. Papanicolaou (Pap) smear
C. Dilation and curettage
D. Culture and smear
E. Cone biopsy
F. Aspiration biopsy
G. Endometrial biopsy
H. Culdoscopy
I. Breast biopsy
J. Colposcopy
K. Laparoscopy
L. Cauterization

Continued next page

Student Name ______________________

(929) **6.** __________ Specimens collected to identify infections

(929) **7.** __________ The procedure that is done to identify ectopic pregnancy or pelvic masses

(929) **8.** __________ A test performed to diagnose uterine cancer

(929) **9.** __________ A procedure in which an instrument is used to inspect the cervix under magnification and to identify abnormal and potentially cancerous tissue

(934) **10.** __________ Deliberate tissue destruction by means of heat, electricity, or chemicals

(931) **11.** __________ Visualization of abdominal organs in order to perform tubal ligation

C. Match the definition or description in the numbered column with the most appropriate term in the lettered column. Some terms may be used more than once, and some terms may not be used.

(953) **1.** __________ The body of the uterus bends backward on itself

(953) **2.** __________ A forward tilt of the uterus at a sharp angle to the vagina

(953) **3.** __________ The uterus bends forward on itself

(953) **4.** __________ A backward tilt of the uterus with the cervix pointed downward toward the anterior vaginal wall

A. Anteflexion
B. Introversion
C. Retroversion
D. Retroflexion
E. Extraversion
F. Anteversion

D. Complete the statement in the numbered column with the most appropriate term in the lettered column. Some terms may be used more than once, and some terms may not be used.

(957) **1.** Mastectomy patients are at risk for injury related to __________.

(955) **2.** The removal of the tumor with a margin of surrounding healthy tissue but preserving most of the breast is called __________.

(955) **3.** A low-incidence cancer of the nipple and areola is __________.

(955, 958) **4.** The implantation of a tissue expander injected with saline is a type of __________

(955) **5.** The removal of all breast tissue, overlying skin, axillary lymph nodes, and underlying pectoral muscles is called __________.

(955) **6.** If breast cancer cells removed during surgery need estrogen for cell replication, they are said to be __________.

(955) **7.** Removal of the entire breast is called __________.

A. Paget's disease
B. ER-negative
C. Radical mastectomy
D. Simple mastectomy
E. Silicone implant
F. ER-positive
G. Lymphedema
H. Breast reconstruction
I. Lumpectomy

E. Match the term in the numbered column with the most appropriate numerical range in the lettered column. (These terms refer to the variations within normal menstrual periods.) Some ranges may be used more than once, and some terms may not be used.

(938) **1.** __________ Length of cycle (days)

(938) **2.** __________ Duration of menstruation (days)

(938) **3.** __________ Amount of blood loss (ml)

A. 2–8
B. 10–14
C. 21–40
D. 40–100
E. 150–200

Student Name____

F. Match the description in the numbered column with the most appropriate term in the lettered column. Some terms may be used more than once, and some terms may not be used.

(940) **1.** __________ Often seen with diabetes

(943) **2.** __________ A sexually transmitted disease that is the primary cause of ectopic pregnancy and infertility

(940) **3.** __________ Includes profuse, frothy, and yellow-gray discharge

(940) **4.** __________ Includes cottage cheese-like discharge

(940) **5.** __________ Protozoal infection

(940) **6.** __________ Fungal infection

(940) **7.** __________ Infection often caused by disruption of the normal vaginal flora

(943) **8.** __________ A sexually transmitted disease that causes most pelvic inflammatory disease

(942) **9.** __________ Associated with mastitis

A. *Trichomonas vaginalis*
B. *Chlamydia trachomatis*
C. *Neisseria gonorrheae*
D. *Candida albicans*
E. *Staphylococcus aureus*

G. Match the definition or description in the numbered column with the most appropriate term in the lettered column. Some terms may be used more than once, and some terms may not be used.

(951) 1. ________ Level of prolapse if the cervix protrudes from the vaginal opening

(950) 2. ________ A vaginal disorder caused by weakness of supportive structures between the vagina and bladder

(951) 3. ________ Level of prolapse if the vagina is inverted and both the cervix and the body of the uterus protrude from the vaginal opening

(951) 4. ________ Method used to diagnose first-degree uterine prolapse

(951) 5. ________ Nonsurgical treatment of uterine prolapse that is aimed at elevating the uterus

(950) 6. ________ A vaginal disorder caused by weakness of supportive structures between the vagina and rectum

(951) 7. ________ A condition in which the uterus descends into the vagina from its usual position in the pelvis

A. Pessary
B. Third-degree
C. Visual inspection
D. First-degree
E. Rectocele
F. Uterine prolapse
G. Second-degree
H. Fourth-degree
I. Cystocele
J. Laparoscopy
K. Pelvic examination

Continued next page

Student Name____

(951) **8.** __________ Method used to diagnose second- and third-degree uterine prolapse

(951) **9.** __________ Level of prolapse if the cervix is above the vaginal opening

H. Match the nursing diagnosis for patients with cystocele and rectocele in the numbered column with the appropriate nursing intervention in the lettered column. Some interventions may be used more than once.

(950) **1.** __________ Stress incontinence

(951) **2.** __________ Constipation

(951) **3.** __________ Risk for infection

(951) **4.** __________ Acute pain

A. Initial application of cold to reduce pain and swelling
B. Teaching the patient Kegel exercises
C. Emphasizing the need for a high-fiber diet
D. Sitz baths and heat lamps
E. Instructing the patient to report signs of urinary frequency, burning, or foul odor
F. Use of indwelling or suprapubic catheter

I. Match the preoperative and postoperative nursing diagnoses in the numbered column for a patient with a hysterectomy with the appropriate nursing interventions in the lettered column.

(947) **1.** __________ Deficient knowledge of information or misinterpretation of effects of HRT

(948) **2.** __________ Risk for deficit fluid volume related to postoperative bleeding

(948) **3.** __________ Urinary retention related to surgical manipulation, local tissue edema, temporary sensory or motor impairment

(947) **4.** __________ Self-esteem disturbance related to perceived potential changes in femininity, effect on sexual relationship

A. Assist patient to bathroom or commode; use bedpan only if absolutely necessary
B. Instruct and assist with foot and leg exercises while the patient is confined to bed; encourage and assist with ambulation when allowed
C. Explain that positions for sexual intercourse should avoid pressure on the abdominal incision for as long as incisional tenderness persists
D. Check mucous membranes for moisture
E. Auscultate abdomen for bowel sounds
F. Explain that estrogen may increase fluid retention, which may make one "feel fat"

Continued next page

(948) **5.** ________ Ineffective tissue perfusion related to reduction of cellular components necessary for delivery of oxygen, hypovolemia, reduction of blood flow, intraoperative trauma

(948) **6.** ________ Constipation related to weakening of abdominal musculature, abdominal pain, decreased physical activity, dietary changes, environmental changes

J. Match the actions and uses of drugs in the numbered column with the drug used to treat disorders of the female reproductive system in the lettered column.

(935) **1.** ________ Enhances bone formation; depresses beta-lipoprotein and cholesterol plasma levels; used to replace natural hormones after menopause and to treat advanced breast cancer and prostate cancer

(935) **2.** ________ Promotes secretory function in endometrium; influences contractile activity of the uterus; used with estrogens as oral contraceptives

(936) **3.** ________ Inhibits production of pituitary gonadotropins; used to treat endometriosis and fibrocystic breast disease

(937) **4.** ________ Initially increases and then decreases testosterone levels; used to treat endometriosis

A. Estrogen-progestin combinations
B. Danazol (Danocrine)
C. Urofollitropin (Metrodin)
D. Conjugated estrogens (Premarin)
E. Leuprolide acetate (Lupron)
F. Oral progestins (Provera)
G. Estrogen only (diethylstilbestrol)
H. SERMS (tamoxifen)
I. Ovulatory stimulants (Clomid)

Continued next page

Student Name ____________________

(937) **5.** __________ Suppresses ovulation to prevent pregnancy

(937) **6.** __________ Prevents implantation of fertilized ovum; used as emergency post-coital contraceptive

(937) **7.** __________ Stimulates ovarian follicular growth; used to treat selected patients who have not responded to clomiphene citrate

(935) **8.** __________ Treats uterine bleeding and endometriosis

(936) **9.** __________ Used to treat breast cancer

(937) **10.** __________ Used as fertility drugs

K. List three parts of the pelvic exam.

(929) **1.** ____________________

(929) **2.** ____________________

(929) **3.** ____________________

L. List two reasons why douching is a potentially dangerous procedure.

(934) **1.** ____________________

(934) **2.** ____________________

M. List four teaching points to include when teaching the patient about appropriate vaginal hygiene.

(934) **1.** ____________________

(934) **2.** ____________________

(934) **3.** ____________________

(934) **4.** ____________________

N. List two groups of women who are especially prone to developing pelvic inflammatory disease not associated with sexually transmitted diseases.

(943) **1.** ____________________

(943) **2.** ____________________

O. List seven signs and symptoms of pelvic inflammatory disease.

(943) **1.** ______________________________

(943) **2.** ______________________________

(943) **3.** ______________________________

(943) **4.** ______________________________

(943) **5.** ______________________________

(943) **6.** ______________________________

(943) **7.** ______________________________

P. List seven common side effects of danazol, which may be given to patients with endometriosis.

(936, 945) **1.** ______________________________

(936, 945) **2.** ______________________________

(936, 945) **3.** ______________________________

(936, 945) **4.** ______________________________

(936, 945) **5.** ______________________________

(936, 945) **6.** ______________________________

(936, 945) **7.** ______________________________

Q. Explain why oral contraceptives may be prescribed for patients with endometriosis. *(946)*

R. In addition to stress incontinence and incomplete bladder emptying, list three symptoms that women with cystoceles are likely to experience.

(950) **1.** ______________________________

(950) **2.** ______________________________

(950) **3.** ______________________________

Student Name ______________________________

S. Indicate how the following categories influence a person's chance for getting breast cancer.

(954) **1.** Gender: ______________________________

(954) **2.** Family history: ______________________________

(954) **3.** Race: White non-Hispanic women ______________________________

African-American women ______________________________

(954) **4.** Age: ______________________________

(954) **5.** Duration of menstruating life stage: ______________________________

(954) **6.** Radiation exposure: ______________________________

T. List six ways the nurse can intervene to prevent or minimize lymphedema in the patient with a mastectomy.

(959) **1.** ______________________________

(959) **2.** ______________________________

(959) **3.** ______________________________

(959) **4.** ______________________________

(959) **5.** ______________________________

(959) **6.** ______________________________

U. List three ways ovarian cancer metastasizes.

(960) **1.** ______________________________

(960) **2.** ______________________________

(960) **3.** ______________________________

V. Internal radiation as a treatment for patients with ovarian cancer poses a nursing challenge; list three conditions related to internal radiation that make nursing interventions a challenge.

(962) **1.** ______________________________

(962) **2.** ______________________________

(962) **3.** ______________________________

W. List three types of medications that may be prescribed for cancer patients receiving internal radiation to moderate radiation side effects and facilitate patient comfort.

(962) **1.** ______________________________

(962) **2.** ______________________________

(962) **3.** ______________________________

X. Indicate how the following structures change after menopause without estrogen present.

(965) **1.** Uterus: ______________________________

(965) **2.** Vagina: ______________________________

(965) **3.** Vaginal tissues: ______________________________

(965) **4.** Breast tissue: ______________________________

(965) **5.** Pubic and axillary hair: ______________________________

(965) **6.** Bone mass: ______________________________

Y. List three contraindications of estrogen replacement therapy.

(965) **1.** ______________________________

(965) **2.** ______________________________

(965) **3.** ______________________________

Student Name ______________________________

Z. Using Figure 45-1 below, label the external female genitalia (A–L) from the terms (1–12) below.

(925)

1. __________ Labia minora

2. __________ Hymen

3. __________ Labia majora

4. __________ Clitoris body

5. __________ Clitoris glans

6. __________ Mons pubis

7. __________ Vaginal orifice (introitus)

8. __________ Urethral meatus

9. __________ Perineum

10. __________ Prepuce

11. __________ Anus

12. __________ Bartholin's glands

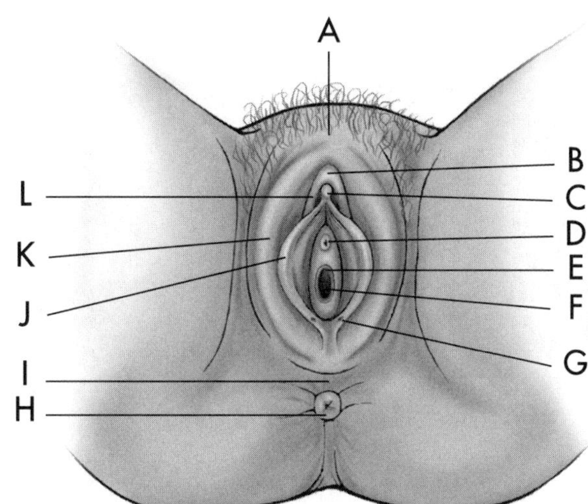

AA. Using Figure 45-9 below, label the sites of endometriosis (A–L) from the terms provided (1–12) below.

(945)

1. __________ Anterior cul-de-sac and bladder
2. __________ Ileum
3. __________ Ovary
4. __________ Cervix
5. __________ Perineum
6. __________ Vulva
7. __________ Posterior surface of uterus
8. __________ Umbilicus
9. __________ Pelvic colon
10. __________ Uterine wall
11. __________ Rectovaginal septum
12. __________ Appendix

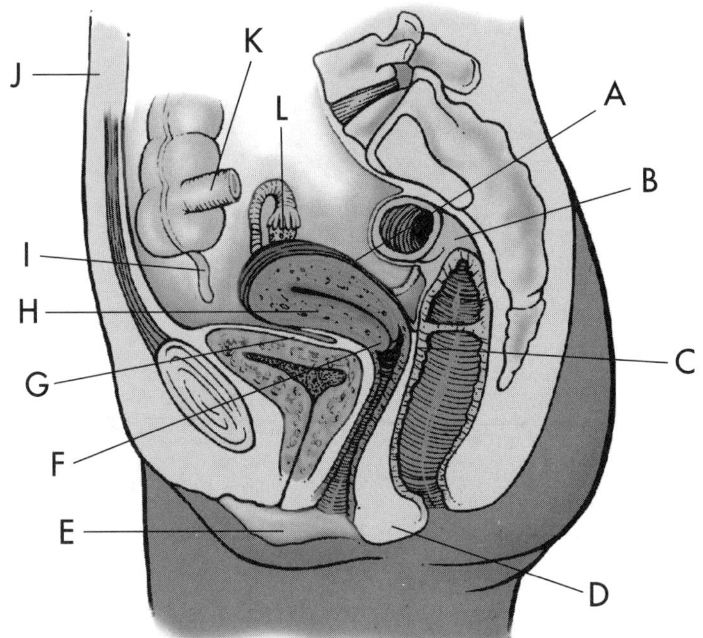

Student Name________________________________

MULTIPLE-CHOICE QUESTIONS

BB. Choose the most appropriate answer.

(927) **1.** The two main hormones produced by the ovaries are:

1. estrogen and progesterone.
2. testosterone and prolactin.
3. thyroxine and oxytocin.
4. follicle-stimulating hormone and luteinizing hormone.

(927) **2.** When a patient comes to a clinic with a female reproductive system problem, the opening question the nurse should ask is:

1. "What is wrong with you today?"
2. "What is the problem that made you come in?"
3. "Why did you come to the clinic today?"
4. "What is the reason for your visit?"

(928) **3.** The physical examination of women with reproductive system problems includes the assessment for the presence of Homans' sign in order to detect possible:

1. vaginal infection.
2. thrombophlebitis.
3. abdominal distention.
4. breast lumps.

(929) **4.** In which position is the patient placed for a pelvic exam?

1. lithotomy
2. right side-lying
3. knee-chest
4. supine

(931) **5.** Advise the patient that air entering the pelvic cavity during the culdoscopy procedure may cause pain in the:

1. abdomen. 2. heart.
3. thigh. 4. shoulder.

(934) **6.** A method of deliberate tissue destruction through use of heat, electricity, or chemicals is called:

1. culdoscopy.
2. colposcopy.
3. cauterization.
4. dilation and curettage.

(934) **7.** A particularly helpful type of heat application for small areas such as the vulva or perineum is:

1. sitz baths.
2. an electric heating pad.
3. aquathermia (K-pad).
4. hot compresses.

(934) **8.** Three signs for which the nurse must observe in patients taking sitz baths are severe pain, shock, and:

1. dyspnea. 2. faintness.
3. dermatitis. 4. headache.

(934) **9.** Dilation of large pelvic vessels during sitz baths may cause:

1. hypertension.
2. hypotension.
3. pneumonia.
4. seizures.

(934) **10.** Following the administration of vaginal suppositories, the patient is asked to remain in which position for at least 15 minutes to allow the medication to be absorbed?

1. prone
2. right side-lying
3. sitting
4. supine

(938) **11.** Deviations from normal menstrual cycles are viewed as:

1. uterine bleeding disorders.
2. vaginal hemorrhage problems.
3. endometrial cancers.
4. pelvic inflammatory diseases.

(940) **12.** The most common characteristics of vulvitis are inflammation and:

1. bleeding.
2. pruritus.
3. cheeselike discharge.
4. pain.

(940) **13.** A significant discharge may be seen in:

1. vulvitis.
2. cystitis.
3. vaginitis.
4. pyelonephritis.

(940) **14.** Signs and symptoms of vaginitis include local swelling, itching, and:

1. redness.
2. pus.
3. hemorrhage.
4. ulcers.

(940) **15.** A potential complication of vulvitis and vaginitis is:

1. hypotension.
2. ascending infection.
3. seizures.
4. thrombophlebitis.

(940) **16.** Bartholin's glands are vulnerable to a wide variety of infectious microorganisms due to their:

1. size. 2. location.
3. structure. 4. secretions.

(940) **17.** When Bartholin's glands are infected, the resultant edema and pus formation occlude the duct and form:

1. tumors. 2. cysts.
3. warts. 4. abscesses.

(940) **18.** The most noticeable symptom of bartholinitis, which causes patients to seek medical attention, is:

1. edema. 2. pain.
3. discharge. 4. itching.

(941) **19.** The most serious complication of a Bartholin's gland abscess is:

1. hypertension.
2. dyspnea.
3. systemic infection.
4. kidney failure.

(941) **20.** Conservative treatment of bartholinitis is sitz baths and oral:

1. diuretics.
2. anticholinergics.
3. antispasmodics.
4. analgesics.

(942) **21.** Cervicitis related to menopause is treated by:

1. estrogens. 2. antiemetics.
3. diuretics. 4. analgesics.

(942) **22.** The portal of entry for organisms that cause mastitis is the:

1. areola.
2. mammary gland.
3. nipple.
4. lactating duct.

(943) **23.** The most serious complication of pelvic inflammatory disease is:

1. peritonitis.
2. pneumonia.
3. hemorrhage.
4. hypertension.

Student Name____

(943) **24.** Treatment of pelvic inflammatory disease includes rest, application of heat, and administration of:

1. antiemetics.
2. antibiotics.
3. diuretics.
4. antispasmodics.

(945) **25.** The major symptom of endometriosis is:

1. hemorrhage.
2. pain.
3. fever.
4. tachycardia.

(945) **26.** Because the uterine endometrial tissue is bleeding simultaneously in endometriosis, pain appears as dysmenorrhea and may extend to a feeling of:

1. stabbing pain.
2. sudden weakness.
3. difficulty breathing.
4. pelvic heaviness.

(945) **27.** Women who are given androgenic steroids for treatment of endometriosis often experience the common side effect of:

1. masculinizing characteristics.
2. palpitations.
3. insomnia.
4. diuresis.

(946) **28.** Surgical management is commonly employed for patients with endometriosis and includes:

1. colposcopy.
2. culdoscopy.
3. laparoscopy.
4. dilation and curettage.

(949) **29.** Severe and sudden abdominal pain may occur as a complication of follicular ovarian cysts due to:

1. infection.
2. rupture.
3. muscle spasms.
4. vaginitis.

(949) **30.** The only procedure for making a definitive diagnosis of cancer from breast cysts is:

1. surgical biopsy.
2. mammography.
3. palpation.
4. ultrasound.

(946) **31.** A serious complication of a very large fibroid tumor is that it may compress the urethra, obstructing urine flow and causing secondary:

1. vaginitis.
2. pelvic inflammatory disease.
3. hydronephrosis.
4. diuresis.

(950) **32.** For women with fibroid tumors who desire to become pregnant, a procedure that can be done by laser surgery to remove only the tumor is:

1. hysterectomy.
2. myomectomy.
3. dilation and curettage.
4. culdoscopy.

(950) **33.** Women at risk for developing rectoceles and cystoceles are those who have experienced a weakened pubococcygeal muscle due to:

1. extended antibiotic treatment.
2. repeated pregnancies.
3. effects of herpes infection.
4. poor nutrition.

(950) **34.** A treatment of small cystoceles that is aimed at improving the tone of the pubococcygeal muscle is:

1. pelvic floor (Kegel's) exercises.
2. surgical intervention (A and P repair).
3. vaginal hysterectomy.
4. increased fluid intake.

(951) **35.** The most common surgical treatment for uterine prolapse is:

1. vaginal hysterectomy.
2. lithotripsy.
3. culdoscopy.
4. dilation and curettage.

(954) **36.** Nearly one half of all malignant breast tumors are located in the:

1. nipple-areolar complex.
2. lower outer quadrant.
3. upper outer quadrant.
4. lower inner quadrant.

(954) **37.** Which of the following is an established risk factor for breast cancer?

1. age over 50
2. age 12 years or older at menarche
3. radiation exposure
4. age of first baby 24 years or older

(931) **38.** It is recommended that yearly mammograms be done every year beginning at age:

1. 35.
2. 40.
3. 50.
4. 65.

(955) **39.** A synthetic nonsteroidal antiestrogen that acts as an estrogen antagonist and blocks circulating estrogen from reaching the cancer receptor cells is:

1. progesterone.
2. tamoxifen.
3. prednisone.
4. doxorubicin (Adriamycin).

(957) **40.** A common nursing diagnosis for mastectomy patients is:

1. Disturbed sleep pattern.
2. Decreased cardiac output.
3. Functional incontinence.
4. Disturbed body image.

(957) **41.** An important aspect of postoperative care after mastectomy is directed toward the prevention and minimization of:

1. lymphedema.
2. hemorrhage.
3. hypertension.
4. nausea.

(959) **42.** Most types of cervical cancer are associated with microbes such as human papillomavirus and herpes simplex virus; therefore, it is thought that cervical cancer is related to:

1. high-fat diets.
2. diabetes mellitus.
3. sexually transmitted diseases.
4. multiple pregnancies.

(960) **43.** The high mortality from ovarian cancer is due to the fact that:

1. symptoms are multiple and serious.
2. it is asymptomatic in early stages.
3. abnormal cell growth occurs in one ovary.
4. it is diagnosed around the time of menopause concurrent with ascites.

Student Name____

(965) **44.** Diminished ovarian function associated with aging causes cessation of ovulation as well as decreased production of:

1. thyroxine.
2. estrogen.
3. epinephrine.
4. prolactin.

(965) **45.** With natural menopause, the woman's first sign may be:

1. increased temperature.
2. loss of memory.
3. menstrual irregularity.
4. bone pain.

(965) **46.** A women is said to be post-menopausal when she has not had a menstrual period for:

1. 3 months.
2. 1 year.
3. 2 years.
4. 5 years.

(965) **47.** Some women experience surgical menopause, which occurs as a result of surgical removal of the:

1. ovaries.
2. uterus.
3. vagina.
4. cervix.

(965) **48.** The type of drug therapy prescribed promptly for surgical menopause to decrease menopausal symptoms is:

1. diuretics.
2. steroids.
3. estrogen.
4. analgesics.

(965) **49.** The symptom of hot flashes that may accompany menopause is due to:

1. increased menstrual bleeding.
2. vasodilation.
3. abdominal cramps.
4. increased body temperature.

(965) **50.** Progesterone is added to estrogen replacement therapy in postmenopausal patients to decrease the risk of:

1. breast cancer.
2. hot flashes.
3. endometrial cancer.
4. insomnia.

(950) **51.** The treatment of choice for large and symptomatic cystoceles and rectoceles is:

1. hysterectomy.
2. myomectomy.
3. Kegel exercises.
4. A and P repair.

(946) **52.** The incidence of fibroid tumors is increased among women who are:

1. African-American.
2. Caucasian.
3. Asian.
4. Hispanic.

(946) **53.** Recent findings from the Women's Health Initiative (2002) indicate that combination estrogen–progestin therapy increases the risk of breast cancer and:

1. osteoporosis.
2. endometriosis.
3. coronary heart disease.
4. amenorrhea.

CHAPTER 46

Student Name ______________________________

Male Reproductive Disorders

Answer Key: Textbook page references are provided as a guide for answering these questions. A complete answer key was provided for your instructor.

OBJECTIVES

1. Describe the major structures and functions of the normal male reproductive system.
2. Identify data to be collected when assessing a male patient with a reproductive system disorder.
3. Discuss commonly performed diagnostic tests and procedures and the nursing implications of each.
4. Identify common therapeutic measures used to treat disorders of the male reproductive system and the nursing implications of each.
5. For selected disorders of the male reproductive system, explain the pathophysiology, signs and symptoms, complications, medical diagnosis, and medical treatment.
6. Assist in developing a nursing care plan for a male patient with a reproductive system disorder.

LEARNING ACTIVITIES

A. Match the description or definition in the numbered column with the most appropriate term in the lettered column. Some terms may be used more than once, and some may not be used.

(968) **1.** __________ Male reproductive organs

(969) **2.** __________ Extends from the bladder to the urinary meatus at the end of the penis

(969) **3.** __________ The production of sperm

A. Testosterone
B. Cryptorchidism
C. Urethra
D. Prostate
E. Vasectomy
F. Spermatogenesis
G. Testes

Continued next page

(969) **4.** __________ Produces alkaline liquid that enhances motility and fertility of sperm

(970) **5.** __________ A hormone necessary for the development of male reproductive organs, descent of the testicles, and production of sperm

(969) **6.** __________ Provides outflow for semen during ejaculation

(970) **7.** __________ The condition when the testes are located outside a dependent scrotal position

(989) **8.** __________ The surgical removal of a portion of the vas deferens

B. Complete the statement in the numbered column with the most appropriate term in the lettered column. Some terms may be used more than once, and some may not be used.

(983) **1.** In erectile dysfunction, arteriosclerosis compromises the ability to fill with blood because of __________.

(984) **2.** Two conditions in patients with diabetes mellitus that may contribute to erectile dysfunction are autonomic neuropathy and __________.

(984) **3.** The type of erectile dysfunction likely to be caused by high blood pressure and its treatment is __________.

(984) **4.** Two treatments that may be recommended for treating erectile dysfunction in the diabetic patient are papaverine self-injection and __________.

(985) **5.** Spinal cord injuries that are more complete and more likely to cause erectile dysfunction are those injuries that are __________.

(985) **6.** The most likely drugs to cause erectile dysfunction are __________.

A. Failure to store
B. Low
C. Antihypertensives
D. Failure to initiate
E. Atherosclerosis
F. Penile implant
G. Vascular surgery
H. High
I. Failure to fill
J. Antibiotics
K. Reduced blood flow
L. Neurologic disorders

Student Name____

C. Match the description or definition in the numbered column with the most appropriate term in the lettered column. Some terms may be used more than once, and some may not be used.

(978) **1.** __________ May be caused by infections, trauma, or the reflux of urine from the urethra through the vas deferens

(987) **2.** __________ May be caused by injury to the penis, sickle cell crisis, medications, or papaverine injections

(978) **3.** __________ Inflammation of one of both testes

(978) **4.** __________ Enlargement of the prostate

(987) **5.** __________ The development of a hard, nonelastic fibrous tissue just under the skin of the penis

(976) **6.** __________ Inflammation of the prostate gland

(978) **7.** __________ Treated with bed rest, ice packs, sitz baths, analgesics, antibiotics, anti-inflammatory drugs, and scrotal support

(978) **8.** __________ Signs and symptoms include fever, tenderness, and scrotal redness

(987) **9.** __________ A prolonged penile erection not related to sexual desire

A. Orchitis
B. Prostatitis
C. Phimosis
D. Epididymitis
E. Benign prostatic hypertrophy
F. Priapism
G. Prostate cancer
H. Peyronie's disease

Continued next page

(976) **10.** ________ Signs and symptoms may include dysuria, frequency, hematuria, and foul-smelling urine

(976) **11.** ________ Treated with antibiotics, analgesics, and sitz baths

(987) **12.** ________ Treatment may include topical or oral medications with vitamin E, oral aminobenzoic acid, radiation, surgical removal, and colchicine

(978) **13.** ________ Signs and symptoms include painful scrotal edema, nausea, vomiting, chills, and fever

(978) **14.** ________ Signs and symptoms include decreasing size and force of the urinary stream, urine retention, and postvoid dribbling

D. Match the nursing diagnosis for the patient with testicular cancer in the numbered column with the "related to" statement in the lettered column.

(991) **1.** ________ Anxiety

(991) **2.** ________ Acute pain

(991) **3.** ________ Impaired urinary elimination

(991) **4.** ________ Risk for injury

(991) **5.** ________ Constipation

(991) **6.** ________ Situational low self-esteem

A. Diminished or absent peristalsis caused by bowel manipulation during surgery
B. Effects of anesthesia and abdominal surgery
C. Diagnosis of cancer or anticipation of side effects of treatments
D. Potential loss of reproductive capacity
E. Surgical incision
F. Surgery

E. On palpation, the epididymis should feel soft and tender. List two characteristics that should *not* normally be present that may indicate epididymitis.

(978) **1.** ______________________________

(978) **2.** ______________________________

Student Name ____________________

F. List four indications for surgical intervention for benign prostatic hypertrophy.

(979) **1.** ____________________

(979) **2.** ____________________

(979) **3.** ____________________

(979) **4.** ____________________

G. Match the nursing interventions for a patient with a prostatectomy in the numbered column with the nursing diagnosis in the lettered column. Some terms may be used more than once, and some may not be used.

(982) **1.** ________ Reposition tubing

(982) **2.** ________ Inspect urine, dressing, and wound drainage for excess bleeding

(982) **3.** ________ Use isotonic fluid for irrigation

(982) **4.** ________ Use strict aseptic technique

(982) **5.** ________ Maintain urine flow

(982) **6.** ________ Assess bladder for distention

(982) **7.** ________ Watch for water intoxication

(982) **8.** ________ Keep closed urinary drainage systems intact

(982) **9.** ________ Monitor output

(982) **10.** ________ Monitor for signs of infection (temperature above 38.3° C; purulent wound drainage, and confusion)

(982) **11.** ________ Give antispasmodics and analgesics

(982) **12.** ________ Irrigate bladder as ordered; notify surgeon if you cannot clear tubing

A. Risk for fluid volume deficit related to hemorrhage

B. Pain related to tissue trauma and bladder spasms

C. Risk for infection related to invasive procedures of the urinary tract or catheterization

D. Risk for injury related to obstructed urine flow, excessive absorption of irrigating fluids, or trauma to urinary sphincter

H. List three parts of the male reproductive system that may be affected by cancer.

(990) **1.** ______________________________

(992) **2.** ______________________________

(990) **3.** ______________________________

I. Match characteristics of drugs used to treat disorders of the male reproductive system in the numbered column with the names of the drugs in the lettered column.

(992) **1.** __________ Prevents production of testosterone

(992) **2.** __________ Inhibits release of pituitary hormones necessary for hormone production

(992) **3.** __________ Luteinizing hormone–releasing hormone (LHRH) analogues

(986) **4.** __________ Prescribed for failure to fill or store

(986) **5.** __________ Used for intracavernosal injection; vasodilator

(986) **6.** __________ Recommended for failure to initiate, fill, or store; injected into erectile chambers

(986) **7.** __________ Replacement for low hormone levels in men

(980) **8.** __________ Decreases testosterone level; used to treat prostate cancer

A. Megestrol acetate (Megace)
B. Testosterone
C. Flutamide (Eulexin)
D. Papaverine
E. Sildenafil (Viagra)
F. Alprostadil
G. Estrogen products (Tace)

Student Name____

J. Using Figure 46-1 below, label the parts of the male reproductive system (A–Q) from the terms (1–17) below.

(969)

1. __________ Sacrum

2. __________ Corpus cavernosum penis

3. __________ Scrotum

4. __________ Seminal vesicle

5. __________ Prostatic urethra

6. __________ Glans penis

7. __________ Bladder

8. __________ Vas deferens

9. __________ Membranous urethra

10. __________ Rectum

11. __________ Pubic symphysis

12. __________ Testis

13. __________ Prostate gland

14. __________ Penile urethra

15. __________ Epididymis

16. __________ Bulbourethral (Cowper's) glands

17. __________ Ejaculatory duct

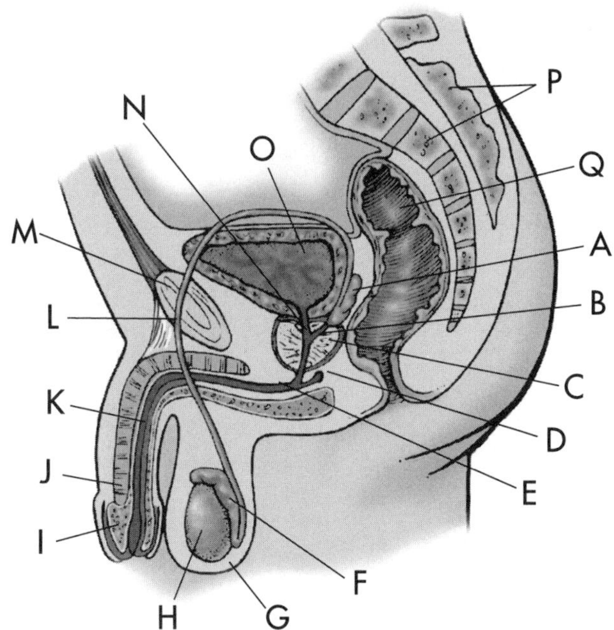

MULTIPLE-CHOICE QUESTIONS

K. Choose the most appropriate answer.

(971) **1.** Three normal changes that may occur in the male reproductive system due to aging are decreased testosterone, a longer refractory period between erections, and:

1. penile discharge.
2. pain with urination.
3. slower arousal.
4. descent of testicles.

(984) **2.** Erectile dysfunction related to diabetes mellitus may be caused by:

1. spinal cord injury.
2. atherosclerosis.
3. low hormone levels.
4. medication side effects.

(984) **3.** Autonomic neuropathy inhibits muscle relaxation of lacunar spaces of the erectile chambers, which may make:

1. the patient anxious about performance.
2. adequate filling of the penis with blood for an erection impossible.
3. testosterone levels abnormally low.
4. the patient sterile.

(972) **4.** Assessment of the male reproductive system may be difficult for some patients because of health beliefs, need for privacy, or:

1. chronic disease.
2. advanced age.
3. defensiveness about sexual behavior.
4. lack of sexual experience.

(989) **5.** Which test is done to document sterilization after a vasectomy?

1. ultrasonography
2. radiography
3. analysis of semen
4. CBC

(972) **6.** Past medical history helps link the current problem with previous problems and should include information about injuries, diseases, surgeries, allergies, treatments, and:

1. marital status.
2. medications.
3. age and health of siblings.
4. age and health of parents.

(972) **7.** The health history should include information about medications the patient is taking because they may:

1. impair his cognitive abilities.
2. make him too tired to participate in the assessment.
3. impair sexual function.
4. impair gastrointestinal function.

(973) **8.** Physical examination of the male reproductive system can be accomplished by inspection and:

1. palpation.
2. auscultation.
3. percussion.
4. radiography.

Student Name____

(986) **9.** Which drug may cause hypotension and cardiovascular collapse in patients who are taking nitrate vasodilators?

1. alprostadil
2. sildenafil
3. papaverine
4. testosterone

(979) **10.** Transurethral prostatectomy is the most common surgical procedure for benign prostatic hypertrophy. In this procedure:

1. the prostate is approached through the bladder by way of a low abdominal incision.
2. portions of the prostate are cut away through a resectoscope inserted into the urethra.
3. access to the prostate is gained through an incision between the scrotum and the anus.
4. the surgeon reaches the prostate through a low abdominal incision and opens the front of the prostate.

(979) **11.** Nursing diagnoses for the patient with benign prostatic hypertrophy include:

1. Risk for infection.
2. Sexual dysfunction.
3. Pain.
4. Impaired urinary elimination.

(981) **12.** Nursing diagnoses for the patient immediately following a prostatectomy may include:

1. Anxiety.
2. Fear.
3. Risk for deficient fluid volume.
4. Impaired urinary elimination.

(972) **13.** Men with low sperm counts should be evaluated for:

1. congestive heart failure.
2. anemia.
3. thyroid function.
4. renal disease.

(978) **14.** A common obstructive symptom of BPH is:

1. urine retention.
2. nocturia.
3. frequency.
4. hematuria.

(981) **15.** The reason for bladder irrigation following a TURP procedure is to:

1. decrease postoperative infection.
2. prevent constriction of the urethra.
3. prevent clot formation and obstruction.
4. decrease urinary retention.

(983) **16.** If postvoid dribbling occurs in a postoperative TURP patient after removal of the catheter, the nurse should:

1. suggest perineal exercises.
2. recommend biofeedback.
3. use isotonic fluid for irrigation.
4. monitor for signs of infection.

(985) **17.** Drugs most likely to interfere with erection are:

1. antihistamines.
2. decongestants.
3. analgesics.
4. antihypertensives.

(992) **18.** Persistent or rising PSA levels in a patient who has undergone treatment for prostatic cancer indicate:

1. a normal change that occurs with aging.
2. an increased risk of infertility.
3. obstruction of the urethra.
4. advancing or recurrent tumor growth.

(986) **19.** Which herb is thought to increase penile blood flow?

1. ginkgo biloba
2. kava kava
3. garlic
4. oil of jasmine

(990) **20.** Which is an established risk factor for testicular cancer?

1. multiple sex partners
2. African-American
3. Caucasian
4. high-fat diet

(992) **21.** A cancer that occurs much more frequently among African-American men than Caucasians is:

1. prostatic cancer
2. testicular cancer
3. penile cancer
4. bladder cancer

(978) **22.** Which is a common symptom of epididymitis?

1. hypertension
2. fever
3. swelling
4. fatigue

(981) **23.** Which intervention is appropriate for a patient with BPH?

1. Place a rolled towel across the patient's thighs to elevate the scrotum and reduce pain.
2. Provide bed rest, scrotal support, and local heat to the scrotum.
3. Drink at least eight glasses of fluids throughout the day.
4. Eat a high-protein diet.

(983) **24.** Postprostatectomy teaching includes which of the following?

1. Consume a low-fiber diet.
2. Limit fluids to four glasses of fluid each day.
3. Use an ice bag and scrotal support.
4. If semen is ejaculated into the bladder, it is not harmful.

(979) **25.** Which extract relieves urinary symptoms associated with BPH and reduces serum levels of PSA?

1. Siberian ginseng
2. ginkgo biloba
3. saw palmetto
4. oil of rose

(978) **26.** Which is an irritative symptom of BPH?

1. nocturia
2. urine retention
3. postvoid dribbling
4. decreased force of urinary stream

(981) **27.** Which drugs may cause urinary retention in patients with BPH?

1. smooth muscle relaxants
2. cold remedies
3. analgesics
4. antacids

Student Name____

(983) **28.** Which drug is given to a postprostatectomy patient to relieve bladder spasms?

1. propantheline bromide (Pro-Banthine)
2. tansudosin (Flomax)
3. phenoxybenzamine HCl (Dibenzyline)
4. finasteride (Proscar)

(979) **29.** Which herb can give a false negative result in patients with prostate cancer?

1. garlic
2. ginkgo biloba
3. Siberian ginseng
4. saw palmetto

CHAPTER 47

Student Name ______________________________

Sexually Transmitted Diseases

Answer Key: Textbook page references are provided as a guide for answering these questions. A complete answer key was provided for your instructor.

OBJECTIVES

1. List infectious diseases classified as sexually transmitted diseases.
2. Explain the importance of the nurse's approach when dealing with patients who have sexually transmitted diseases.
3. Discuss tests used to diagnose sexually transmitted diseases and the nursing considerations associated with each.
4. Explain why sexually transmitted diseases must be reported to the health department.
5. For selected sexually transmitted diseases, describe the pathophysiology, signs and symptoms, complications, and medical treatment.
6. Design a teaching plan on the prevention of sexually transmitted diseases.
7. List nursing considerations when a patient is on drug therapy for a sexually transmitted disease.
8. Identify data to be collected when assessing a patient with a sexually transmitted disease.
9. Assist in developing a nursing care plan for a patient with a sexually transmitted disease.

LEARNING ACTIVITIES

A. Match the definition in the numbered column with the most appropriate term in the lettered column.

(1001)	**1.** ________	A papule that breaks down into a painless ulcer at the site of entry of the organism that causes syphilis	A. Vaginitis B. Cautery C. Opportunistic infection D. HIV-positive E. Sexually transmitted disease F. Pelvic inflammatory disease G. Chancre H. Latent
(1009)	**2.** ________	A condition in which the blood has antibodies for the human immunodeficiency virus (HIV), meaning that the individual has been infected with this virus	
(996)	**3.** ________	Inflammation of the vagina; can be caused by chemical irritants, dryness, estrogen deficiency, or infectious agents	
(996)	**4.** ________	An infection of the ovaries, fallopian tubes, and pelvic area	
(1001)	**5.** ________	Dormant; during this period of a disease, there are no signs or symptoms of the disease	
(1004)	**6.** ________	Burning of tissue	

Continued next page

Student Name ______________________________

(995) **7.** __________ A disease that can be transmitted by intimate genital, oral, or rectal contact

(1004) **8.** __________ An infection caused by an organism that usually does not cause a disease but becomes pathogenic when body defenses are impaired

B. Complete the statement in the numbered column with the most appropriate term in the lettered column. Some terms may be used more than once, and some terms may not be used.

(1000) **1.** Erythromycin ophthalmic ointment may be ordered for the newborn to prevent eye infection caused by exposure during delivery to __________.

(1001) **2.** A papule that becomes a painless red ulcer within a week is a sign of __________.

(1000) **3.** Treatment with ceftriaxone sodium (Rocephin) and doxycycline calcium (Vibramycin) or tetracycline cures most cases of __________.

(1001) **4.** __________ is caused by the spirochete *Treponema pallidum.*

(1000) **5.** If gonorrhea is untreated, the bacteria remain in the body and the person remains __________.

(1001) **6.** When the chancre disappears, patients may erroneously assume that they are cured; in fact, the infecting organism has moved into the __________.

(1000) **7.** Infections that may lead to heart tissue and joint damage are complications of ________.

A. Gonorrhea
B. Sterility
C. Infectious
D. Digestive system
E. Syphilis
F. *Chlamydia trachomatis*
G. Blood
H. Gonococci
I. Liver failure
J. *Treponema pallidum*

Continued next page

(1001) **8.** Pustules, fever, sore throat, and generalized aching are symptoms that occur in the secondary stage of __________.

(1001) **9.** A typical lesion, called a chancre, is the first sign of __________.

(1000) **10.** If untreated, gonorrhea can cause __________.

C. Complete the statement in the numbered column with the most appropriate term in the lettered column. Some terms may be used more than once, and some terms may not be used.

(998) **1.** An eye ointment that is recommended because it is effective against chlamydia as well as gonorrhea is __________.

(1003) **2.** An antibody test called the Herp-Check can detect active __________.

(1004) **3.** In females, venereal warts generally appear around the urethra, vagina, cervix, perineum, anal canal, and __________.

(996) **4.** A penile discharge that is initially thin and then creamy, accompanied by painful urination, is a symptom of __________.

(1003) **5.** A sexually transmitted disease caused by a protozoan parasite is __________.

(1003) **6.** The drug of choice for the treatment of trichomoniasis is __________.

(996) **7.** If left untreated, chlamydia can result in __________.

(1003) **8.** A condition caused by the human papillomavirus is __________.

(1003) **9.** There is an increased risk of cervical cancer in women who have __________.

A. *Chlamydia trachomatis*
B. Condylomata acuminata (venereal warts)
C. Erythromycin
D. Metronidazole (Flagyl)
E. Heart damage
F. Vulva
G. Acyclovir (Zovirax)
H. Trichomoniasis
I. Tetracycline
J. Herpes
K. Sterility

Continued next page

Student Name____

(1004) **10.** The drug of choice for treatment of bacterial vaginosis is __________.

(1004) **11.** Premature births and miscarriages are high among women with __________.

(996) **12.** The most common STD in the United States is __________.

D. Complete the statement in the numbered column with the most appropriate term in the lettered column. Some terms may be used more than once, and some terms may not be used.

(1002) **1.** Complaints of flulike symptoms and a burning sensation during urination are symptoms of __________.

(1004) **2.** Venereal warts are generally pink and soft with a __________ mass.

(1003) **3.** A frothy, yellowish vaginal discharge with a foul odor is a sign of __________.

(1004) **4.** Males with venereal warts generally present with warts on the glans, foreskin, urethral opening, penile shaft, or __________.

(996) **5.** __________ is transmitted by contact with the mucous membranes in the mouth, eyes, urethra, vagina, or rectum.

(1002) **6.** Painful, itchy sores on or around the genitals that appear about 2 to 20 days after infection are symptoms of __________.

(1004) **7.** Genital irritation; a thin, gray discharge; and a fishy odor are symptoms of __________.

(996) **8.** Newborns with eye damage or infant pneumonia may have been exposed to __________.

(1003) **9.** A drug that is helpful in minimizing symptoms of herpes simplex virus is the antiviral drug called __________.

(1004) **10.** Cryosurgery may be used in the treatment of __________.

A. Acyclovir (Zovirax)
B. Trichomoniasis
C. *Chlamydia trachomatis*
D. Strawberrylike
E. Metronidazole (Flagyl)
F. Herpes
G. Bacterial vaginosis
H. Cauliflowerlike
I. Anus
J. Condylomata acuminata (venereal warts)
K. Scrotum

E. List the key points to teach the patient with an STD regarding the following topics.

(1009) **1.** Antibiotic therapy:

(1009) **2.** Transmission of STDs:

(1009) **3.** Sexual activity:

(1010) **4.** Condoms:

(1009) **5.** Patients with HSV infections:

Student Name____

MULTIPLE-CHOICE QUESTIONS

F. Choose the most appropriate answer.

(995) **1.** What percentage of all cases of sexually transmitted diseases involve people between the ages of 15 and 30?

1. 55% 2. 65%
3. 75% 4. 85%

(995) **2.** Serologic tests for STDs are designed to detect infectious diseases by measuring:

1. white blood cells.
2. red blood cells.
3. clotting factors.
4. antigens or antibodies.

(996) **3.** Patients with gonococcal, chlamydial, herpes simplex, trichomonal, or yeast infections often have:

1. vaginal or penile discharge.
2. increased temperature or tachycardia.
3. generalized infection and rash.
4. mouth sores and pharyngitis.

(996) **4.** When collecting a sample of vaginal discharge for culture and sensitivity tests, the person collecting the sample always wears:

1. goggles. 2. a mask.
3. gloves. 4. a gown.

(1000) **5.** If males have a whitish or greenish colored discharge from the penis and complain of a burning sensation during urination, this is suggestive of:

1. HSV infection.
2. chlamydia.
3. gonorrhea.
4. syphilis.

(1000) **6.** Female patients with gonorrhea are apt to have vaginal discharge, a burning sensation during urination, abnormal menstruation, and:

1. dyspnea.
2. abdominal pain.
3. hypotension.
4. edema.

(1001) **7.** Paralysis, mental illness, blindness, and heart disease may occur as complications of:

1. HSV infection.
2. cervicitis.
3. syphilis.
4. gonorrhea.

(1001) **8.** Two screening tests for syphilis include the rapid plasma reagin (RPR) and the:

1. VDRL. 2. RBC.
3. WBC. 4. BUN.

(1001) **9.** The treatment of choice for syphilis is:

1. doxycycline calcium (Vibramycin).
2. erythromycin.
3. tetracycline.
4. penicillin.

(1002) **10.** After completing treatment for primary or secondary syphilis, the patient is advised not to engage in sexual activity for:

1. 5 days. 2. 2 weeks.
3. 1 month. 4. 6 months.

(1000) **11.** If untreated, sterility, prostatitis in males, and pelvic inflammatory disease in females may result from:

1. syphilis.
2. gonorrhea.
3. HSV infection.
4. venereal warts.

(1004) **12.** HIV gradually destroys cells that are essential for resisting pathogens; these cells are called:

1. neutrophils.
2. T4 cells.
3. B cells.
4. eosinophils.

(1005) **13.** HIV is passed from person to person primarily through:

1. air droplet contact.
2. hand-to-mouth contact.
3. sexual contact.
4. mouth-to-mouth contact.

(1005) **14.** Early symptoms of HIV include fever, night sweats, anorexia, and:

1. edema.
2. hypertension.
3. confusion.
4. weight loss.

(1005) **15.** The most common infection seen in persons with AIDS is:

1. herpes zoster.
2. dermatitis.
3. *Pneumocystis carinii* pneumonia.
4. Kaposi's sarcoma.

(1005) **16.** For many women, one of the first symptoms of HIV infection is:

1. vaginal candidiasis.
2. burning on urination.
3. menstrual irregularities.
4. hemorrhoids.

(1005) **17.** A type of skin cancer that has dramatically increased as a result of AIDS is:

1. *Pneumocystis carinii* pneumonia.
2. melanoma.
3. Kaposi's sarcoma.
4. venereal warts.

(1001) **18.** Which STD can be transmitted through the placenta, causing an infant to be born with the disease?

1. HSV infection
2. gonorrhea
3. syphilis
4. chlamydia

(1005) **19.** The medical treatment of HIV infection includes the use of zidovudine (AZT, Retrovir), which is given to:

1. cure AIDS.
2. prevent transmission to sexual partners.
3. treat the secondary infections of AIDS.
4. slow the progress of AIDS.

(998) **20.** Drugs such as pentamidine isethionate (Pentam) and trimethoprim and sulfamethoxazole (Septra) are used to:

1. prevent or treat opportunistic infections.
2. slow the progress of AIDS.
3. decrease the dermatitis associated with AIDS.
4. increase T4 lymphocytes.

(1006) **21.** The best way to prevent transmission of HIV is to:

1. use condoms during all sexual contact.
2. wash hands thoroughly following contact with HIV-positive persons.
3. abstain from sexual contact.
4. get plenty of rest and eat a nutritious diet.

Student Name____

(1006) **22.** The risk of transmission of HIV during sexual contact is reduced by the use of:

1. antibiotics.
2. condoms.
3. antiviral agents.
4. birth control pills.

(996) **23.** It is recommended that gloves be worn when handling body fluids of:

1. HIV-positive patients.
2. infectious patients.
3. patients with opportunistic infections.
4. all patients.

(996) **24.** Confirmed cases of HIV must be reported to the:

1. hospital administrator.
2. family.
3. local health department.
4. legal guardian.

(1006) **25.** A discussion of sexual behavior can be awkward for the nurse and the patient; before nurses can deal with patients' sexuality, they must:

1. present the patient with written information.
2. be aware of their own values.
3. ask the patient to demonstrate understanding of the material presented by stating information in their own words.
4. check the patient's chart to see whether the patient has a sexually transmitted disease.

(1006) **26.** With a sexually transmitted disease, common reasons that patients give for seeking medical care include pain, fever, lesions, or genital:

1. itching. 2. edema.
3. bleeding. 4. discharge.

(1007) **27.** Specimens collected during a pelvic exam are handled as:

1. infective material.
2. clean specimens.
3. sterile specimens.
4. chemically unstable material.

(1008) **28.** A nursing diagnosis related to lesions or inflammation for patients with STDs is:

1. Anxiety.
2. Acute pain.
3. Situational low self-esteem.
4. Ineffective management of therapeutic regimen: noncompliance.

(1008) **29.** A nursing diagnosis related to possible effects of STD or partner reaction to the STD is:

1. Pain.
2. Risk for injury.
3. Anxiety.
4. Impaired tissue integrity.

(1009) **30.** A nursing diagnosis related to stigma associated with STDs, shame, or anger is:

1. Sexual dysfuntion.
2. Pain.
3. Ineffective coping.
4. Risk for infection.

(1008) **31.** Some STDs are painless, but patients may have pain associated with oral lesions, rectal lesions, or:

1. vaginal bleeding.
2. genital edema.
3. nerve irritation.
4. pelvic infection.

(1008) **32.** Untreated STDs can lead to serious complications such as PID and:

1. edema.
2. sterility.
3. shock.
4. kidney failure.

(1008) **33.** The patient with AIDS is at high risk for secondary infections because of impaired:

1. skin integrity.
2. immune function.
3. physical mobility.
4. airway clearance.

(1006) **34.** Patients with AIDS pose a threat to their:

1. children.
2. parents.
3. sexual partners.
4. siblings.

(1008) **35.** Emergency drugs for possible hypersensitivity reactions that need to be kept on hand when administering drug therapy to patients with STDs include epinephrine, corticosteroids, and:

1. acyclovir (Zovirax).
2. diphenhydramine hydrochloride (Benadryl).
3. didanosine (Videx).
4. pentamidine isethionate (Pentam).

(1009) **36.** Chronic infections, such as HSV and HIV, require permanent alterations in:

1. sexual activity.
2. menstrual periods.
3. skin integrity.
4. nutritional habits.

(1009) **37.** Related to altered sexuality patterns in patients with STDs, the nurse explains that sexual dysfunction may be overcome by dealing with:

1. the adverse drug effects of prescribed medications.
2. the need for more exercise.
3. emotional reactions to the disease.
4. conflict resolution.

(1009) **38.** The nurse can show support for patients with HIV infection by being sensitive, courteous, and:

1. reassuring.
2. positive.
3. nonjudgmental.
4. authoritarian.

(1003) **39.** Females with HSV infections are advised to have annual Papanicolaou smears because they are at increased risk of:

1. pyelonephritis.
2. cervical cancer.
3. kidney failure.
4. AIDS.

(1002) **40.** The herpes simplex virus can be transmitted by sexual contact, but unlike most other STDs, it can also be transmitted by:

1. air droplets.
2. mouth-to-nose contact.
3. fecal contamination.
4. hand contact.

(1003) **41.** Most STDs respond to antimicrobial agents, but an exception is HSV, which is minimized but not cured by:

1. penicillin G.
2. tetracycline hydrochloride (Achromycin).
3. acyclovir (Zovirax).
4. metronidazole (Flagyl).

Student Name____

(996) **42.** Which STD has symptoms similar to those of gonorrhea?

1. syphilis
2. herpes simplex
3. chlamydia
4. HIV

(996) **43.** In order to identify and treat infected individuals so that transmission of the STD can be slowed, partners may be notified and confirmed cases of certain STDs must be reported to the:

1. United States Department of Health.
2. hospital administrator.
3. Department of Public Safety.
4. local public health department.

(996) **44.** In children between the ages of 10 and 14, more than 10,000 cases of which STD are reported annually?

1. herpes simplex
2. chlamydia
3. gonorrhea
4. trichomoniasis

(996) **45.** Gonorrhea can be found in the pharynx. urethra, uterus, and:

1. kidney.
2. rectum.
3. heart.
4. lungs.

(996) **46.** Gonorrhea is transmitted most often by:

1. infected mothers to newborn infants.
2. direct sexual contact.
3. skin lacerations of medical personnel.
4. toilet seats and doorknobs.

(1001) **47.** The heart, joints, skin, and meninges may become involved with which systemic infection?

1. gonorrhea
2. syphilis
3. chlamydia
4. genital warts

(1000) **48.** The treatment for gonorrhea is a single dose of IM ceftriaxone sodium (Rocephin), followed by 7 days of oral:

1. erythromycin
2. vibramycin
3. penicillin
4. tetracycline

(1004) **49.** As the number of T4 lymphocytes decreases, that patient becomes increasingly susceptible to:

1. myelosuppression.
2. anemia.
3. thrombocytopenia.
4. opportunistic infections.

(1005) **50.** Which is the most common cancer seen with HIV infection?

1. Kaposi's sarcoma
2. *Pneumocystis carinii*
3. herpes zoster
4. liver cancer

(1003) **51.** What is the correct treatment for a patient who has trichomoniasis?

1. penicillin
2. metronidazole (Flagyl)
3. acyclovir
4. tetracycline

(1003) **52.** An antiviral drug used to treat symptoms of herpes simplex is:

1. acyclovir
2. erythromycin
3. penicillin
4. metronidazole (Flagyl)

Student Name ____________________

CHAPTER 48

Skin Disorders

Answer Key: Textbook page references are provided as a guide for answering these questions. A complete answer key was provided for your instructor.

OBJECTIVES

1. Describe the structure and functions of the skin.
2. List the components of the nursing assessment of the skin.
3. Define terms used to describe the skin and skin lesions.
4. Explain the tests and procedures used to diagnose skin disorders.
5. Explain the nurse's responsibilities regarding the tests and procedures for diagnosing skin disorders.
6. Explain the therapeutic benefits and nursing considerations for patients who receive dressings, soaks and wet wraps, phototherapy, and drug therapy for skin problems.
7. For selected skin disorders, describe the pathophysiology, signs and symptoms, diagnostic tests, and medical treatment.
8. Assist in developing a nursing care plan for the patient with a skin disorder.

LEARNING ACTIVITIES

A. Complete the statement in the numbered column with the most appropriate term in the lettered column. Some terms may be used more than once, and some terms may not be used.

(1012) **1.** The secretion that coats the skin and creates an oily barrier that holds in water is __________.

(1013) **2.** A result of the thinning of the skin layers and degeneration of elastin fibers is __________.

(1012) **3.** The dissipation of heat from the skin occurs through __________.

A. Evaporation
B. Vasoconstriction
C. Sebum
D. Melanin
E. Vasodilation
F. Sweat
G. Lymph
H. Wrinkling
I. Pressure
J. Lactic acid
K. Vitamin D

Continued next page

(1012) **4.** Sweating helps cool the body through __________.

(1013) **5.** Ultraviolet rays in sunlight activate a substance in the skin that is eventually converted into __________.

(1012) **6.** Heat is retained through __________.

(1012) **7.** Two skin secretions are sweat and __________.

(1013) **8.** The skin is endowed with sensory receptors for touch, pain, temperature, and __________.

B. Match the description or definition in the numbered column with the most appropriate term in the lettered column. Some terms may be used more than once, and some terms may not be used.

(1017) **1.** __________ A test used to diagnose viral skin infections

(1017) **2.** __________ Used to diagnose fungal infections by studying a skin specimen

(1017) **3.** __________ An examination in which the patient's skin is inspected under a black light in a darkened room

(1017) **4.** __________ A test used to identify allergens in which common irritants are applied to the skin

(1017) **5.** __________ The removal of skin for microscopic examination

(1017) **6.** __________ A specimen no deeper than the dermis is obtained with a scalpel

(1017) **7.** __________ The type of biopsy in which a circular tool cuts around the lesion, which is then lifted and severed

A. Biopsy
B. Aspiration biopsy
C. Scalpel
D. Punch biopsy
E. Gram's stain
F. Wood's light
G. Shave biopsy
H. Surgical excision
I. Tzanck's smear
J. Patch testing
K. Scabies scraping
L. KOH examination

Continued next page

Student Name____

(1017) **8.** __________ The type of biopsy indicated for deep specimens in which sutures are required to close the site

(1017) **9.** __________ Used to detect mites

C. Complete the statement in the numbered column with the most appropriate term in the lettered column. Some terms may be used more than once, and some terms may not be used.

(1026) **1.** Candidiasis infections, which are manifested as red lesions with white plaques, are found on the __________.

(1026) **2.** Lesions with scaly patches and raised borders along with pruritus are associated with __________ infections.

(1026) **3.** Three common sites for candidiasis include the mouth, skin, and __________.

(1026) **4.** Moist red lesions associated with *Candida albicans* are seen on the __________.

(1026) **5.** A yeast infection caused by *C. albicans* is known as __________.

(1026) **6.** Oral candidiasis is treated with __________.

(1026) **7.** In addition to the mouth and vagina, an area that is susceptible to candidiasis, owing to the constant moisture found there, is __________.

A. Nystatin
B. Vagina
C. Candidiasis
D. Toes
E. Mucous membranes
F. Skin
G. Ostomy site
H. Tinea
I. Scalp

D. Complete the statement in the numbered column with the most appropriate term in the lettered column. Some terms may be used more than once, and some terms may not be used.

(1027) **1.** Mild cases of acne respond well to antibiotics and __________.

(1027) **2.** A serious adverse effect of isotretinoin (Accutane) is __________.

(1027) **3.** A drug that may be prescribed to counteract the effects of androgenic hormones in acne patients is __________.

(1027) **4.** Comedones (whiteheads and blackheads), pustules, and cysts are characteristics of __________.

(1027) **5.** Two oral antibiotics that are frequently given for acne are tetracycline and __________.

(1027) **6.** If acne is severe and unresponsive to antibiotics, __________ may be prescribed.

(1027) **7.** A condition in which androgenic hormones cause increased sebum production and bacteria proliferate, causing hair follicles to block and become inflamed, is __________.

A. Herpes simplex
B. Acne
C. Tretinoin (Retin-A)
D. Acyclovir (Zovirax)
E. Estrogen
F. Erythromycin
G. Fetal deformities
H. Isotretinoin (Accutane)

E. Complete the statement in the numbered column with the most appropriate term in the lettered column. Some terms may be used more than once, and some terms may not be used.

(1029) **1.** The elderly are especially susceptible to complications from herpes zoster, which include __________ involvement.

(1028) **2.** The first symptoms of herpes zoster are heightened sensitivity along a nerve pathway, pain, and __________.

A. Genitalia
B. Crusts
C. Ophthalmic
D. Acyclovir (Zovirax)
E. Itching
F. Burow's solution
G. Ulcers
H. Immunosuppressed
I. HSV
J. Shingles
K. Tzanck smear

Continued next page

Student Name____

(1027) **3.** Cold sores or fever blisters are oral lesions caused by __________.

(1027) **4.** Sites most often infected by the herpes simplex virus (HSV) are the nose, lips, cheeks, ears, and __________.

(1029) **5.** Wet dressings soaked in __________ may be used to treat lesions associated with herpes zoster.

(1029) **6.** Diagnostic tests used to identify herpes infections include __________.

(1028) **7.** When the mucous membranes are affected with the varicella-zoster virus, __________ develop.

(1029) **8.** Herpes simplex infections are treated with __________.

(1028) **9.** Herpes zoster is commonly called __________.

(1028) **10.** When the skin is infected with the varicella-zoster virus, __________ form.

(1029) **11.** __________ patients are especially susceptible to herpes infections and must be protected from infected people.

F. Complete the statement in the numbered column with the most appropriate term in the lettered column.

(1031) **1.** Squamous cell carcinomas, unlike basal cell carcinomas, grow rapidly and __________.

(1029) **2.** A chronic autoimmune condition in which bullae (blisters) develop on the face, back, chest, groin, and umbilicus is __________.

(1031) **3.** The use of liquid nitrogen to freeze and destroy lesions found in actinic keratosis is called __________.

(1031) **4.** A condition with painless, nodular lesions that have a pearly appearance is __________.

(1031) **5.** The drug of choice for actinic keratosis is __________.

(1032) **6.** __________ arises from the pigment-producing cells in the skin.

(1031) **7.** Scaly ulcers or raised lesions are characteristics of __________.

A. Melanoma
B. Sun
C. Kaposi's sarcoma
D. Metastasize
E. Squamous cell carcinoma
F. Cryotherapy
G. Actinic keratosis
H. 5-FU
I. Pemphigus
J. Tobacco
K. Tissue destruction
L. Basal cell carcinoma
M. Cutaneous T-cell lymphoma
N. Melanoma

Continued next page

(1031) **8.** Although basal cell carcinomas grow slowly and rarely metastasize, they should be removed because they can cause local __________.

(1032) **9.** A malignancy of the blood vessels with red, blue, or purple macules is __________.

(1031) **10.** A precancerous lesion most often found on areas exposed to sunlight, such as the face, neck, forearms, and backs of the hands, is __________.

(1030) **11.** A condition in which malignant T cells migrate to the skin is __________.

(1031) **12.** Skin cancers are most common among light-skinned people who have had repeated __________ exposure.

(1031) **13.** Squamous cell carcinomas are usually caused by overuse of alcohol and __________.

(1032) **14.** Mohs' surgery is used to determine margins of malignancy for ________.

G. Match the description in the numbered column with the type of burn in the lettered column.

(1033) **1.** __________ Pink to red and painful, like a sunburn

(1033) **2.** __________ Large, thick-walled blisters or edema

(1033) **3.** __________ Burned tissue lacking sensation

(1033) **4.** __________ Burn affecting only the epidermis

(1033) **5.** __________ Burn involving the epidermis, dermis, and underlying tissues, including fat, muscle, and bone

(1033) **6.** __________ Burned tissue is painful and sensitive to cold air

(1033) **7.** __________ Blistered and weepy and pale to red or pink

A. Superficial burn
B. Superficial partial-thickness burn
C. Deep partial-thickness burn
D. Full-thickness burns

Continued next page

Student Name ____________________

(1033) **8.** __________ Dry, leathery, and sometimes red, white, brown, or black

(1033) **9.** __________ Weeping, cherry-red, exposed dermis

(1033) **10.** __________ A severe sunburn

H. Match the example or description in the numbered column with the appropriate type of lesion in the lettered column.

(1015) **1.** __________ Freckle, petechia, hypopigmentation

(1015) **2.** __________ Mole, wart

(1015) **3.** __________ Herpes simplex, herpes zoster

(1015) **4.** __________ Acne, impetigo

(1015) **5.** __________ Vitiligo

(1015) **6.** __________ Psoriasis

(1015) **7.** __________ Fibroma, xanthone

(1015) **8.** __________ Allergic response, insect bite

A. Plaque
B. Wheal
C. Papule
D. Patch
E. Pustule
F. Vesicle
G. Nodule
H. Macule

I. Match the actions and uses in the numbered column with the appropriate drug classification in the lettered column.

(1020) **1.** __________ Interfere with viral replication

(1021) **2.** __________ Decrease proliferation of epidermal cells in psoriasis

(1020) **3.** __________ Reduce inflammation in various skin disorders

(1021) **4.** __________ Kill parasites and their eggs; used to treat pediculosis (lice) and scabies (mite) infestations

A. Keratolytics (for example, coal tar)
B. Topical anti-infectives (for example, bacitracin)
C. Antiviral agents (for example, acyclovir)
D. Photosensitivity drugs (for example, methoxsalen)
E. Topical antifungal agents (for example, nystatin)
F. Topical anti-inflammatories (for example, hydrocortisone)
G. Vitamin A derivatives (for example, tretinoin[Retin-A])
H. Pediculicides and scabicides (for example, lindane [Kwell])
I. Antipsoriatics (for example, anthralin)

Continued next page

(1020) **5.** __________ Dissolve keratin and slow bacterial growth; used to treat acne and psoriasis

(1020) **6.** __________ Effective against fungi; used to treat fungal infections

(1021) **7.** __________ Used to treat psoriasis

(1020) **8.** __________ Destroy microorganisms; used to treat skin infections

(1021) **9.** __________ Reduce formation of comedones; increase mitosis of epithelial cells; used to treat acne

J. Match the signs or symptoms in the numbered column with the most appropriate skin infection in the lettered column.

(1030) **1.** __________ Vesicle or pustule that ruptures, leaving a thick crust

(1030) **2.** __________ Inflamed hair follicles with white pustules

(1030) **3.** __________ Inflamed skin and subcutaneous tissue with deep, inflamed nodules

(1030) **4.** __________ Clustered, interconnected furuncles

(1030) **5.** __________ Local tenderness and redness at first, then malaise, chills, and fever; site becomes more erythematous; nodules and vesicles may form; vesicles may rupture, releasing purulent material

(1030) **6.** __________ At first, small shiny lesions; they enlarge and become rough

A. Furuncle (boil)
B. Verruca (wart)
C. Folliculitis
D. Cellulitis
E. Impetigo
F. Carbuncle

Student Name____

K. Match the appearance characteristics in the numbered column with the sensations experienced (in the same depth of burn) in the lettered column.

(1033) **1.** __________ Large, thick-walled blisters covering extensive areas (vesiculation); edema; mottled red base; broken epidermis; wet, shiny, weeping surface

(1033) **2.** __________ Variable, for example, deep red, black, white, brown; dry surface; edema; fat exposed; tissue disrupted

(1033) **3.** __________ Mild to severe erythema; skin blanches with pressure

A. Little pain; insensate
B. Painful; sensitive to cold air
C. Painful; hyperesthetic; tingling; pain eased by cooling

L. Match the definition or description in the numbered column with the most appropriate term in the lettered column. Some terms may be used more than once, and some terms may not be used.

(1037) **1.** __________ Removal of necrotic tissue from a wound

(1037) **2.** __________ Covering a wound with skin

(1038) **3.** __________ Can be reduced by use of pressure dressings in early stages of care

(1037) **4.** __________ May be accomplished by mechanical means, surgical excision, or enzymes

(1038) **5.** __________ Can be reduced by use of custom-fitted garments that apply continuous pressure 24 hours a day

A. Skin grafting
B. Scarring
C. Débridement

M. Match the conditions treated with plastic surgery in the numbered column with the type of surgery used in the lettered column. Answers may be used more than once.

(1041)	**1.**	__________	Birthmarks	A.	Aesthetic surgery
				B.	Reconstructive surgery
(1040)	**2.**	__________	Excess tissue around the eyes		
(1041)	**3.**	__________	Developmental defects		
(1041)	**4.**	__________	Disfiguring scars		
(1040)	**5.**	__________	Receding chin		
(1040)	**6.**	__________	Facial wrinkles		

N. Match the signs and symptoms of skin infestations in the numbered column with infestation in the lettered column.

(1031)	**1.**	__________	Thin, red lines on skin; itching	A.	Lice
				B.	Scabies
(1031)	**2.**	__________	Itching of hairy areas of body (head, pubis); nits (eggs) seen as tiny white particles attached to hair shafts		

Student Name____

O. Using Figure 48-1, label the parts of the skin (A–L) from the terms provided (1–12).

(1013)

1. __________ Sebaceous gland

2. __________ Hair follicle

3. __________ Dermis

4. __________ Hair shaft

5. __________ Stratum corneum

6. __________ Artery

7. __________ Vein

8. __________ Epidermis

9. __________ Arrector pili muscle

10. __________ Sweat gland

11. __________ Adipose tissue

12. __________ Subcutaneous tissue

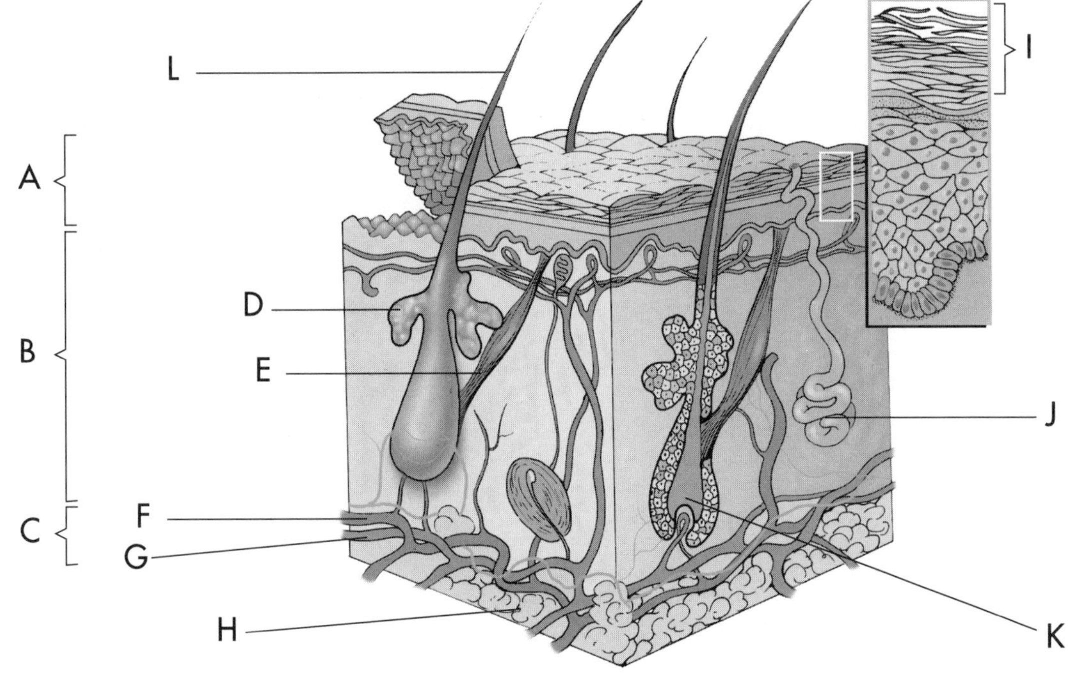

MULTIPLE-CHOICE QUESTIONS

P. Choose the most appropriate answer.

(1012) **1.** Epidermal cells produce a dark pigment that helps determine the color of the skin called:

1. sebum.
2. cerumen.
3. keratin.
4. melanin.

(1014) **2.** Scalp hair thins in older men and women, but there may be an increase in:

1. elastic tissue.
2. facial hair.
3. subcutaneous tissue.
4. capillaries.

(1014) **3.** Nevi (moles) are carefully inspected for pigmentation, ulcerations, changes in surrounding skin, and:

1. vascular irregularities.
2. amount of edema.
3. amount of pus.
4. irregularities in shape.

(1015) **4.** When assessing capillary refill, after applying pressure to cause blanching and then releasing the pressure, the nurse should observe that the color returns to normal within:

1. 1–2 minutes.
2. 3–5 seconds.
3. 30–40 seconds.
4. 50–60 seconds.

(1017) **5.** The potassium hydroxide (KOH) examination is used in combination with a culture to diagnose infections of the skin, hair, or nails that are:

1. viral.
2. bacterial.
3. caused by parasites.
4. fungal.

(1018) **6.** When a skin biopsy is scheduled, the physician may advise the patient to avoid which drug before the procedure to reduce bleeding?

1. diphenhydramine
2. tetracycline
3. aminophylline
4. aspirin

(1015) **7.** Two assessments of the fingernails and toenails include noting the color of the nail bed and assessing:

1. capillary refill.
2. edema.
3. hemorrhage.
4. mobility.

(1019) **8.** The most common nursing diagnosis for patients with pruritus is Risk for:

1. poisoning.
2. impaired skin integrity.
3. injury.
4. infection.

(1028) **9.** Nursing diagnoses for the patient with atopic dermatitis may include Impaired skin integrity related to:

1. decreased resistance to infection.
2. self-care practices.
3. hypertension.
4. excessive dryness.

(1023) **10.** Patients with any break in the skin are at risk for infection because the break in the skin presents a portal for:

1. pathogens. 2. blood.
3. pus. 4. sweat.

(1023) **11.** The assessment of patients with seborrheic dermatitis includes inspecting affected areas for:

1. bleeding and exudate.
2. edema and redness.
3. scales and crusts.
4. yellow skin and ascites.

(1026) **12.** An important risk factor for developing candidiasis is:

1. hypertension.
2. antibiotic therapy.
3. emotional stress.
4. tachycardia.

(1026) **13.** A primary nursing diagnosis for patients with candidiasis is:

1. Activity intolerance.
2. Altered oral mucous membrane.
3. Decreased cardiac output.
4. Self-care deficit.

Student Name____

(1027) **14.** Acne is caused by:

1. eating too much chocolate.
2. fatty foods.
3. poor hygiene.
4. blocked hair follicles.

(1028) **15.** The nurse advises the patient with shingles that the condition is communicable to people who have never been exposed to:

1. measles. 2. pertussis.
3. chickenpox. 4. polio.

(1032) **16.** The most serious form of skin cancer is:

1. basal cell carcinoma.
2. melanoma.
3. squamous cell carcinoma.
4. cutaneous T-cell lymphoma.

(1034) **17.** Following a burn injury, plasma leaks into the tissue due to increased capillary:

1. constriction.
2. dilation.
3. production.
4. permeability.

(1034) **18.** After a burn injury, shifts in fluids and electrolytes cause local edema and a decrease in:

1. respiratory rate.
2. CNS stimulation.
3. cardiac output.
4. red blood cell production.

(1034) **19.** The shift of plasma proteins from the capillaries may result in:

1. hypoproteinemia.
2. increased blood volume.
3. dehydration.
4. increased urine output.

(1034) **20.** A complication of untreated fluid shifts in burn patients is:

1. hypovolemic shock.
2. kidney failure.
3. pneumonia.
4. convulsions.

(1019) **21.** A type of therapy used in the treatment of psoriasis, vitiligo, and chronic eczema is:

1. phototherapy.
2. soaks.
3. wet wraps.
4. débridement.

(1043) **22.** Vitamin A is essential for:

1. blood clotting.
2. bone formation.
3. wound healing.
4. healthy skin.

(1022) **23.** Food allergies can cause:

1. scabies.
2. basal cell carcinoma.
3. psoriasis.
4. atopic dermatitis.

(1019) **24.** Which is a topical herbal preparation used as an emollient?

1. aloe
2. angelica
3. balm of Gilead
4. ginseng

(1022) **25.** When a patient has an allergic dermatitis, the nurse should be sure to assess for the topical use of:

1. corticosteroids.
2. aloe.
3. antihistamines.
4. emollients.

(1027) **26.** Acne lesions develop when there is:

1. increased fatty food intake.
2. increased sebum production.
3. increased chocolate intake.
4. poor hygiene.

(1024) **27.** Which drug, used to remove heavy scales in patients with psoriasis, can stain normal skin and hair?

1. tazarotene (Tazorac)
2. glucocorticoids
3. methotrexate sodium
4. anthralin (Anthra-Derm)

(1025) **28.** Cornstarch should not be used in patients with intertrigo because it supports the growth of:

1. *S. aureus.*
2. *C. albicans.*
3. *E. coli.*
4. streptococci.

(1025) **29.** Which skin disorder, characterized by irritation and redness in body folds, is fairly common among patients in long-term care facilities?

1. intertrigo
2. impetigo
3. candidiasis
4. pemphigus

(1031) **30.** Who is at greatest risk for skin cancer?

1. Caucasians
2. African-Americans
3. Native Americans
4. Hispanics

(1019) **31.** A prominent symptom of psoriasis, dermatitis, eczema, and insect bites is:

1. fever.
2. pain.
3. pruritus.
4. edema.

(1033) **32.** If one arm and one leg are burned, what is the estimated burn size, according to the rule of nines?

1. 18%
2. 27%
3. 36%
4. 54%

(1034) **33.** The burn patient is at great risk for:

1. hyperthermia.
2. paralysis.
3. edema.
4. infection.

CHAPTER 49

Student Name ______________________________

Eye and Vision Disorders

Answer Key: Textbook page references are provided as a guide for answering these questions. A complete answer key was provided for your instructor.

OBJECTIVES

1. Identify the data to be collected in the nursing assessment of the eye and vision.
2. Identify the nursing responsibilities for patients having diagnostic tests or procedures to diagnose eye disorders.
3. List measures to reduce the risk of eye injuries.
4. Describe the nursing care of patients who require common therapeutic measures for eye disorders: irrigation, application of ophthalmic drugs, and surgery.
5. Describe the pathophysiology, signs and symptoms, diagnosis, and treatment of selected eye conditions.
6. Assist in developing a nursing care plan for the patient with an eye disorder.

LEARNING ACTIVITIES

A. Match the definition in the numbered column with the most appropriate term in the lettered column. Some terms may be used more than once, and some terms may not be used.

(1051) **1.** __________ Measurement of pressure, such as intraocular pressure

(1054) **2.** __________ Agent that causes the pupil to constrict

(1062) **3.** __________ Error of refraction caused by uneven curvature of the cornea or lens; causes visual distortion

A. Keratitis
B. Myopia
C. Tonometry
D. Cycloplegic
E. Conjunctivitis
F. Refraction
G. Presbyopia
H. Miotic
I. Mydriatic
J. Cataract
K. Astigmatism
L. Hyperopia

Continued next page

(1060) **4.** __________ Inflammation of the cornea

(1060) **5.** __________ Inflammation of the membrane lining the eyelids and the eyeball

(1063) **6.** __________ Clouding or opacity of the normally transparent lens within the eye; causes blurred vision and objects to take on a yellowish hue

(1065) **7.** __________ Agent that paralyzes the ciliary muscle so that the eye does not accommodate

(1050) **8.** __________ Bending of light rays

(1062) **9.** __________ Farsightedness

(1062) **10.** __________ Agent that causes the pupil to dilate

(1062) **11.** __________ Visual impairment associated with older age

(1062) **12.** __________ Nearsightedness

B. Complete the statement in the numbered column with the most appropriate term in the lettered column. Some terms may be used more than once, and some terms may not be used.

(1066) **1.** Timolol maleate (Timoptic) is a __________ used in glaucoma to lower intraocular pressure.

(1066) **2.** A condition in which intraocular pressure is increased above normal is __________.

(1066) **3.** Excess pressure impairs blood flow to the optic nerve, resulting in __________.

(1066) **4.** __________ vision is lost first in glaucoma.

(1066) **5.** Patients with glaucoma have fields of vision that gradually narrow until the patient has __________.

(1067) **6.** A type of acute glaucoma that is considered a medical emergency is __________.

(1067) **7.** Acetazolamide (Diamox) is a __________ used to reduce intraocular pressure by decreasing the production of aqueous humor.

(1067) **8.** __________ is a surgical procedure for glaucoma.

A. Open-angle glaucoma
B. Iridotomy
C. Intraocular pressure
D. Miotic(s)
E. Carbonic anhydrase inhibitor (s)
F. Peripheral
G. Phacoemulsification
H. Glaucoma
I. Angle-closure glaucoma
J. Tunnel vision
K. Trabeculoplasty
L. Vision impairment
M. Beta blocker(s)

Continued next page

Student Name ______________________________

(1066) **9.** Chronic glaucoma is also called __________.

(1066) **10.** A person who can only see a small circle, as if looking through a tube, has __________.

(1067) **11.** A surgical procedure in which a window is cut to permit aqueous humor to flow through the pupil normally in patients with angle-closure glaucoma is __________.

(1067) **12.** Open-angle glaucoma is usually treated first with drug therapy, which includes __________.

(1066) **13.** Adrenergics decrease __________ by decreasing the formation of aqueous humor and increasing its outflow.

C. Complete the statement in the numbered column with the most appropriate term in the lettered column. Some terms may be used more than once, and some terms may not be used.

(1063) **1.** Cataracts may be congenital, degenerative, or __________.

(1063) **2.** The __________ is located behind the iris and changes shape to focus on images of various sizes.

(1063) **3.** When the lens becomes opaque so that it is no longer transparent, it is called a __________.

(1064) **4.** Once the lens is removed, the eye is said to be __________.

(1063) **5.** __________ cataracts are more common with aging but may occur earlier in patients with diabetes or Down syndrome.

(1064) **6.** Signs and symptoms of cataracts include cloudy vision, seeing spots, and __________.

(1064) **7.** The only treatment for cataracts is removal of the __________.

(1064) **8.** The surgical treatment for cataracts that involves the use of sound waves to break up the lens is __________.

A. Floaters
B. Cataract
C. Degenerative
D. Phacoemulsification
E. Traumatic
F. Lithotripsy
G. Aphakic
H. Lens
I. Cornea

D. Match the actions and uses in the numbered column with the most appropriate drug classification in the lettered column.

(1055) **1.** ________ Used to treat or prevent eye infections

(1055) **2.** ________ Used to treat herpes simplex keratitis

(1054) **3.** ________ Dilate pupil; used in open-angle glaucoma; decreases corneal congestion; controls hemorrhage

(1055) **4.** ________ Prevent redness and swelling caused by inflammation due to causes other than bacterial infection

(1067) **5.** ________ Used primarily to treat glaucoma

(1055) **6.** ________ Block sensation in external eye for tonometry; used in removal of sutures or foreign bodies and in some surgical procedures

(1055) **7.** ________ Are effective against some fungal infections of eye

(1054) **8.** ________ Dilate pupil; used before eye exams and for uveitis; decrease lacrimal gland secretion

A. Antibiotics
B. Anti-inflammatory agents
C. Miotics
D. Antifungals
E. Topical anesthetics
F. Antimuscarinics
G. Antivirals
H. Sympathomimetics

Student Name____

E. Match the most appropriate nursing diagnosis for patients following eye surgery in the numbered column with the "related to" statement in the lettered column.

(1055) **1.** __________ Pain

(1055) **2.** __________ Anxiety

(1055) **3.** __________ Risk for injury

(1055) **4.** __________ Disturbed sensory perception (visual)

A. Tissue trauma
B. Temporary vision impairment
C. Disease process, trauma to the eye, patching
D. Pressure or trauma

F. List interventions in the following areas that relate to lighting for patients who are partially sighted.

(1058) **1.** Glare: ____

(1058) **2.** Windows: ____

(1058) **3.** Floors: ____

(1058) **4.** Furniture color: ____

(1058) **5.** Light switches, handrails, and steps: ____

(1058) **6.** Dishes and cups: ____

G. Match the actions and uses in the numbered column with the classification of drugs used to treat glaucoma in the lettered column. Some classifications may be used more than once, and some classifications may not be used.

(1067) **1.** __________ Treatment of acute glaucoma

(1066) **2.** __________ Initial treatment of acute and chronic glaucoma

(1067) **3.** __________ Preoperative preparation for glaucoma surgery

(1066) **4.** __________ Treatment of chronic glaucoma

A. Direct-acting miotics
B. Osmotic diuretics
C. Beta-adrenergic blockers

H. List the associated eye/vision disorders that may be present in patients with the following diseases.

(1048) **1.** Diabetes

a. Elevated blood glucose: ____________________

b. Changes in retina due to diabetes: ____________________

(1048) **2.** Neurologic disorders (brain tumors, head injuries, and strokes)

a. Vision: ____________________

b. Movement of eyes: ____________________

(1048) **3.** Thyroid disease

a. Hyperthyroidism: ____________________

(1048) **4.** Hypertension

a. Changes in blood vessels of the eye: ____________________

Student Name____

I. Using Figure 49-2, label the internal structures of the eye (A–O) by using the terms (1–15) below.

(1046)

1. __________ Anterior chamber

2. __________ Choroid

3. __________ Ciliary muscle

4. __________ Conjunctiva

5. __________ Cornea

6. __________ Fovea

7. __________ Iris

8. __________ Lens

9. __________ Optic disk

10. __________ Vitreous body

11. __________ Optic nerve

12. __________ Posterior chamber

13. __________ Pupil

14. __________ Retina

15. __________ Sclera

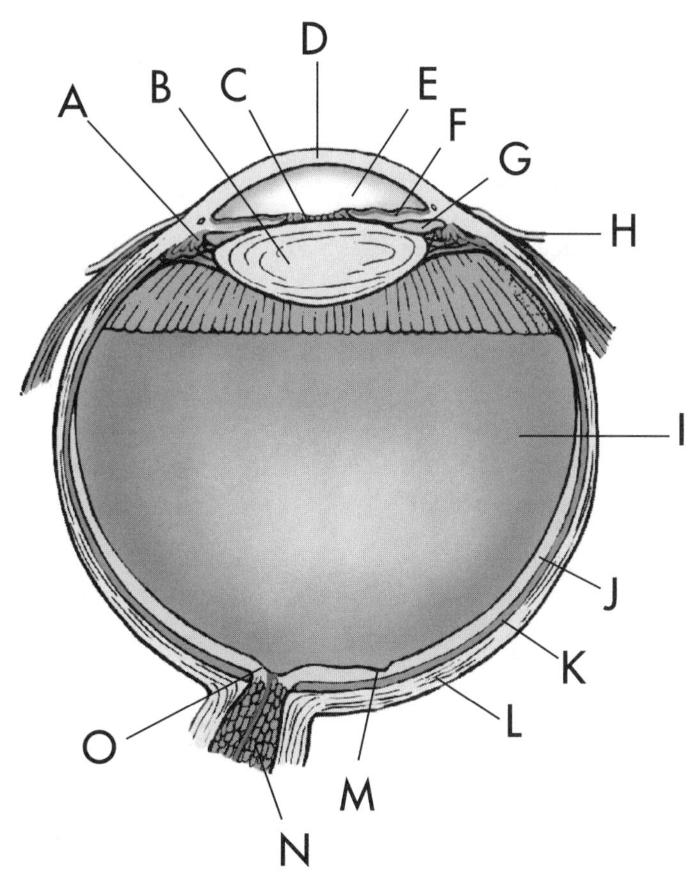

MULTIPLE-CHOICE QUESTIONS

J. Choose the most appropriate answer.

(1047) **1.** As light enters the eye, it passes through the transparent cornea, aqueous humor, lens, and:

1. conjunctiva.
2. sclera.
3. vitreous humor.
4. lacrimal glands.

(1048) **2.** Dark spots that are actually bits of debris in the vitreous are called:

1. flashes.
2. floaters.
3. blind spots.
4. cataracts.

(1048) **3.** Sensitivity to light is called:

1. photophobia.
2. presbyopia.
3. myopia.
4. hyperopia.

(1048) **4.** When the nurse is performing a physical assessment of the eyes, the lids should cover the eyeball completely when closed; when the eyes are open, the lower lid should be at the level of the:

1. conjunctiva.
2. retina.
3. iris.
4. lacrimal gland.

(1048) **5.** The eyeball is inspected for color and moisture; the sclera should be clear:

1. yellow.
2. white.
3. gray.
4. black.

(1048) **6.** Excessive redness of the sclera may be an indication of:

1. hypertension.
2. exophthalmos.
3. liver dysfunction.
4. irritation.

(1048) **7.** The pupils are assessed for size, equality, and reaction to light; pupils that are unequal, dilated, or do not respond to light suggest:

1. diabetes.
2. liver dysfunction.
3. inflammation.
4. neurologic problems.

(1048) **8.** When you ask the patient to focus on the nurse's finger as it is moved slowly toward the patient's nose, the nurse is assessing:

1. presbyopia.
2. astigmatism.
3. accommodation.
4. refraction.

(1049) **9.** Visual acuity is commonly tested using:

1. the Snellen chart.
2. the accommodation test.
3. tonometry.
4. fluorescein angiography.

(1053) **10.** If more than one eye medication is being given, the nurse must wait how long between each medication?

1. 60 seconds
2. 5 minutes
3. 30 minutes
4. 60 minutes

(1053) **11.** Eye surgery may involve surgical incisions, the application of cold probes (cryotherapy), or the use of:

1. tonometry.
2. lasers.
3. fluorescein angiography.
4. topical dyes.

Student Name____

(1055) **12.** Following eye surgery, the patient is usually positioned:

1. flat in bed.
2. prone.
3. side-lying on affected side.
4. with the head of bed elevated.

(1056) **13.** An important aspect of the care of postoperative eye patients is to prevent increased:

1. blood pressure.
2. cardiac output.
3. intraocular pressure.
4. ocular movement.

(1056) **14.** Nurses can teach people how to care for their eyes in order to protect their vision; it is important to tell people that:

1. burning sensations in the eyes should be reported to the physician.
2. watching too much television or sitting too close to the television injures the eyes.
3. eating foods with high vitamin A content will improve vision.
4. eyes need to be rinsed regularly to protect vision.

(1064) **15.** The most frequently performed eye operation in the United States is:

1. enucleation.
2. cryotherapy.
3. cataract extraction.
4. vitrectomy.

(1066) **16.** Medications prescribed after cataract surgery usually include antibiotics and:

1. miotics.
2. antihistamines.
3. anticholinergics.
4. corticosteroids.

(1066) **17.** One of the leading causes of blindness in the United States is:

1. conjunctivitis.
2. retinal detachment.
3. glaucoma.
4. cataracts.

(1048) **18.** Which drug has a side effect of vision disturbances?

1. digitalis
2. Lasix
3. aspirin
4. Synthroid

(1049) **19.** A vision of 20/30 on the Snellen chart means that the person can:

1. read at 20 feet from the left eye and 30 feet from the right eye what a normal person reads at these distances.
2. read at 20 feet what a normal person reads at 50 feet.
3. read at 30 feet what a person with normal vision reads at 20 feet.
4. read at 20 feet what a person with normal vision reads at 30 feet.

(1051) **20.** The measurement of pressure in the anterior chamber of the eye is:

1. refraction.
2. electroretinopathy.
3. tonometry.
4. angiography.

(1056) **21.** The nurse should treat nausea promptly in the postoperative eye surgery patient in order to prevent:

1. infection.
2. hemorrhage.
3. pain.
4. increased intraocular drainage.

(1057) **22.** Which is correct patient teaching regarding protection of health of the eyes?

1. Watching too much TV or sitting too close to the TV can injure your eyes.
2. Gently cleanse your eyelids each time you wash your face.
3. Eating foods that contain large amounts of vitamin A improves vision.
4. Eyes need to be rinsed on a daily basis.

(1057) **23.** A primary consideration of the patient with visual impairment is:

1. safety.
2. infection.
3. hemorrhage.
4. nutrition.

(1059) **24.** Which is an inflammation of hair follicles along the eyelid?

1. hordeolum (stye).
2. conjunctivitis.
3. blepharitis.
4. keratitis.

(1065) **25.** Corticosteroids are contraindicated in patients with conjunctivitis caused by:

1. herpes.
2. bacteria.
3. fungi.
4. chlamydia.

(1065) **26.** Which drug is ordered before surgery for a patient with cataracts?

1. an analgesic
2. a mydriatic
3. a miotic
4. an anticholinergic

(1066) **27.** Following cataract surgery, the nurse should:

1. advised the patient to sleep on the affected side.
2. have the patient cough and deep-breathe.
3. administer mydriatic agents.
4. keep the bed low.

(1066) **28.** In which eye condition is peripheral vision lost first?.

1. cataracts
2. macular degeneration
3. conjunctivitis
4. glaucoma

(1067) **29.** Which drugs are used to treat glaucoma?

1. anticholinergics (Atropine)
2. carbonic anhydrase inhibitors (Diamox)
3. anticonvulsants (Dilantin)
4. antihistamines (Benadryl)

(1070) **30.** Which herb should not be taken by patients with glaucoma because it increases intraocular pressure?

1. kava kava
2. garlic
3. ginkgo
4. Ephedra

(1070) **31.** A patient sees floaters and states: "It is like a curtain has come down across my vision." This is a symptom of:

1. cataracts.
2. macular degeneration.
3. retinal detachment.
4. glaucoma.

(1071) **32.** Which antioxidant is believed to slow the progression of age-related macular degeneration?

1. vitamin A
2. vitamin B
3. vitamin E
4. vitamin K

CHAPTER 50

Student Name ______________________________

Ear and Hearing Disorders

Answer Key: Textbook page references are provided as a guide for answering these questions. A complete answer key was provided for your instructor.

OBJECTIVES

1. Identify the data to be collected when assessing a patient with a disorder affecting the ear, hearing, or balance.
2. Describe the tests and procedures used to diagnose disorders of the ear, hearing, or balance.
3. Explain the nursing considerations for each of the tests and procedures.
4. Explain the nursing involvement for patients receiving common therapeutic measures for disorders of the ear, hearing, or balance.
5. For selected disorders, describe the pathophysiology, signs and symptoms, complications, and medical or surgical treatment.
6. Assist in the development of a nursing care plan for a patient with a disorder of the ear, hearing, or balance.
7. Identify measures the nurse can take to reduce the risk of hearing impairment and to detect problems early.

LEARNING ACTIVITIES

A. Match the definition in the numbered column with the most appropriate term in the lettered column.

(1075) **1.** __________ Eardrum; the structure that separates the external and middle portions of the ear

(1078) **2.** __________ Waxy secretion in the external auditory canal; earwax

A. Tinnitus
B. Cerumen
C. Tympanic membrane
D. Otalgia
E. Equilibrium
F. Vertigo
G. Dizziness
H. Ototoxic
I. Presbycusis

Continued next page

(1077) **3.** __________ Ringing, buzzing, or roaring noise in the ears

(1075) **4.** __________ State of balance needed for walking, standing, and sitting

(1084) **5.** __________ Feeling of unsteadiness

(1084) **6.** __________ Sensation that one's body or one's surroundings are rotating

(1077) **7.** __________ Capable of injuring the eighth cranial nerve (acoustic) of hearing and balance structures in the ear

(1077) **8.** __________ Pain in the ear

(1077) **9.** __________ Hearing loss associated with age

B. Complete the statement in the numbered column with the most appropriate term in the lettered column. Some terms may be used more than once, and some terms may not be used.

(1084) **1.** Patients who hear better in noisy settings than in quiet settings have __________.

(1084) **2.** Congenital problems, noise trauma, aging, Meniere's syndrome, ototoxicity, diabetes, and syphilis may all be causes of __________.

(1084) **3.** A condition in which the stapes in the middle ear does not vibrate is __________.

(1084) **4.** A hearing loss that results from interference with the transmission of sound waves from the external or middle ear to the inner ear is __________.

(1084) **5.** A disturbance of the neural structures in the inner ear or the nerve pathways to the brain results in __________.

(1084) **6.** Patients who either cannot perceive or cannot interpret sounds that are heard may have __________.

A. Mixed hearing loss
B. Otosclerosis
C. Cochlear implants
D. Nerve deafness
E. Central hearing loss
F. Otitis media
G. Cholesteatoma
H. Sensorineural hearing loss
I. Hearing aids
J. Labyrinthitis
K. Conductive hearing loss
L. Bone conduction
M. Stapedectomy

Continued next page

Student Name____

(1084) **7.** Otosclerosis can be treated surgically with a procedure called __________.

(1084) **8.** A combination of conductive and sensorineural losses results in __________.

(1084) **9.** Persons with conductive hearing losses are usually helped to hear by __________.

(1084) **10.** Otosclerosis or obstruction of the external canal or eustachian tube may cause __________.

(1084) **11.** Sensorineural hearing loss is sometimes called __________.

(1084) **12.** Problems in the central nervous system may result in __________.

(1084) **13.** Patients who can hear sounds but have difficulty understanding speech have __________.

C. Complete the statement in the numbered column with the most appropriate term in the lettered column. Some terms may be use more than once, and some terms may not be used.

(1087) **1.** A type of ear infection that usually develops with colds is __________.

(1088) **2.** The treatment for cholesteatoma is __________.

(1087) **3.** Soreness, headache, malaise, and an elevated white blood cell count are symptoms of __________.

(1087) **4.** If fluid remains in the middle ear following serous otitis media, __________ may develop.

(1088) **5.** A very serious infection that can lead to a brain abscess, meningitis, or paralysis of the facial muscles is __________.

(1087) **6.** The usual treatment for acute otitis media is __________.

(1087) **7.** An infection of the middle ear is called __________.

(1088) **8.** A condition that produces disturbances in both hearing and balance is __________.

A. Meningitis
B. Mastoiditis
C. Serous otitis media
D. Labyrinthitis
E. Anti-inflammatories
F. Chronic otitis media
G. Eustachian tube
H. Acute otitis media
I. Electronystagmography
J. Antibiotics
K. Adhesive otitis media
L. Cholesteatoma
M. Chemotherapy
N. Surgical removal
O. Myringotomy
P. Otitis media

Continued next page

(1087) **9.** An ear infection characterized by hearing loss and continuous or intermittent drainage is __________.

(1087) **10.** Sterile fluid accumulates behind the tympanic membrane in __________.

(1087) **11.** __________ is the creation of a small opening in the tympanic membrane to reduce pressure and allow fluid to drain.

(1087) **12.** __________ is characterized by thickening and scarring in the middle ear structures.

(1087) **13.** An ear infection that is usually not painful but in which the eardrum is usually perforated is __________.

(1087) **14.** Edema in acute otitis media leads to blockage of the __________.

(1088) **15.** Inflammation of the labyrinth is __________.

(1088) **16.** A growth in the middle ear is called a __________.

D. Complete the statement in the numbered column with the most appropriate term in the lettered column. Some terms may be used more than once, and some terms may not be used.

(1087) **1.** "Swimmer's ear" is also called __________.

(1087) **2.** An inflamed area in the external auditory canal caused by infection of a hair follicle is a __________.

(1087) **3.** Treatment of otitis externa includes topical corticosteroids and __________.

(1087) **4.** Infection or inflammation of the lining of the external ear canal is called __________.

(1087) **5.** Swimming can lead to otitis by washing out protective __________.

(1087) **6.** Drainage in otitis externa may be blood-tinged or __________.

(1087) **7.** __________ may be caused by scratching or cleaning the ear with sharp objects.

(1087) **8.** When infection is present in otitis externa, it is frequently caused by streptococci or __________.

(1087) **9.** The most characteristic symptom of otitis externa is __________.

A. Cerumen
B. Pain
C. Furuncle
D. Otitis media
E. Purulent
F. Antibiotics
G. Redness
H. Staphylococci
I. Otitis externa

Student Name____

E. Match the nursing intervention in the numbered column with the nursing diagnoses in the lettered column for patients who have had ear surgery.

A. Risk for infection
B. Disturbed sensory perception
C. Pain
D. Risk for injury

(1084) **1.** __________ Encourage patient to avoid crowds and people with colds for several weeks

(1084) **2.** __________ Position patient and offer massage to promote relaxation

(1084) **3.** __________ Instruct patient not to shampoo for 2 weeks

(1084) **4.** __________ Advise patient to avoid straining; give stool softeners as ordered

(1084) **5.** __________ Have patient keep ear canal dry for 2 to 4 weeks

(1084) **6.** __________ Advise patient to avoid nose blowing, coughing, and sneezing

(1084) **7.** __________ Raise side rails and leave bed in low position

(1084) **8.** __________ Encourage balanced diet with adequate protein and vitamin C

(1084) **9.** __________ Assist with ambulation as long as dizziness occurs

F. Match the ototoxic drugs in the numbered column with their most appropriate classification in the lettered column. Some classifications may be used more than once, and some classifications may not be used.

(1092)	**1.**	________	Aspirin	A. Antiarrhythmics
				B. Antibiotics
(1092)	**2.**	________	Erythromycin estolate (Ilosone)	C. Antineoplastics
				D. Antihistamines
				E. Anti-inflammatories/analgesics
(1092)	**3.**	________	Furosemide (Lasix)	F. Diuretics
(1092)	**4.**	________	Cisplatin (Platinol-AQ)	
(1092)	**5.**	________	Indomethacin (Indocin)	
(1092)	**6.**	________	Streptomycin sulfate	
(1092)	**7.**	________	Ethacrynic acid (Edecrin)	
(1092)	**8.**	________	Quinidine	
(1092)	**9.**	________	Tetracycline	
(1092)	**10.**	________	Bleomycin (Blenoxane)	

G. List four potential complications of surgery for Meniere's disease.

(1090) **1.** ________________________________

(1090) **2.** ________________________________

(1090) **3.** ________________________________

(1090) **4.** ________________________________

H. List four signs and symptoms of ototoxicity.

(1092) **1.** ________________ *(1092)* **3.** ________________

(1092) **2.** ________________ *(1092)* **4.** ________________

Student Name____

I. Using Figure 50-1 below, label all parts of the ear (A–L) from the terms (1–12) below.

(1076)

1. __________ Auricle

2. __________ External ear

3. __________ Stapes

4. __________ Malleus

5. __________ Inner ear

6. __________ Semicircular canals

7. __________ Eustachian tube

8. __________ Incus

9. __________ Middle ear

10. __________ Tympanic membrane

11. __________ Cochlea

12. __________ Ear canal

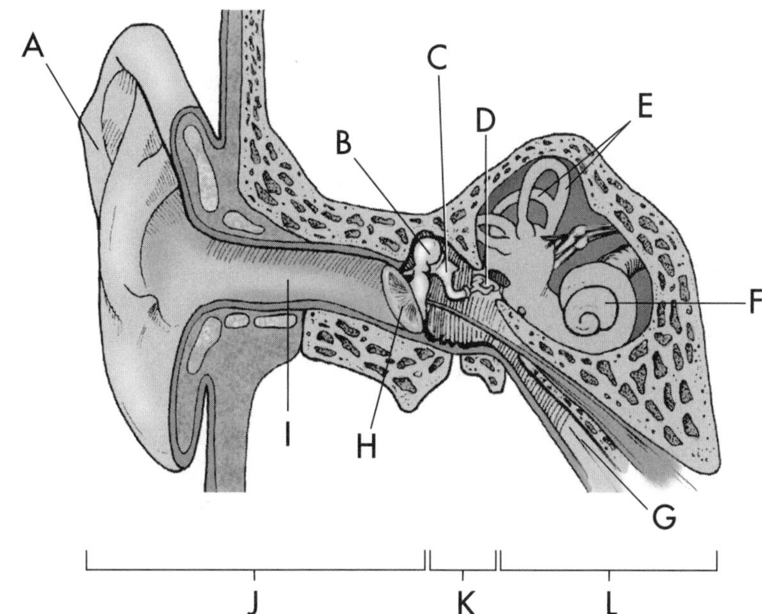

J. Trace the sound waves from the external ear to the brain in Figure 50-3 below. Label each step (A–F) from the terms (1–6) below.

(1077)

1. __________ Oval window

2. __________ Sensory receptors in inner ear

3. __________ External canal

4. __________ Tympanic membrane

5. __________ Acoustic nerve

6. __________ Malleus, incus, and stapes

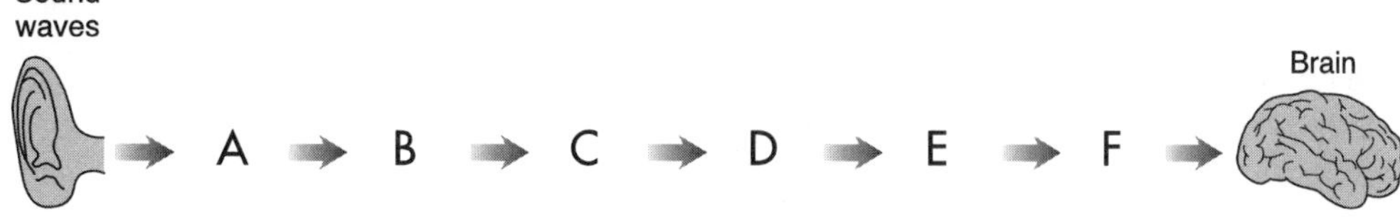

MULTIPLE-CHOICE QUESTIONS

K. Choose the most appropriate answer.

(1077) **1.** Age-related changes in the inner ear affect sensitivity to sound, understanding of speech, and:

1. balance.
2. infection.
3. cerumen production.
4. blood pressure.

(1077) **2.** The type of hearing loss usually associated with aging is:

1. otitis media.
2. cholesteatoma.
3. otosclerosis.
4. presbycusis.

(1077) **3.** Pain in the ear is called:

1. otosclerosis. 2. otitis.
3. ototoxicity. 4. otalgia.

(1077) **4.** Ototoxicity means that a drug can damage the eighth cranial nerve or the organs of:

1. hearing and balance.
2. vision and sight.
3. smell and taste.
4. movement and coordination.

(1077) **5.** Examples of drugs that can have ototoxic effects are:

1. aspirin and antibiotics.
2. anticoagulants and corticosteroids.
3. central nervous system stimulants and adrenergics.
4. diuretics and antihypertensives.

(1078) **6.** When assessing the position of the auricles, the nurse should observe that the top of the auricle normally will be at about the level of the:

1. nostrils. 2. forehead.
3. eye. 4. mouth.

(1078) **7.** The external auditory canal is inspected for obvious obstructions or:

1. edema. 2. cyanosis.
3. drainage. 4. jaundice.

(1078) **8.** The only normal secretion in the external auditory canal is:

1. sebum.
2. purulent drainage.
3. cerumen.
4. mucus.

(1080) **9.** Otic drops, or ear drops, are intended to be placed directly into the:

1. middle ear canal.
2. inner ear canal.
3. tympanic membrane.
4. external ear canal.

(1081) **10.** The use of a solution to cleanse the external ear canal or to remove something from the canal is called:

1. audiometry.
2. irrigation.
3. débridement.
4. electronystagmography.

(1081) **11.** A common indication for irrigation is:

1. clot formation.
2. impacted cerumen.
3. purulent drainage.
4. bleeding.

(1081) **12.** A device that amplifies sound is:

1. an audiometer.
2. a tuning fork.
3. a hearing aid.
4. an otoscope.

Student Name____

(1081) **13.** Persons who benefit the most from hearing aids are those with:

1. sensorineural loss.
2. mixed hearing loss.
3. conductive hearing loss.
4. hearing loss due to Meniere's disease.

(1083, 1084) **14.** Postoperative dizziness or vertigo following ear surgery may put the patient at risk for:

1. injury.
2. impaired skin integrity.
3. infection.
4. pain.

(1084) **15.** Patients who have had ear surgery may have altered auditory sensory perception as a result of:

1. dizziness or vertigo.
2. knowledge deficit.
3. self-care deficit.
4. packing and edema in affected ear.

(1084) **16.** Following ear surgery, patients often complain of the sensation that the room is spinning or that their bodies are spinning; this is charted as:

1. dizziness. 2. otalgia.
3. edema. 4. vertigo.

(1084) **17.** After ear surgery, patients are advised to move slowly and carefully to avoid sudden movement, which may cause:

1. hemorrhage.
2. vertigo.
3. infection.
4. edema.

(1086) **18.** Of all patients with sensory disorders, people who probably suffer the most severe social isolation are those with:

1. hearing impairment.
2. sight impairment.
3. smell impairment.
4. taste impairment.

(1085) **19.** To prevent one form of congenital hearing impairment, all women of childbearing age should be immunized for:

1. pertussis. 2. influenza.
3. rubella. 4. hepatitis B.

(1086) **20.** One of the most common causes of obstruction of the external ear canal is:

1. hemorrhage.
2. infection.
3. impacted cerumen.
4. blood clots.

(1086) **21.** Patients with impacted cerumen may complain of hearing loss or:

1. sharp pain.
2. tinnitus.
3. bloody discharge.
4. headache.

(1088) **22.** A very common problem after mastoidectomy or middle ear surgery is:

1. nausea. 2. constipation.
3. oliguria. 4. seizures.

(1088) **23.** Because the fixed stapes cannot vibrate in patients with otosclerosis, sound waves cannot be transmitted to the:

1. middle ear.
2. tympanic membrane.
3. inner ear.
4. external auditory canal.

(1088) **24.** Slow progressive hearing loss in the absence of infection is the primary symptom of:

1. acute otitis media.
2. labyrinthitis.
3. perforated eardrum.
4. otosclerosis.

(1088) **25.** The most common treatment for otosclerosis is a surgical procedure called:

1. myringotomy.
2. stapedectomy.
3. mastoidectomy.
4. incision and drainage.

(1088) **26.** A hereditary condition in which an abnormal growth causes the footplate of the stapes to become fixed is:

1. cholesteatoma.
2. otosclerosis.
3. labyrinthitis.
4. conductive hearing loss.

(1089) **27.** An inner ear infection that usually follows an upper respiratory infection and that may lead to Meniere's disease is:

1. otitis media.
2. otosclerosis.
3. mastoiditis.
4. labyrinthitis.

(1089) **28.** The treatment for labyrinthitis is:

1. antiemetics.
2. analgesics.
3. corticosteroids.
4. beta blockers.

(1084) **29.** A major concern for a patient with vertigo is:

1. infection. 2. safety.
3. nutrition. 4. edema.

(1092) **30.** The primary symptom of ototoxicity with salicylates is:

1. vertigo. 2. tinnitus.
3. dizziness. 4. anorexia.

(1089) **31.** A low buzzing sound that sometimes becomes a roar and that is a symptom of Meniere's disease is documented as:

1. vertigo. 2. tinnitus.
3. dizziness. 4. otitis.

(1090) **32.** When the caloric test or electronystagmography is done in patients with Meniere's disease, they will experience severe:

1. vertigo. 2. seizures.
3. headache. 4. flushing.

(1090) **33.** Following surgery for Meniere's disease, the nurse needs to assess the patient for:

1. facial nerve damage.
2. fluid volume excess.
3. decreased cardiac output.
4. urinary retention.

(1077) **34.** Presbycusis is the result of changes in one or more parts of the:

1. middle ear.
2. external auditory canal.
3. eustachian tube.
4. cochlea.

(1089) **35.** A labyrinth disorder in which there is an accumulation of fluid in the inner ear is:

1. otosclerosis.
2. otitis media.
3. Meniere's disease.
4. presbycusis.

Student Name____

(1092) **36.** Drugs that can cause permanent hearing loss are:

1. antihypertensives.
2. aminoglycosides (antibiotics).
3. anticholinergics.
4. diuretics.

(1092) **37.** Patients who are at special risk of developing ototoxicity because their bodies excrete drugs more slowly are those with:

1. renal failure.
2. pneumonia.
3. myocardial infarction.
4. liver disease.

(1080) **38.** Rinne's and Weber's tests use a tuning fork to assess the:

1. ability of persons to hear whispers.
2. presence of lesions in the vestibule.
3. conduction of sound by air and bone.
4. function of the eighth cranial nerve.

(1084) **39.** The correct postoperative intervention for a patient who has had ear surgery is as follows:

1. Position yourself on the unaffected side to promote drainage.
2. Keep your mouth closed, if you need to cough or sneeze.
3. Increase vitamin K and protein intake in your diet.
4. Avoid shampooing for 2 weeks.

(1086) **40.** A nursing intervention related to patients with impaired verbal communication is:

1. provide adequate lighting away from the patient's face.
2. raise the tone your voice.
3. if the patient has a good ear, speak to that side.
4. explain the use of the call button and bedside intercom.

(1089) **41.** Which problem for patients with inner ear disorders may be worsened by taking certain herbal products?

1. sedation
2. dry mouth
3. confusion
4. constipation

(1090) **42.** Which diet may be recommended for patients with Meniere's disease?

1. increased calcium
2. increased vitamin K
3. Increased potassium
4. low sodium

CHAPTER 51

Student Name ______________________________

Nose, Sinus, and Throat Disorders

Answer Key: Textbook page references are provided as a guide for answering these questions. A complete answer key was provided for your instructor.

OBJECTIVES

1. Describe the nursing assessment of the nose, sinuses, and throat.
2. Identify nursing responsibilities for patients undergoing tests or procedures to diagnose disorders of the nose, sinuses, or throat.
3. Describe the nurse's role when the following common therapeutic measures are instituted: administration of topical medications, irrigations, humidification, suctioning, tracheostomy care, and surgery.
4. Explain the pathophysiology, signs and symptoms, complications, and medical or surgical treatment of selected disorders of the nose, sinuses, and throat.
5. Assist in developing nursing care plans for patients with disorders of the nose, sinuses, or throat.

LEARNING ACTIVITIES

A. Complete the statement in the numbered column with the most appropriate term in the lettered column. Some terms may be used more than once, and some terms may not be used.

(1095) **1.** The terms maxillary, frontal, ethmoid, and sphenoid refer to __________.

(1095) **2.** __________ are projections that increase the surface area that inspired air crosses.

(1097) **3.** In __________, the nurse shines a special light into the patient's mouth to see whether the sinus cavities are filled with air.

(1095) **4.** Mucus protects the nasal airway because it is __________.

A. Acidic
B. Optic nerve
C. Cilia
D. Nasal cavity
E. Olfactory nerve
F. Turbinates
G. Nares
H. Mucous membrane
I. Moisturizes
J. Sinuses
K. Alkaline
L. Tonsils
M. Transillumination
N. Olfactory

Continued next page

(1095) **5.** Spaces in the bones of the skull are called __________.

(1095) **6.** The sinuses are lined with __________.

(1095) **7.** Particles that are trapped in the mucus are swept toward the throat by __________.

(1095) **8.** The __________ cells line the roof of the nasal cavity.

(1095) **9.** Specialized sensory cells detect odors and relay information about odors to the brain by way of the __________.

(1095) **10.** A layer of mucus covers the membrane inside the nose; this layer traps particles and __________ dry air.

(1095) **11.** The sinuses produce mucus that drains into the __________.

(1095) **12.** The __________ are air spaces that act as sound chambers for the voice and reduce the weight of the skull.

B. Complete the statement in the numbered column with the most appropriate term in the lettered column. Some terms may be used more than once, and some terms may not be used.

(1103) **1.** Pain or a feeling of heaviness over the frontal or maxillary area is a common symptom of __________.

(1103) **2.** Sinus infection usually spreads into the sinuses from the __________.

(1103) **3.** __________ sinusitis follows obstruction of the flow of secretions from the sinus.

(1097) **4.** Two findings related to assessment of the sinuses, which may be observed during palpation of the frontal and maxillary sinuses, include __________.

(1103) **5.** Toothache-like pain is a common symptom of sinusitis that involves the __________.

(1103) **6.** Potential complications of sinusitis include brain abscess, osteomyelitis, orbital cellulitis, and __________.

(1103) **7.** Repeated infections often result in __________.

A. Pain and tenderness
B. Chronic
C. Meningitis
D. Pharynx
E. Nasal passages
F. Chronic sinusitis
G. Redness and fever
H. Acute
I. Skull
J. Acute sinusitis
K. Sinusitis
L. Streptococci
M. Maxillary sinuses

Continued next page

Student Name____

(1103) **8.** Inflammation of the sinuses, usually the maxillary and frontal sinuses, is called __________.

(1103) **9.** The most common causative organisms of sinusitis are staphylococci and __________.

(1103) **10.** __________ sinusitis is a permanent thickening of the mucous membranes in the sinuses.

(1103) **11.** The possibility of brain infection exists in patients with sinusitis because the sinuses are located in the __________.

(1103) **12.** Allergic rhinitis, deviated septum, nasal polyps, tumors, airborne pollution, and inhaled drugs such as cocaine are causes of __________.

C. Complete the statement in the numbered column with the most appropriate term in the lettered column. Some terms may be used more than once, and some terms may not be used.

(1104) **1.** To decrease the patient's reaction to offending allergens, the allergist may recommend injections for __________.

(1104) **2.** Nasal polyps tend to grow, and they eventually obstruct the __________.

(1106) **3.** Medical treatment for epistaxis includes the use of silver nitrate or __________.

(1106) **4.** The priority assessment when a patient has severe epistaxis is for evidence of excessive __________.

(1104) **5.** A common respiratory condition, which is classified as acute (seasonal) or chronic (perennial), is __________.

(1104) **6.** The drugs used to treat allergic rhinitis are primarily decongestants and __________.

(1106) **7.** Two methods used to apply pressure in patients with epistaxis include placement of a nasal balloon catheter and __________.

A. Numbness
B. Allergic rhinitis
C. Hypovolemia
D. Nasal airways
E. Antihistamines
F. Airway obstruction
G. Nasal packing
H. Electric cautery
I. Desensitization
J. Coryza
K. Aspirin
L. House dust
M. Blood loss

Continued next page

(1104) **8.** Three symptoms that are normal following the Caldwell-Luc operation are swelling, bruising, and __________.

(1104) **9.** Following nasal polyp surgery, the patient is advised not to take __________.

(1104) **10.** Complications related to posterior packing include infection, blockage of the eustachian tube, and __________.

(1104) **11.** Chronic allergic rhinitis is often due to exposure to allergens in the environment such as __________.

(1106) **12.** Nursing care of patients with epistaxis includes monitoring vital signs to detect signs of __________.

D. Complete the statement in the numbered column with the most appropriate term in the lettered column. Some terms may be used more than once, and some terms may not be used.

(1104) **1.** In an effort to limit new growth of polyps, sinus surgery is done; two surgical procedures include the Caldwell-Luc operation or __________.

(1104) **2.** The release of chemicals, including histamine, following exposure to an allergen causes increased capillary permeability and __________.

(1104) **3.** __________ resemble white grapes in size and shape.

(1104) **4.** Acute allergic rhinitis is most often due to exposure to __________.

(1104) **5.** Patients with triad disease have asthma, aspirin allergy, and __________.

(1104) **6.** Removing allergens or treating the allergic responses may reduce the size of __________.

(1104) **7.** The overuse of decongestant nose drops or sprays may result in __________.

A. Allergic rhinitis
B. Vasodilation
C. Vasoconstriction
D. Capillaries
E. Pollens
F. Rhinitis
G. Coryza
H. Nasal polyps
I. Functional fundoscopic sinus surgery (FESS)

Continued next page

Student Name____

(1104) **8.** A condition that follows exposure to an allergen is __________.

(1104) **9.** Swelling of the nasal mucosa occurs as a result of fluid leaks from the __________.

(1104) **10.** The cause of nasal polyps is unknown, but patients often have a history of infections or __________.

E. Complete the statement in the numbered column with the most appropriate term in the lettered column.

(1105) **1.** Growths that may develop in the nasal passages and sinuses and that may be benign or malignant are called __________.

(1105) **2.** The primary symptom of nasal tumors is __________.

(1105) **3.** External nasal tumors are usually either basal cell or __________ carcinomas.

(1105) **4.** The common cold is known as __________.

(1105) **5.** Acute viral coryza is contagious and spread by __________.

(1105) **6.** Signs and symptoms of the common cold include fever, fatigue, sore throat, and __________.

(1105) **7.** Complications of acute viral coryza include otitis media, sinusitis, bronchitis, and __________.

(1105) **8.** Septal deviations are corrected by a surgical procedure called a submucosal resection or nasal __________.

(1105) **9.** The two major complications of submucosal resection are tears of the septum and __________.

(1105) **10.** A diagnosis of cancer of the nose is made by taking a __________.

A. Nasal discharge
B. Resistance
C. Septoplasty
D. Biopsy
E. Squamous cell
F. Viruses
G. Droplet infection
H. Acute viral coryza
I. Septum
J. Nasal obstruction
K. Bacteria
L. Pneumonia
M. Decongestants
N. Tumors
O. Saddle deformity

Continued next page

(1105) **11.** The nose is divided into two passages by a cartilaginous wall called the __________.

(1105) **12.** Complications of acute viral coryza are more common in people with lowered __________.

(1105) **13.** Drug therapy for acute common coryza includes antipyretics, antihistamines, and __________.

(1105) **14.** Antibiotics are not effective against infections caused by __________.

(1105) **15.** Inappropriate use of antibiotics promotes the development of resistant strains of __________.

F. Complete the statement in the numbered column with the most appropriate term in the lettered column.

(1107) **1.** Pharyngitis is treated with rest, fluids, analgesics, and __________.

(1107) **2.** As long as the patient has a fever, the level of activity that is often recommended is __________.

(1107) **3.** A soft or liquid diet may be ordered because of __________.

(1107) **4.** A treatment that may be ordered to increase moisture in the room air is __________.

(1108) **5.** The recommended daily fluid intake for patients with pharyngitis is __________.

(1108) **6.** Fluids must be increased slowly in the elderly because they do not adjust well to sudden changes in __________.

(1107) **7.** Inflammation of the mucous membranes of the throat is called __________.

(1107) **8.** __________ is a complication of bacterial pharyngitis that occurs 7–10 days after the throat infection.

A. 48 hours
B. Humidification
C. Acute glomerulonephritis
D. Dysphagia
E. Blood volume
F. Culture specimen
G. Rheumatic fever
H. Bed rest
I. 10 days
J. Pharyngitis
K. Throat gargles (irrigations)
L. Penicillin
M. 2000–3000 ml

Continued next page

Student Name ____________________

(1107) **9.** A usual course of antibiotic therapy is __________.

(1107) **10.** If bacterial infection is confirmed, the antibiotic is usually continued for __________ after all signs and symptoms disappear.

(1107) **11.** The physician often orders antibiotics for pharyngitis, usually erythromycin or __________.

(1107) **12.** Before an antibiotic is ordered, a __________ should be taken.

(1107) **13.** __________ is a complication of bacterial pharyngitis that occurs 3–5 weeks after the initial throat infection.

G. Complete the statement in the numbered column with the most appropriate term in the lettered column.

(1108) **1.** Common causative organisms of tonsillitis include streptococcus, staphylococcus, *Haemophilus influenzae,* and __________.

(1108) **2.** Tonsillitis is a contagious infection spread by food or __________.

(1108) **3.** A patient with tonsillitis usually reports a sore throat, difficulty swallowing, fever, chills, muscle aches, and __________.

(1108) **4.** If swollen tissue blocks the eustachian tubes in patients with tonsillitis, there may also be pain in the __________.

(1108) **5.** An elevated white blood cell count in patients with tonsillitis suggests a __________.

(1108) **6.** The medical treatment of tonsillitis usually includes the use of __________.

(1108) **7.** A serious complication of tonsillitis caused by streptococcus is __________.

A. Headache
B. Peritonsillar abscess
C. Airborne routes
D. Bacterial infection
E. Ears
F. Antibiotics
G. Pneumococcus

H. Complete the statement in the numbered column with the most appropriate term in the lettered column.

(1115) **1.** Following laryngectomy, many patients are able to learn to control and use air to produce sounds, which is called __________.

(1115) **2.** Following laryngectomy, some patients use an electronic device to produce sound, which is called a(n) __________.

(1115) **3.** A procedure performed during total laryngectomy to create a connection between the pharynx and trachea is called __________.

(1115) **4.** A procedure in which the surgeon creates a fistula between the trachea and the esophagus is called __________.

A. Laryngoplasty
B. Artificial larynx
C. Esophageal speech
D. Tracheoesophageal prosthesis

I. Match the actions and uses of the drugs in the numbered column with the classification of drugs in the lettered column.

(1100) **1.** __________ Anesthetic effect on skin and mucous membranes

(1100) **2.** __________ Reduce body temperature, treat fever

(1100) **3.** __________ Decongestion, vasoconstriction

(1100) **4.** __________ Treat allergic reactions, prevent motion sickness

(1100) **5.** __________ Reduce pain

(1100) **6.** __________ Kill or suppress growth of microorganisms

(1100) **7.** __________ Decrease salivary and respiratory secretions

A. Sympathomimetics
B. Anticholinergics
C. Antihistamines
D. Antipyretics
E. Analgesics
F. Anesthetics
G. Anti-infectives

Student Name____

J. Indicate for each characteristic below whether it refers to (A) viral or (B) bacterial pharyngitis.

A. Viral
B. Bacterial

(1108) **1.** __________ Positive culture

(1108) **2.** __________ Dysphagia

(1108) **3.** __________ Normal CBC

(1108) **4.** __________ Rhinorrhea

(1108) **5.** __________ Abrupt onset of symptoms

(1108) **6.** __________ Malaise

(1108) **7.** __________ Mild elevation of temperature

(1108) **8.** __________ Gradual onset of symptoms

(1108) **9.** __________ Joint and muscle pain

(1108) **10.** __________ Rare complica-tions

K. List 10 age-related changes of the nose, throat, and sinuses in the following areas.

(1097) **1.** Size of nose: ____________________________

(1097) **2.** Nasal obstruction: ____________________________

(1097) **3.** Cartilage of the external nose: ____________________________

(1097, 1098) **4.** Effect of nasal decongestants: ____________________________

(1097) **5.** Mucous membrane: ____________________________

(1097) **6.** Production of mucus: ____________________________

(1098) **7.** Occurrence of epistaxis (nosebleed): ____________________________

(1098) **8.** Sense of smell: ____________________________

(1098) **9.** Tissues of the larynx: ____________________________

(1098) **10.** Esophageal sphincter: ____________________________

L. Using Figure 51-2 below, label the structures of the nose and throat (A–J) by using the terms (1–10) below.

(1096)

1. ________ Nasal cavity

2. ________ Sinuses

3. ________ Area of pharynx

4. ________ Auditory tube orifice

5. ________ Vocal cord

6. ________ Esophagus

7. ________ Pharyngeal tonsils (adenoids)

8. ________ Epiglottis

9. ________ Nasopharynx

10. ________ Larynx

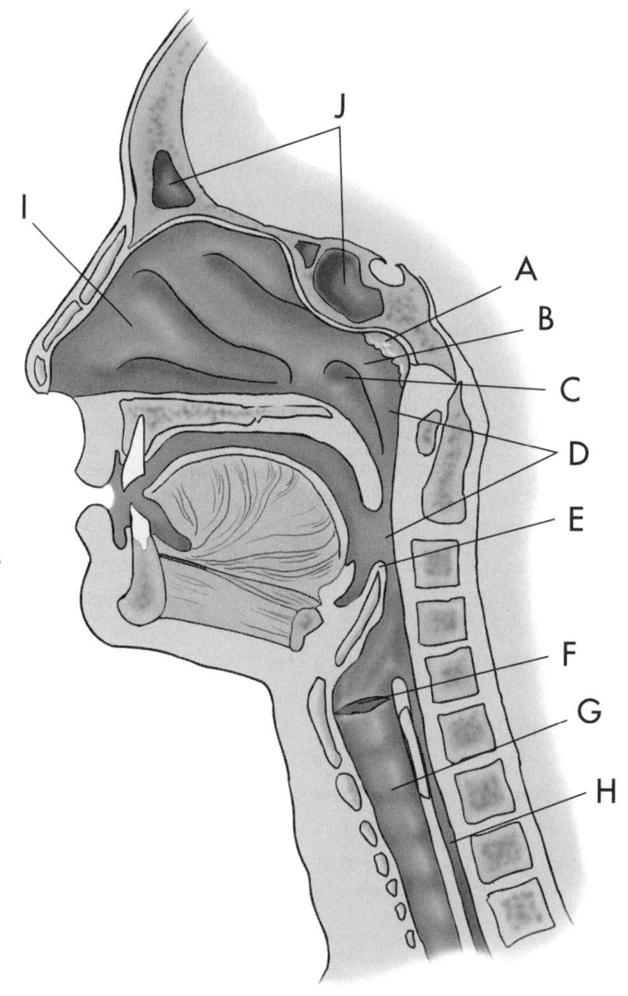

Student Name______________________________

MULTIPLE-CHOICE QUESTIONS

M. Choose the most appropriate answer.

(1097) **1.** The mucous membranes and tonsils of the throat are inspected for redness, drainage, swelling, or:

1. cyanosis.
2. lesions.
3. pallor.
4. coolness.

(1097) **2.** Inspection and palpation of the neck may reveal enlarged:

1. lymph nodes.
2. tonsils.
3. adenoids.
4. vocal cords.

(1098) **3.** Epistaxis (nosebleed) is more common in older people, especially in those taking:

1. antibiotics.
2. analgesics.
3. anticoagulants.
4. diuretics.

(1098) **4.** A weakened esophageal sphincter allows gastric contents to flow back into the throat when the patient lies down. The patient experiences a burning sensation in the:

1. larynx.
2. nares.
3. trachea.
4. stomach.

(1099) **5.** Following laryngoscopy, the patient takes nothing by mouth until:

1. respirations are normal.
2. vomiting has stopped.
3. the gag reflex returns.
4. 24 hours after surgery.

(1099) **6.** Before suctioning a patient, it is important to:

1. administer antiemetics as ordered.
2. ambulate the patient.
3. oxygenate the patient.
4. administer antibiotics as ordered.

(1100) **7.** A key point to remember when suctioning a patient is to:

1. keep the vent closed when inserting the catheter.
2. apply suction continuously as the catheter is withdrawn.
3. suction for no longer than 30 seconds.
4. use of sterile procedure.

(1100) **8.** A key point to remember when providing tracheostomy care is to:

1. use universal precautions.
2. suction the tracheostomy after removing the old dressings.
3. use a sterile solution of iodine to clean the inner cannula.
4. cut a new pad to fit around the tracheostomy site.

(1102) **9.** After nasal surgery, the nurse assesses for pain, pressure, anxiety, and:

1. tachycardia.
2. dyspnea.
3. hypotension.
4. pallor.

(1102) **10.** After nasal surgery, the patient's vital signs are monitored to detect signs of:

1. hypokalemia.
2. hypernatremia.
3. hypovolemia.
4. inadequate circulation.

(1103) **11.** The patient who has had nasal surgery may be at risk for decreased cardiac output because of:

1. blood loss from nasal passageways.
2. nasal packing.
3. airway obstruction.
4. facial bruising.

(1103) **12.** Because the nasal cavity has an extensive blood supply, following nasal surgery there is a risk of:

1. hemorrhage.
2. infection.
3. hypertension.
4. confusion.

(1103) **13.** Laxatives or stool softeners may be ordered for patients after nasal surgery in order to prevent:

1. diarrhea.
2. vomiting.
3. hypertension.
4. straining.

(1103) **14.** The best position for patients after nasal surgery to help control swelling is:

1. lying flat in bed.
2. lying with the head of bed elevated.
3. side-lying.
4. supine.

(1103) **15.** When the nasal cavity is packed following surgery, the patient breathes through the mouth; a measure that helps decrease dryness of the mucous membranes is use of:

1. frequent oral hygiene.
2. humidifiers.
3. oral fluids high in vitamin C.
4. ice packs.

(1103) **16.** Patients may experience disturbed body image following nasal surgery due to:

1. airway obstruction.
2. blood loss.
3. hypovolemia.
4. facial bruises.

(1103) **17.** Serious neurologic complications should be suspected in patients with sinusitis if the patient develops:

1. tachycardia and restlessness.
2. high fever and seizures.
3. confusion and cyanosis.
4. dyspnea and anxiety.

(1104) **18.** The type of surgery performed for chronic maxillary sinusitis is:

1. laryngoscopy.
2. tonsillectomy and adenoidectomy.
3. the Caldwell-Luc operation.
4. nasal septoplasty.

(1104) **19.** Desensitizing injections, or "allergy shots," are composed of dilute solutions of:

1. allergens.
2. histamines.
3 antihistamines.
4. plasma.

(1105) **20.** A deviated septum may obstruct the nasal passage and block:

1. sinus drainage.
2. eustachian tube drainage.
3. pharyngeal drainage.
4. jugular vein drainage.

(1105) **21.** Patients with a deviated septum may complain of epistaxis, sinusitis, and:

1. palpitations.
2. headaches.
3. insomnia.
4. sweating.

Student Name ____________________

(1106) **22.** When epistaxis occurs, the patient should sit down and lean forward and direct pressure should be applied for:

1. 1–2 minutes.
2. 3–5 minutes.
3. 7–10 minutes.
4. 15–20 minutes.

(1106) **23.** With facial trauma or nasal fracture, the recommended treatment initially is application of:

1. an ice pack.
2. a warm compress.
3. direct pressure.
4. heat.

(1105) **24.** Patients with severe epistaxis may be at high risk for infection due to:

1. possible airway obstruction.
2. nasal packing.
3. hypotension.
4. hypovolemia.

(1110) **25.** The two major problems that may develop in the postoperative phase of tonsillectomy are respiratory distress and:

1. infection.
2. hemorrhage.
3. hypersensitivity reaction.
4. cardiac dysrhythmia.

(1110) **26.** Early signs of inadequate oxygenation in the postoperative tonsillectomy patient include restlessness, increased pulse rate, and:

1. cyanosis.
2. pallor.
3. numbness.
4. confusion.

(1110) **27.** Following a tonsillectomy, a treatment that may be applied to the neck to decrease swelling and pain is:

1. a heating pad.
2. a TENS unit.
3. antibiotic ointment.
4. an ice collar.

(1110) **28.** Which foods should be avoided in patients after a tonsillectomy?

1. frozen liquids
2. ice cream
3. applesauce
4. citrus juices

(1110) **29.** Which symptoms should be reported to the physician if the nurse observes them in the postoperative tonsillectomy patient who is ready to be discharged?

1. bleeding
2. earache
3. white patches in the throat (surgical site)
4. sore throat

(1110) **30.** In order to reduce irritation of the larynx in patients with laryngitis, a treatment usually prescribed is:

1. surgery.
2. voice rest.
3. intravenous fluids.
4. application of heat.

(1110) **31.** A primary nursing diagnosis for patients with larymgytis due to aphonia is:

1. Risk for infection.
2. Risk for injury.
3. Impaired verbal communication.
4. Altered tissue perfusion.

(1111) **32.** Benign masses of fibrous tissue that result primarily from overuse of the voice but that can also follow infections are called:

1. nodules. 2. myomas.
3. fibromas. 4. tumors.

(1111) **33.** The only symptom of laryngeal nodules is:

1. pain.
2. fever.
3. dysphagia.
4. hoarseness.

(1111) **34.** A swollen mass of mucous membrane attached to the vocal cord is called a:

1. nodule. 2. tumor.
3. cancer. 4. polyp.

(1111) **35.** Individuals who both smoke and use alcohol are at particularly high risk for:

1. tonsillitis.
2. pneumonia.
3. cancer of the larynx.
4. nasal polyps.

(1111) **36.** Malignancies in the larynx tend to spread fairly early; the most common site of metastasis is the:

1. liver. 2. colon.
3. lung. 4. brain.

(1112) **37.** Total laryngectomy causes permanent loss of:

1. the voice.
2. cough.
3. the sternocleidomastoid muscle.
4. the swallow reflex.

(1113) **38.** A total laryngectomy involves removal of the entire larynx, vocal cords, and:

1. pharynx. 2. epiglottis.
3. tonsils. 4. esophagus.

(1097) **39.** Gently closing one naris at a time and instructing the patient to breathe through the other naris is a way to assess:

1. lung sounds.
2. aphonia.
3. sense of smell.
4. patency of the nostrils.

(1095) **40.** Normally, the frontal and maxillary sinuses are filled with:

1. fluid. 2. air.
3. polyps. 4. cysts.

(1114) **41.** In the immediate postoperative period after total laryngectomy, the nurse's assessment focuses on comfort, circulation, and:

1. fluid balance.
2. oxygenation.
3. infection.
4. hypovolemia.

(1114) **42.** In the patient with a laryngectomy, the nurse assesses the need for suctioning by observing audible or visible mucus, increased pulse, and:

1. pallor. 2. swelling.
3. pain. 4. restlessness.

(1114) **43.** Factors that affect the respiratory status of patients with laryngectomies include positioning, fluids, and:

1. nutrition.
2. verbal communication.
3. humidification.
4. personal hygiene.

(1114) **44.** A position that promotes maximal lung expansion in the patient with a laryngectomy is:

1. semiprone.
2. flat.
3. semi-Fowler's.
4. side-lying.

Student Name____

(1114) **45.** To prevent pooling of secretions in the lungs of patients with laryngectomies, the nurse should encourage:

1. coughing and deep breathing.
2. increased fluid intake.
3. early ambulation.
4. avoidance of dusty places.

(1105) **46.** Which herb is used to boost the immune system and is taken by some to decrease the severity of a cold?

1. ginseng
2. Ephedra
3. Echinacea
4. St. John's wort

(1100) **47.** Suctioning is limited to 10 seconds because prolonged suctioning may lead to:

1. hypoxia.
2. hypertension.
3. increased intracranial pressure.
4. bradycardia.

CHAPTER 52

Student Name ______________________________

Psychological Responses to Illness

Answer Key: Textbook page references are provided as a guide for answering these questions. A complete answer key was provided for your instructor.

OBJECTIVES

1. Define mental health.
2. Discuss the concepts of stress, anxiety, adaptation, and homeostasis.
3. Discuss how age and cultural and spiritual beliefs affect an individual's ability to cope with illness.
4. Identify some basic coping strategies (defense mechanisms).
5. Discuss the concepts of anxiety, fear, stress, loss, grief, hopelessness, and powerlessness in relation to illness.
6. Describe several factors that may precipitate adaptive or maladaptive coping behaviors in response to illness.
7. Discuss implementation of the nursing process to enhance a patient's mental health as the patient deals with the stresses of illness.

LEARNING ACTIVITIES

A. Complete the statement in the numbered column with the most appropriate term in the lettered column. Some terms may be used more than once.

(1124) **1.** When a woman finds a suspicious lump in her breast and does not keep appointments for a breast biopsy, this action could be called __________.

(1124) **2.** When anxiety intensifies to an excessive level, perception of reality becomes solely focused on the __________.

A. Introjection
B. Rationalization or intellectualization
C. Compensation
D. Denial
E. Identification
F. Isolation
G. Displacement
H. Crisis
I. Anxiety

Continued next page

(1124) **3.** When a student fails to complete an assignment correctly and complains about the objectives for the assignment, this action is __________.

(1124) **4.** Transferring feelings associated with one person or event to another that is considered less threatening is __________.

(1124) **5.** An attempt to make up for real or imagined weakness is __________.

(1124) **6.** The use of logic, reasoning, and analysis to avoid unacceptable feelings is __________.

(1124) **7.** A painful emotion that results from one's perception of danger is __________.

(1124) **8.** Internalizing or taking on the values and beliefs of another person is __________.

(1124) **9.** A boy who is angry with a teacher comes home and yells at his dog; this is an example of __________.

(1125) **10.** When a man appears apathetic as he discusses a fire fight in which he participated in Vietnam, it is an example of __________.

(1124) **11.** When a child dresses and uses mannerisms similar to those of a movie star, this action is called __________.

(1124) **12.** Refusal to acknowledge a real situation is __________.

(1124) **13.** When an adolescent perceived as unattractive becomes an outstanding athlete, this action could be called __________.

(1124) **14.** When a child takes on the values and beliefs of a parent, it is called __________.

(1124) **15.** Emulation of admirable qualities in another to enhance one's self-esteem is __________.

(1125) **16.** The separation of emotion from an associated thought or memory is __________.

B. Complete the statement in the numbered column with the most appropriate term in the lettered column. Some terms may be used more than once.

(1125) **1.** The transformation of unacceptable impulses or drives into constructive or more acceptable behavior is __________.

(1125) **2.** Actually or symbolically attempting to cancel out an action that was unacceptable is __________.

(1125) **3.** When the individual who witnesses a murder then experiences sudden blindness without an organic cause, it is called __________.

A. Substitution
B. Projection
C. Sublimation
D. Repression
E. Regression
F. Reaction formation
G. Undoing
H. Suppression
I. Isolation
J. Conversion

Continued next page

Student Name____

(1125) **4.** When a patient who unconsciously hates his father continuously tells the nurses how great his father is, it is an example of __________.

(1125) **5.** Unacceptable feelings or impulses are transferred to another in __________.

(1125) **6.** __________ is a conscious or voluntary inhibition of unacceptable ideas, impulses, and memories.

(1125) **7.** Sprinkling salt over one's left shoulder to prevent bad luck after spilling salt on the table is an example of __________.

(1125) **8.** When the person who has a strong unconscious sexual attraction to a parent marries someone who resembles that parent, it is called __________.

(1125) **9.** When a child starts sucking her thumb when her new baby brother comes home from the hospital, it is an example of __________.

(1125) **10.** When a child who fails an algebra class forgets to show his report card to his parents, this action is called __________.

(1125) **11.** An emotional conflict is turned into a physical symptom, which provides the individual with some sort of benefit (secondary gain), in __________.

(1125) **12.** Avoidance of unacceptable thoughts and behaviors by expressing opposing thoughts or behaviors is __________.

(1125) **13.** When a wife who is jealous of her husband accuses him of jealousy, this is called __________.

(1125) **14.** An unconscious defense mechanism in which unacceptable ideas, impulses, and memories are kept out of consciousness is __________.

(1125) **15.** In __________, an individual replaces a highly valued, unattainable object with a less valued, attainable object.

(1125) **16.** __________ is withdrawing to an earlier level of development to benefit from the associated comfort levels.

(1125) **17.** When a person cannot remember a sexual assault, it is an example of __________.

(1125) **18.** When a person who has aggressive tendencies becomes a football star, it is an example of __________.

C. Match the descriptions in the numbered column with the coping strategy in the lettered column. Some strategies may be used more than once, and some strategies may not be used.

(1125) **1.** ________ Imagery, therapeutic touch, and music therapy

(1125) **2.** ________ The use of imagination to develop sensory pictures that focus away from the stressful experience and emphasize other sensory experiences and pleasant memories

(1125) **3.** ________ Use of earphones with audio cassettes

(1125) **4.** ________ Discussion with clients about a higher power or their beliefs

(1125) **5.** ________ Biofeedback, meditation, yoga, and Zen practices

(1125) **6.** ________ A process by which the therapist acts as a channel for environmental and universal energy through the therapist's mental concentration

A. Therapeutic touch
B. Relaxation techniques
C. Spiritual dimension
D. Music therapy
E. Art therapy
F. Role-playing
G. Imagery

D. List 12 characteristics of healthy individuals, according to Maslow.

(1120) **1.** ____________________

(1120) **2.** ____________________

(1120) **3.** ____________________

(1120) **4.** ____________________

(1120) **5.** ____________________

(1120) **6.** ____________________

(1120) **7.** ____________________

(1120) **8.** ____________________

(1120) **9.** ____________________

(1121) **10.** ____________________

(1121) **11.** ____________________

(1121) **12.** ____________________

Student Name____

MULTIPLE-CHOICE QUESTIONS

E. Choose the most appropriate answer.

(1124) **1.** Defense mechanisms are adapted by the individual as protective measures to allow the ego relief from:

1. rationalization.
2. denial.
3. anxiety.
4. repression.

(1127) **2.** A factor that is basic to helping the patient cope with illness is the nurse's:

1. caring attitude.
2. educational background.
3. professionalism.
4. organization.

(1127) **3.** Effective nursing interventions can be made only after patients have been assessed as:

1. members of a particular culture.
2. members of a particular sex.
3. members of a certain race.
4. unique individuals.

(1122) **4.** A group's affiliation because of a shared language, race, and values is:

1. culture. 2. behavior.
3. morality. 4. ethnicity.

(1123) **5.** People subjected to prolonged stressors eventually become:

1. defensive. 2. exhausted.
3. cognitive. 4. emotional.

(1124) **6.** An early response to illness is often:

1. grief. 2. depression.
3. anxiety. 4. loss.

(1124) **7.** When a person with a severe illness is forced to relinquish original hopes, this process is called:

1. mourning. 2. grief.
3. anxiety. 4. fear.

(1124) **8.** The experience of loss is related to the individual's:

1. self-concept.
2. sense of belonging.
3. anxiety.
4. depression.

(1121) **9.** Any changes in a person's life create:

1. fear. 2. anxiety.
3. stress. 4. mourning.

(1124) **10.** Unconscious coping mechanisms are referred to as:

1. stressors.
2. defense mechanisms.
3. self-concepts.
4. illusions.

(1126) **11.** Passivity and verbal expression of loss of control over situations are characteristics of:

1. gratification.
2. denial.
3. intellectualization.
4. powerlessness.

(1126) **12.** Denial of obvious problems and weaknesses is related to the nursing diagnosis of:

1. Ineffective individual coping.
2. Activity intolerance.
3. Altered growth and development.
4. Ineffective management of therapeutic regimen: individual.

(1126) **13.** Passivity and dependence on others are characteristics of:

1. helplessness.
2. powerlessness.
3. denial.
4. displacement.

(1124) **14.** Minimizing the severity of an illness by a patient is an example of:

1. denial.
2. repression.
3. compensation.
4. regression.

(1126) **15.** Ineffective coping mechanisms may evolve from a sense of:

1. isolation.
2. projection.
3. powerlessness.
4. reaction formation.

Student Name ______________________________

Psychiatric Disorders

Answer Key: Textbook page references are provided as a guide for answering these questions. A complete answer key was provided for your instructor.

OBJECTIVES

1. Describe the differences between social relationships and therapeutic relationships.
2. Describe key strategies in communicating therapeutically.
3. Describe the components of the mental status examination.
4. Identify target symptoms, behaviors, and potential side effects for the following types of medications: antianxiety (anxiolytic), antipsychotic, and antidepressant drugs.
5. Summarize current thinking about the etiology of schizophrenia and the mood disorders.
6. Identify key features of the mental status examination and their relevance in: anxiety disorders, schizophrenia, mood disorders, cognitive disorders, and personality disorders.
7. Identify common nursing diagnoses, goals, and interventions for persons with: anxiety disorders, schizophrenia, mood disorders, cognitive disorders, and personality disorders.

LEARNING ACTIVITIES

A. Match the definition or description in the numbered column with the most appropriate term in the lettered column.

(1136) **1.** __________ Frequently irreversible side effect of antipsychotic medication that develops after years of use; symptoms include involuntary movements of face, jaw, and tongue, leading to grimacing; jerky movements of upper extremities; and tonic contractions of neck and back

(1135) **2.** __________ A state in which a person's perception of reality is impaired, thereby interfering with the capacity to function and to relate to others

(1129) **3.** __________ Assumes that mental disorders are related to physiologic changes within the central nervous system

(1132) **4.** __________ Level of consciousness and orientation to time, place, person, and self

A. Sensorium
B. Depersonalization
C. Projection
D. Psychosis
E. Syndrome
F. Psychoanalytic approach
G. Disorder
H. Tardive dyskinesia
I. Extrapyramidal effects
J. Interpersonal approach
K. Biologic approach
L. Denial

Continued next page

Student Name ____________________

(1129) **5.** __________ Based on the theory that people function at different levels of awareness (conscious to unconscious) and that ego defense mechanisms, such as denial and repression, are used to prevent anxiety

(1129) **6.** __________ A defense mechanism in which particular feelings or specific aspects of reality are excluded from awareness

(1129) **7.** __________ A defense mechanism in which one sees others as a source of one's own unacceptable thoughts, feelings, or impulses

(1136) **8.** __________ Side effects of antipsychotic drugs on the portion of the central nervous system controlling involuntary movements

(1136) **9.** __________ Refers to behaviors and symptoms

(1134) **10.** __________ A state of feeling outside of oneself, that is, watching what is happening as if it were happening to someone else

(1129) **11.** __________ The patient learns new ways to behave in a therapeutic relationship built on trust

(1138) **12.** __________ A term used when a definite organic cause, such as delirium or dementia, is established for behaviors and symptoms

B. Match the definition or description in the numbered column with the most appropriate term in the lettered column.

(1145) **1.** ________ Uses behavior modification (positive and negative reinforcement) and recognizes that particular thoughts influence emotional states

(1131) **2.** ________ Observations and descriptions regarding appearance, mood and effect, speech and language, thought content, perceptual disturbances, insight and judgment, sensorium, and memory and attention

(1143) **3.** ________ Involves deficits in orientation, memory, language comprehension, and judgment

(1140) **4.** ________ Class of antidepressant drugs; patients taking these drugs must be carefully monitored to avoid life-threatening food and drug interactions

A. Dissociative disorder
B. Dementia
C. Organic mental disorder
D. Borderline personality disorder
E. Parkinsonian syndrome
F. Monoamine oxidase inhibitor
G. Electroconvulsive therapy
H. Bipolar disorder
I. Mood
J. Mental status examination
K. Panic disorder
L. Effect
M. Cognitive behavioral approach
N. Agoraphobia
O. Schizophrenia

Continued next page

Student Name____

(1131) **5.** __________ Briefly occurring feelings such as happiness, sadness, or worry; when inappropriate, there is incongruence between the feeling appropriate to the situation and the way the feeling is expressed

(1135) **6.** __________ A very serious group of usually chronic thought disorders in which patients' ability to interpret the world around them is severely impaired

(1134) **7.** __________ A mental disorder that involves a change in identity, memory, or consciousness that enables patients to remove themselves from anxiety-provoking situations

(1141) **8.** __________ Periods of elevated mood (manic episodes) and depression

(1133) **9.** __________ Fear of situations outside the home

(1136) **10.** __________ Possible side effect after years of antipsychotic drug therapy; patient exhibits masklike face, shuffling gait, resting tremor, and rigid posture

(1143) **11.** __________ A mental state that is characterized by cognitive and intellectual deficits severe enough to impair social or occupational functioning (memory, abstract thinking, and judgment)

(1133) **12.** __________ Patient experiences intense episodes of apprehension to the point of terror

(1144) **13.** __________ Patient exhibits unstable relationships, unstable self-image, and unstable mood

(1131) **14.** __________ Feeling state experienced by the patient over a period of time

(1140) **15.** __________ Controversial therapy that uses electric current to the brain to evoke a grand mal seizure

C. Match the definition or description in the numbered column with the most appropriate term in the lettered column.

(1134)	**1.**	________	Person exhibits two or more distinct personalities	A.	Post-traumatic stress disorder
				B.	Major depression
				C.	Dissociative identity disorder
				D.	Hypochondriasis
(1136)	**2.**	________	Effect of medication that can develop after one dose or after years of drug therapy; the first symptom usually is muscular rigidity accompanied by akinesia and respiratory distress; the cardinal sign is hyperthermia (body temperature 101–103° F or higher)	E.	Obsessions
				F.	Anxiety
				G.	Affect
				H.	Neuroleptic malignant syndrome
				I.	Somatoform disorder
				J.	Personality disorder
				K.	Compulsions
				L.	Akathisia
				M.	Obsessive-compulsive disorder
				N.	Conversion disorder
(1143)	**3.**	________	Incessant behaviors, such as hand washing, that interfere with normal functioning		
(1133)	**4.**	________	Loss of body function (e.g., paralysis) without physiologic cause		
(1133)	**5.**	________	A disorder that is characterized by vague, multiple, recurring physical complaints that are not caused by real physical illness		
(1143)	**6.**	________	Pervasive, chronic, and maladaptive personality characteristics that interfere with normal functioning		

Continued next page

Student Name____

(1133) **7.** __________ A psychological disorder experienced following a traumatic event that is characterized by flashbacks, detachment, and sleeping and eating difficulties

(1136) **8.** __________ A reversible condition of restlessness manifested as an urge to pace

(1131) **9.** __________ Emotional responsiveness and feeling state

(1133) **10.** __________ Recurrent intrusive thoughts that interfere with normal functioning

(1133) **11.** __________ Recurrent obsessions or compulsions, or both, that produce distress and interfere with daily functioning

(1134) **12.** __________ Belief that a serious medical condition exists when medical findings are absent

(1138) **13.** __________ Depressed mood

(1132) **14.** __________ State of being uneasy, apprehensive, or nervous in response to a vague, nonspecific threat

D. Complete the statement in the numbered column with the most appropriate term in the lettered column. Some terms may be used more than once, and some terms may not be used.

(1144) **1.** A frequently utilized mechanism by patients with borderline personality disorder that is caused by problems with separation-individuation is called __________.

(1132) **2.** Asking the patient to interpret proverbs, such as asking "What does 'a rolling stone gathers no moss' mean?", is a way to assess __________.

(1132) **3.** The four levels of consciousness are alert, drowsy, stuporous, and __________.

(1132) **4.** When a spot on the wall is perceived as a bug, this is called __________.

A. Illusion
B. Multiple personality disorder(s)
C. Sensorium
D. Comatose
E. Recent memory
F. Personality disorder(s)
G. Insight
H. Hallucination
I. Splitting
J. Mood
K. Attention
L. Remote memory
M. Judgment
N. Abstract thinking
O. Phobia(s)

Continued next page

(1132) **5.** Asking a patient to spell the word *world* backwards is a way to measure __________.

(1143) **6.** Paranoid, schizoid, antisocial, borderline, avoidant, obsessive-compulsive, and passive-aggressive are examples of __________.

(1132) **7.** Important factors in relation to suicide potential are insight and __________.

(1132) **8.** Asking the patient "What day is today?" is a way to assess __________.

(1143) **9.** The person with borderline personality disorder has patterns involving unstable relationships, unstable self-image, and unstable __________.

(1132) **10.** Asking a patient what was eaten at the previous meal is one way to measure __________.

(1132) **11.** The soundness of proposed actions in relation to one's particular background is __________.

(1132) **12.** When a person sees nonexistent bugs crawling on the floor or feels nonexistent bugs crawling on the skin, this is called __________.

(1132) **13.** A clear understanding of the significance of one's own symptoms and behavior is __________.

E. Match the description in the numbered column with (A) therapeutic or (B) social relationship.

(1130) **1.** __________ May or may not be clear boundaries and a clear ending

(1130) **2.** __________ Focus is on personal and emotional needs of patient

(1130) **3.** __________ Purpose is to benefit both participants in the relationship

(1130) **4.** __________ Participants are not formally responsible for evaluating their interaction

(1130) **5.** __________ Helper has responsibility for evaluating the interaction and the changing behavior

A. Therapeutic relationship
B. Social relationship

Continued next page

Student Name ____________________

(1130) **6.** ________ Relationship has some boundaries (purpose, place, time) and clear ending

(1130) **7.** ________ Relationship develops spontaneously

F. Match the description in the numbered column with the appropriate interpersonal strategy in the lettered column. Some strategies may be used more than once, and some strategies may not be used.

(1130) **1.** ________ "Experiencing" the patient and refraining from thinking of responses to the patient when the patient is speaking

(1130) **2.** ________ When with the patient, the nurse's attention should be directed completely toward him or her

(1130) **3.** ________ The nurse asks the patient, "What do you mean when you say, 'The world is falling apart'?"

(1130) **4.** ________ This approach allows patients time to consider their own thoughts as well as the communication of the nurse

(1130) **5.** ________ Patients benefit from knowing what nurses see and hear while listening

(1130) **6.** ________ If nurses are aware of their own feelings, they will be able to control their own responses

A. Sharing observations
B. Accepting silence
C. Listening
D. Clarifying
E. Being available

Continued next page

(1130) **7.** ________ The nurse makes a statement that lets the patient know that verbal and nonverbal behaviors are not congruent

(1130) **8.** ________ The nurse says, "You are saying that your life is falling apart, and you are also smiling."

(1130) **9.** ________ Asking questions of the patient

G. Match the description in the numbered column with the most appropriate term in the lettered column.

(1132) **1.** ________ A continual shifting from topic to unrelated topic

(1132) **2.** ________ Minimal or very little speech

(1132) **3.** ________ A patient starts out toward a particular point but veers away and never reaches the point

(1132) **4.** ________ Stopping speaking before reaching the point

(1132) **5.** ________ Loud and insistent speech

(1132) **6.** ________ Shifting topics to the point of incoherence

(1131) **7.** ________ Not speaking

A. Tangential
B. Word salad
C. Pressured speech
D. Paucity
E. Loose associations
F. Mutism
G. Blocking

Student Name____

H. Match the nursing intervention in the numbered column with the appropriate nursing diagnosis for the patient with schizophrenia in the lettered column. Some diagnoses may be used more than once, and some diagnoses may not be used.

(1132) **1.** __________ Encourage involvement in activities

(1132) **2.** __________ Focus on reality

(1138) **3.** __________ Make brief, frequent contacts with the patient to interrupt hallucinatory experiences

(1138) **4.** __________ Let the patient know that the nurse does not share the delusion

(1132) **5.** __________ Connect delusions with anxiety-provoking situations

(1132) **6.** __________ Encourage the patient to pay attention to what is occurring in the environment (instead of external stimuli)

(1132) **7.** __________ Inform the patient that hallucinations are part of the disease process

(1138) **8.** __________ Encourage the patient to express feelings and anxiety

A. Disturbed thought processes
B. Self-care deficit
C. Disturbed sensory perception
D. Impaired verbal communication

I. List nine features assessed during the mental status examination.

(1131) **1.** ______________ *(1131)* **6.** ______________

(1131) **2.** ______________ *(1131)* **7.** ______________

(1131) **3.** ______________ *(1131)* **8.** ______________

(1131) **4.** ______________ *(1131)* **9.** ______________

(1131) **5.** ______________

J. List eight common physical signs and symptoms of anxiety.

(1132) **1.** ______________ *(1132)* **5.** ______________

(1132) **2.** ______________ *(1132)* **6.** ______________

(1132) **3.** ______________ *(1132)* **7.** ______________

(1132) **4.** ______________ *(1132)* **8.** ______________

K. List four side effects of antianxiety medications that are associated with sedation.

(1134) **1.** ______________

(1134) **2.** ______________

(1134) **3.** ______________

(1134) **4.** ______________

L. In addition to counseling the patient, list four ways to prevent and manage increasing anxiety in patients.

(1135) **1.** ______________

(1135) **2.** ______________

(1135) **3.** ______________

(1135) **4.** ______________

M. List five typical symptoms of schizophrenia.

(1135) **1.** ______________

(1135) **2.** ______________

(1135) **3.** ______________

(1135) **4.** ______________

(1135) **5.** ______________

Student Name____

N. List five side effects of drug therapy (antipsychotic and antiparkinsonian medications) used for patients with schizophrenia.

(1136) **1.** ________________________________

(1136) **2.** ________________________________

(1136) **3.** ________________________________

(1136) **4.** ________________________________

(1136) **5.** ________________________________

O. List three probable etiologic factors of mood disorders.

(1136) **1.** ________________________________

(1136) **2.** ________________________________

(1136) **3.** ________________________________

P. List three types of antidepressant medications used for mood disorders.

(1138) **1.** ________________________________

(1138) **2.** ________________________________

(1138) **3.** ________________________________

MULTIPLE-CHOICE QUESTIONS

Q. Choose the most appropriate answer.

(1133) **1.** Intense episodes of apprehension, at times to the point of terror, that are often accompanied by the feeling of impending doom are characteristic of:

1. panic disorder.
2. obsessive-compulsive disorder.
3. somatoform disorder.
4. personality disorder.

(1133) **2.** A type of anxiety disorder in which the individual is extremely fearful of situations outside the home from which escape may be difficult is:

1. somatoform disorder.
2. borderline personality disorder.
3. agoraphobia.
4. hypochondriasis.

(1133) **3.** Repeated checking to see whether the door is locked is an example of:

1. obsessions.
2. hallucinations.
3. delusions.
4. compulsions.

(1133) **4.** Many people with obsessive-compulsive disorders have become symptom-free once therapeutic levels of which drug have been reached?

1. analgesics
2. antihistamines
3. antidepressants
4. anticonvulsants

(1133) **5.** Conversion disorders and hypochondriasis are examples of:

1. mood disorders.
2. somatoform disorders.
3. panic disorders.
4. obsessive-compulsive disorders.

(1134) **6.** Amnesia and multiple personality disorder are examples of:

1. somatoform disorders.
2. dissociative disorders.
3. panic disorders.
4. post-traumatic stress disorders.

(1134) **7.** A symptom of dissociative disorders is:

1. depersonalization.
2. hypochondriasis.
3. agitation.
4. hallucinations.

(1134) **8.** Most patients with multiple personality disorder report severe:

1. agoraphobia.
2. hallucinations.
3. delusions.
4. childhood abuse.

(1134) **9.** The primary antianxiety medications are the:

1. benzodiazepines.
2. antihistamines.
3. thiazides.
4. salicylates.

(1134) **10.** Withdrawal from antianxiety medications should be medically supervised because of the effect(s) of:

1. amnesia and confusion.
2. negative feedback.
3. hormones and histamines.
4. physical and psychological dependence.

(1135) **11.** The two key nursing diagnoses for patients with anxiety disorders are anxiety and:

1. Disturbed body image.
2. Powerlessness.
3. Spiritual distress.
4. Ineffective coping.

(1138) **12.** One of the most common psychiatric disorders is:

1. bipolar disorder.
2. unipolar depression.
3. post-traumatic stress disorder.
4. conversion disorder.

(1140) **13.** As patients respond to antidepressant medications and their energy level increases, what risk may increase?

1. mutism
2. panic
3. suicide
4. hypertension

(1140) **14.** A type of therapy that may be used for patients with severe depression when other forms of therapy have failed is:

1. antidepressants.
2. electroconvulsive therapy.
3. psychotherapy.
4. isolation therapy.

Student Name____

(1140) **15.** Possible side effects of electroconvulsive therapy are temporary memory loss and:

1. orthostatic hypotension.
2. confusion.
3. tardive dyskinesia.
4. parkinsonian syndrome.

(1140) **16.** A patient who exhibits psychomotor retardation, no spontaneous movements, a downcast gaze, and occasional agitated movements of hand wringing is exhibiting signs of:

1. unipolar depression.
2. agoraphobia.
3. schizophrenia.
4. post-traumatic stress syndrome.

(1141) **17.** Frequently assessing a patient's suicidal potential and maintaining continuous one-to-one contact, if indicated, are interventions for depressed patients who are at risk for:

1. sleep pattern disturbance.
2. anxiety.
3. self-directed violence.
4. self-esteem disturbance.

(1141) **18.** Learning to limit self-criticism and to give and receive compliments are interventions for the nursing diagnosis of:

1. Risk for self-directed violence.
2. Chronic low self-esteem.
3. Anxiety.
4. Dysfunctional grieving.

(1141) **19.** Offering small snacks and warm baths and teaching relaxation exercises to be used before retiring for the evening are interventions for patients with:

1. Chronic low self-esteem.
2. Risk for self-directed violence.
3. Hopelessness.
4. Disturbed sleep pattern.

(1138) **20.** The key medication for patients with manic episodes is:

1. alprazolam (Xanax).
2. fluoxetine hydrochloride (Prozac).
3. lithium.
4. benztropine mesylate (Cogentin).

(1135) **21.** The key problems for people with organic mental disorders stem from:

1. speech and language impairments.
2. anxiety disorders.
3. conversion disorders.
4. cognitive impairments.

(1140) **22.** Which herbal preparation is used by many people to relieve depression?

1. Ephedra
2. ginkgo
3. ginseng
4. St. John's wort

CHAPTER 54

Student Name ______________________________

Substance-Related Disorders

Answer Key: Textbook page references are provided as a guide for answering these questions. A complete answer key was provided for your instructor.

OBJECTIVES

1. Discuss the biologic, sociocultural, behavioral, and interpersonal theories of the etiology of substance abuse or dependence.
2. Describe the components of the nursing assessment of a patient with substance abuse or dependence.
3. Describe alcohol dependence, alcohol withdrawal syndrome, medical complications of alcohol dependence, and treatment of alcohol abuse and dependence.
4. Discuss the pathophysiologic effects of frequently abused drugs.
5. Describe disorders associated with substance abuse and dependence.
6. Differentiate between drug abuse treatment and alcohol abuse treatment.
7. Describe the nursing diagnoses and interventions associated with substance abuse and dependence.
8. Discuss populations who present special problems in relation to drug abuse and dependency.

LEARNING ACTIVITIES

A. Match the definition in the numbered column with the most appropriate term in the lettered column.

(1147) **1.** ________ Maladaptive pattern of substance use that differs from generally accepted cultural norms; sometimes referred to as chemical abuse or drug abuse

(1151) **2.** ________ Self-help support process outlining 12 steps to overcoming a physical or psychological dependence on something outside oneself that has a destructive impact on one's life

(1154) **3.** ________ Intense cravings for the substance on which one is dependent without physical withdrawal symptoms

(1150) **4.** ________ Effect of habitual ingestion of a substance to the point of physical dependence; used interchangeably with the term dependence

(1150) **5.** ________ Occurs when body cells are dependent on alcohol to carry out metabolic processes

A. Substance dependence
B. Substance abuse
C. Tolerance
D. Physical addiction
E. Dual diagnosis
F. Codependence
G. Psychological dependence
H. Withdrawal
I. Twelve-step program
J. Recovery
K. Addiction

Continued next page

Student Name ____________________

(1147) **6.** __________ Ingestion of substances in gradually increasing amounts due to a physical need; used interchangeably with the terms chemical dependence and drug dependence

(1150) **7.** __________ Unpleasant and sometimes life-threatening physical substance-specific syndrome occurring after stopping or reducing the habitual dose or frequency of an abused drug

(1163) **8.** __________ Simultaneous existence of a major psychiatric condition and a medical condition

(1153) **9.** __________ Lifelong process of maintaining abstinence from the substance to which one is addicted; a return to moderate substance use is never the end result

(1151) **10.** __________ Exaggerated dependent pattern of self-defeating behaviors, beliefs, and feelings learned as a result of pathologic relationship to a chemically dependent, or otherwise dysfunctional, person

(1147) **11.** __________ Need for increasing amounts of a substance to achieve the same effect brought about by the original amount

B. Complete the statement in the numbered column with the most appropriate term in the lettered column. Some terms may be used more than once, and some terms may not be used.

(1149) **1.** A recent addition to the methods for the detection of abused substances is __________.

(1150) **2.** A complication of chronic alcoholism that is due to thiamine and niacin deficiencies, which contribute to the degeneration of the cerebrum and the peripheral nervous system, is __________.

(1149) **3.** The preferred way of screening for the recent use of an unknown drug is __________.

A. Urine drug screening
B. Hypertension
C. 0.1%
D. Withdrawal
E. Hair analysis
F. Fetal alcohol syndrome
G. Hallucinations
H. Physical addiction
I. 0.05%
J. Korsakoff's psychosis
K. Blood alcohol
L. 1.0%

Continued next page

(1150) **4.** __________ occurs when alcohol becomes integrated into physiologic processes at the cellular level.

(1149) **5.** Legal intoxication in most states occurs when a person's blood alcohol level is __________.

(1149) **6.** __________ requires sensitive technology and can detect drugs for up to 1 year after use.

(1150) **7.** Bugs, snakes, and rats are commonly described by patients with __________.

(1149) **8.** A critical sign of withdrawal in substance abusers is __________.

(1150) **9.** __________ is a medical complication that may cause low birth weight and heart defects in newborn babies.

(1149) **10.** The detection of amphetamines, barbiturates, marijuana, narcotics, and benzodiazepines can be identified with __________.

(1149) **11.** The most accurate type of test available to measure the degree of intoxication on initiation of treatment for alcohol abuse is __________.

C. Complete the statement in the numbered column with the most appropriate term in the lettered column. Some terms may be used more than once, and some terms may not be used.

(1157) **1.** Oversedation, respiratory depression, impaired coordination, and brain damage are symptoms of overdose of __________.

(1154) **2.** Amphetamines and cocaine are __________.

(1157) **3.** Once a person is dependent on depressants, such as barbiturates, abruptly stopping any of these drugs may trigger __________.

(1157) **4.** Runny nose, sniffles, weight loss, and hyperactivity are symptoms of chronic inhalation of __________.

(1154) **5.** Overdose of __________ is life-threatening because no drug is available to counteract the overstimulation, resulting in respiratory failure.

A. Psychosis
B. "Ice"
C. Crack
D. Amphetamines
E. "Bad trip"
F. Stimulants
G. "Snow"
H. Physical dependence
I. Narcotics
J. Depressants
K. Anxiolytics
L. Cocaine
M. Hallucinogens
N. "Crashing"

Continued next page

Student Name____

(1157) **6.** Regular use of depressants results in __________.

(1157) **7.** A drug that may cause strokes, seizures, and heart attacks, even in first-time users, is __________.

(1154) **8.** There are no physical withdrawal symptoms following amphetamine use, but the user typically experiences a profound depression and sense of exhaustion commonly called __________.

(1154) **9.** Hyperactivity, irritability, combativeness, and paranoia are symptoms of use of __________.

(1157) **10.** Depressants that are misused include the sedatives, hypnotics, and __________.

(1156) **11.** __________ is a stimulant that is commonly misused among middle to upper socioeconomic classes owing to its status and expense; it is typically inhaled nasally or mixed with other drugs

(1157) **12.** LSD, PCP, MDMA, and marijuana are examples of __________.

(1156) **13.** A form of methamphetamine ingested by smoking with effects that last as long as 14 hours is __________.

(1157) **14.** A smokable form of cocaine is called __________.

D. Match the description in the numbered column with the appropriate defense mechanism in the lettered column. Some mechanisms may be used more than once, and some mechanisms may not be used.

(1149) **1.** __________ Drug abusers insist that they became addicted to alcohol as a result of pressure to drink socially with colleagues so that colleagues would not think they were prudes

(1149) **2.** __________ Abusers attempt to justify the reasons for their abuse of substances, making an excuse for their addiction

A. Intellectualization
B. Rationalization
C. Denial
D. Regression
E. Projection

Continued next page

(1149) **3.** _________ Persons focus only on objective facts as a way of avoiding dealing with unconscious conflicts and the emotions they evoke

(1149) **4.** _________ Patients state that they do not have a problem with drug abuse despite evidence to the contrary

(1149) **5.** _________ Persons state that they must use heroin because the drugs their doctor gave them for their back injuries were not working

(1149) **6.** _________ People shift blame for their behavior on someone else

(1149) **7.** _________ Individuals may minimize their substance abuse problems by maintaining that they can stay sober by themselves

E. Match the description in the numbered column with the most appropriate drug in the lettered column. Some drugs may be used more than once, and some drugs may not be used.

(1157) **1.** _________ Abusers may possess enormous strength and may feel no pain

(1157) **2.** _________ When this drug is smoked, the inner experience of patients is altered so that individuals have a sense of heightened awareness, distortion of space and time, heightened sensitivity to sound, and depersonalization

(1157) **3.** _________ Individuals taking this drug often experience depersonalization

A. LSD
B. Amphetamines
C. PCP
D. Heroin
E. Marijuana

Continued next page

Student Name ______________________________

(1157) **4.** __________ Very high temperature, hypertensive crisis, and renal failure, in addition to the risk of injuring oneself or others, are symptoms of its use

(1157) **5.** __________ Chronic smoking of this drug irritates the lungs and may lead to lung cancer

(1157) **6.** __________ This drug produces physical symptoms of altered perceptions that are dreamlike

(1157) **7.** __________ Abusers experience a psychotic state similar to that observed in schizophrenics

(1157) **8.** __________ Psychosis, depression, and flashbacks are chronic long-term effects

(1157) **9.** __________ Acute adverse reactions are most often described as a "bad trip"

(1157) **10.** __________ This drug is apt to have a sedative rather than stimulant effect and is unlikely to produce true hallucinations

(1157) **11.** __________ Paranoia, depression, frightening hallucinations, and confusion may be acute adverse reactions

(1157) **12.** __________ Users' motions are intensified and labile

F. Match the classification of common mood-altering chemicals in the numbered column with the most appropriate effects in the lettered column. Some effects may be used more than once, and some classifications may have more than one effect.

(1155) **1.** __________ Hallucinogens

(1155) **2.** __________ Cannabinoids

(1155) **3.** __________ Opiates

(1155) **4.** __________ Sedative-hypnotics and anxiolytics

(1156) **5.** __________ Stimulants

(1156) **6.** __________ Phencyclidines

(1156) **7.** __________ Inhalants

(1156) **8.** __________ Alcohol

(1156) **9.** __________ Xanthines

(1156) **10.** __________ Nicotine

A. Stimulation
B. Emotional swings/lability
C. Dilated pupils
D. Increased blood pressure
E. Analgesia
F. Restlessness
G. Illusions of superhuman strength
H. Paranoia
I. Euphoria
J. Pupillary constriction
K. Sexual arousal
L. Sedation

G. A few patients may not experience any physical withdrawal symptoms despite a history of prolonged, frequent, and heavy substance abuse; list four factors that may affect the incidence of withdrawal effects.

(1148) 1. ______________ (1148) 3. ______________

(1148) 2. ______________ (1148) 4. ______________

H. List four physical characteristics of the appearance of the average substance abuser.

(1149) 1. ______________

(1149) 2. ______________

(1149) 3. ______________

(1149) 4. ______________

I. List four neurologic signs that are significant and that may be associated with nutritional deficits in the substance abuser.

(1161) 1. ______________ (1161) 3. ______________

(1161) 2. ______________ (1161) 4. ______________

J. List six typical stressors of aging that may cause the elderly to use or abuse alcohol for the first time.

(1162) 1. ______________

(1162) 2. ______________

(1162) 3. ______________

(1162) 4. ______________

(1162) 5. ______________

(1162) 6. ______________

K. List four goals of an intervention for an impaired nurse.

(1163) 1. ______________

(1163) 2. ______________

(1163) 3. ______________

(1163) 4. ______________

Student Name____________________

L. Usually there is a 2-year time period after intervention for an impaired nurse to comply with the peer assistance process. List four steps in this 2-year period.

(1163) 1. ____________________

(1163) 2. ____________________

(1163) 3. ____________________

(1163) 4. ____________________

MULTIPLE-CHOICE QUESTIONS

M. Choose the most appropriate answer.

(1148) **1.** The least likely way to alienate an already defensive patient is to use a manner that is matter-of-fact and:

1. nonjudgmental.
2. assertive.
3. reassuring.
4. positive.

(1150) **2.** It is believed that the cause of hangover symptoms is related to the buildup of acetaldehyde and lactic acid in the blood and to:

1. hyperkalemia.
2. hyponatremia.
3. hypoglycemia.
4. hyperthyroidism.

(1153) **3.** When patients abusing alcohol state that they can quit easily and that they do not have a problem, they may be experiencing:

1. Chronic low self-esteem.
2. Ineffective denial.
3. Risk for injury.
4. Impaired verbal communication.

(1153) **4.** Substance abusers who are overly sensitive and use critical self-talk may be experiencing:

1. Ineffective coping.
2. Risk for injury.
3. Knowledge deficit.
4. Chronic low self-esteem.

(1161) **5.** Substance abusers who have driven under the influence of drugs and who engage in excessive drug use are at high risk for:

1. infection.
2. injury.
3. aspiration.
4. activity intolerance.

(1161) **6.** The biggest issue to be addressed at first during rehabilitation is:

1. rationalization.
2. sublimation.
3. denial.
4. compensation.

(1161) **7.** Overtiredness, argumentativeness, depression, self-pity, and decreased participation in AA or NA meetings are symptoms that often lead to:

1. relapse.
2. detoxification.
3. withdrawal.
4. rehabilitation.

(1162) **8.** Elderly individuals who abuse substances over an extended period of time may experience significant medical problems as a result of decreased ability to:

1. circulate and absorb drugs.
2. utilize and react to drugs.
3. metabolize and excrete drugs.
4. transport and detoxify drugs.

(1162) **9.** Intravenous drug use and the likelihood of sexual activity without precautions in the adolescent age group have led to an increased risk of:

1. injuries and falls.
2. HIV infection.
3. altered self-esteem.
4. ineffective individual coping.

(1163) **10.** Dually diagnosed patients usually have psychiatric illnesses of schizophrenia, bipolar illness, or:

1. depression.
2. panic.
3. conversion disorder.
4. somatoform disorder.

(1163) **11.** Patients taking antianxiety or antidepressant agents with alcohol may risk accidental overdose due to:

1. antagonist effects.
2. idiosyncratic effects.
3. stimulant effects.
4. additive effects.

(1163) **12.** Programs designed to offer a supportive alternative to health professionals addicted to a substance so that they do not have to have their licenses removed are called:

1. Alcoholics Anonymous.
2. peer assistance programs.
3. Codependents Anonymous.
4. Al-Anon.

(1164) **13.** Substance abusers frequently have erratic and unprovoked mood swings, blackouts, significant work problems, and damaged:

1. relationships.
2. circulation.
3. grieving.
4. activity levels.

(1163) **14.** Individuals with chronic alcoholism may require supplements of:

1. vitamin C.
2. vitamin K.
3. vitamin B_6.
4. Vitamin E.